Families Across the Life Cycle:
Studies for Nursing

Families Across

the Life Cycle
Studies for Nursing

Kathleen Astin Knafl, Ph.D.
Assistant Professor, College of Nursing,
University of Illinois at the Medical Center,
Chicago

Helen K. Grace, Ph.D.
Professor and Dean, College of Nursing,
University of Illinois at the Medical Center,
Chicago

Little, Brown and Company   Boston

Contents

Contributing Authors

Jeanie Snodgrass Almo, R.N., M.S.N.
Supervisory Psychiatric Nurse, Richardson Division—Youth Program, Department of Health, Education, and Welfare, St. Elizabeth's Hospital, Washington, D.C.

Beverly J. Bernstein, R.N., M.S.N.
Assistant Professor, Department of Psychiatric–Mental Health Nursing, College of Nursing, University of Illinois at the Medical Center, Chicago

Dorothy D. Camilleri, R.N., M.A.
Ph.D. candidate, Department of Sociology, University of Illinois at Chicago Circle, Chicago

Katherine A. Cavallari, R.N., M.S.
Ph.D. candidate, Department of Sociology, University of Illinois at Chicago Circle, Chicago

Dale S. Cohen, R.N., M.S.N.

Susan H. Colgate, R.N., M.S.
Instructor, Maternal-Child Health, Harvard University Project at the University Centre for the Health Sciences, Yaounde, Cameroun, Africa

Norma Traub Cox, R.N., M.S.N.
Formerly Instructor, Department of General Nursing, College of Nursing, University of Illinois at the Medical Center, Chicago

Norma Link Curley, R.N., B.S.N.
Clinical Nurse Specialist—Mental Health, Alexian Brothers Medical Center, Elk Grove Village, Illinois

Donna M. Dixon, B.S.N.
Research Assistant, College of Nursing, University of Illinois at the Medical Center, Chicago

Anne Flickinger, R.N., M.S.N.
Clinical Nurse Specialist—Alcoholism, Edward J. Hines Jr. Veterans Administration Hospital, Hines, Illinois

Mary M. Glenn, R.N., M.S.N.
Formerly Assistant Professor of Nursing, Department of Psychiatric–Mental Health Nursing, College of Nursing, University of Illinois at the Medical Center, Chicago

Helen K. Grace, R.N., Ph.D.
Professor, Department of Psychiatric–Mental Health Nursing, and Dean, College of Nursing, University of Illinois at the Medical Center, Chicago

Janice K. Janken, R.N., M.S.N.
Ph.D. candidate, Department of Nursing Science, College of Nursing, University of Illinois at the Medical Center, Chicago

Joan M. King, R.N., D.N.Sc.
Professor, Department of Psychiatric–Mental Health Nursing, College of Nursing, University of Illinois at the Medical Center, Chicago

Kathleen Astin Knafl, Ph.D.
Assistant Professor, Department of General Nursing, College of Nursing, University of Illinois at the Medical Center, Chicago

Barbara Bryan Logan, R.N., M.S.N.
Assistant Professor, Department of Psychiatric–Mental Health Nursing, College of Nursing, University of Illinois at the Medical Center, Chicago

Bette L. Morrison, R.N., M.S.N.
Instructor, Department of Psychiatric–Mental Health Nursing, College of Nursing, University of Illinois at the Medical Center, Chicago; Nurse Consultant—Psychiatry, Jackson Park Sanitarium, Chicago

Hildy Heine Reiter, R.N., M.S.N.
Trainee, Family Institute of Chicago

Constance Ritzman, R.N., M.S.N.
Instructor, Psychiatric–Community Health Department, School of Nursing, Loyola University, Chicago

Karen Skerrett, R.N., M.S.
Assistant Professor, Department of Psychiatric–Mental Health Nursing, College of Nursing, University of Illinois at the Medical Center, Chicago

Preface

The research reported herein grew out of a series of informal meetings attended by nursing faculty and graduate students interested in family studies. The graduate students were seeking advice and encouragement while writing their master's theses. The faculty members viewed the sessions as an efficient and pleasant way to advise students. Thus the initial concerns of both groups attending the original sessions were pragmatic. Both wanted to get the theses written and the advising done in the most satisfying and positive manner possible.

The group continued in this vein for almost two years, meeting weekly and dealing primarily with the problems of thesis research. Gradually, over this period of time, its focus expanded as its commitment to facilitating thesis research gave rise to a genuine enthusiasm for the various family topics being studied.

In the course of sharing their research difficulties, the students also shared many of their research findings with the group. The data were so fascinating that faculty members not actively involved in family research were inspired to initiate a research project of their own. Thus two years ago, almost two years after the original sessions began, some of us faculty members involved in the group began to investigate socialization into adult family roles by studying couples as they moved from their engagement through their first three years of marriage.

In addition to discussing the various student research projects and planning the study of socialization into adult family roles, we began to consider how nurses interact with families and the bases for these interactions. Clearly, nurses already deal with families, whatever the setting — medical, surgical, pediatric, public health, obstetrical, or psychiatric care. Moreover, as nurses increasingly seek out advanced preparation in programs emphasizing family practice and family counseling or therapy, their involvement with families will become even greater in the future. In short, nurses at all levels and in a wide variety of settings are being and will be called upon to assess family units and to intervene on the basis of these assessments. In their dealings with individual patients and clients, nurses are and will be expected to take into account the individual's various family roles and relationships.

Recognizing the close ties between nursing and the family, we decided to begin a systematic study of all available literature pertaining to the family. Once completed, this review allowed us to evaluate the knowledge base upon which nurses could make family assessments and interventions. It also provided background information for our ongoing studies of family life.

In reviewing the numerous empirical studies and theoretical formulations about the family, we found ourselves comparing this "official" body of knowledge with our own clinical and personal experiences. Through this comparative process we came gradually and reluctantly to the conclusion that in several very important ways the official body of knowledge misrepresents families and family life. Specifically, we identified two main sources of distortion.

In the first place, much of what has been written about families, particularly those studies emanating from psychiatry, predicates intervention on a model of abnormality. Because the majority of these studies are based on data drawn from families that have been labeled disturbed, or that at least have one member so identified, little research is directed toward developing baseline data about the ongoing development of normal families. Clearly, the majority of families and family members seen by nurses do not conform to a disturbed family model. For the most part, nurses see families undergoing a circumscribed health crisis or in need of some sort of health care teaching or counseling. It is wholly inappropriate for nurses dealing with these essentially normal families to base their intervention on a pathological model.

Secondly, we were troubled by an apparent lack of concern for studying families on their own terms. Few investigations have attempted to view the processes involved in moving into and sustaining adult family roles from the perspectives of the family members themselves. As a result, although we have a very large amount of valuable data pertinent to discrete factors associated with family life, we have only scant, disjointed information concerning the ways in which family members interrelate and develop their views of the issues that researchers have so carefully measured. Even more important, we have little insight into whether the topics we have been studying are really crucial issues for the family members themselves. Moreover, we practitioners have often had difficulty translating the highly conceptual, theoretical findings of many such studies into useful clinical applications.

It is a serious matter when in an applied field such as nursing we proceed from an invalid or inappropriate knowledge base. To do so often causes us to deal with people according to how we think they should be rather than how they are. We find ourselves labeling our patients and clients as abnormal, unmotivated, or uncooperative. We look to our textbooks and journals for clues regarding the complexities of human behavior, and we judge the individuals we deal with by presumably scientific standards. Of course, if years of practical experience, common sense, or gut-level feelings lead us to question some of these scientific bases for intervention, we can always fall back on a more intuitive approach and justify it as reliance on the "art" of nursing. Yet, neither approach is wholly acceptable. Invalid scientific findings are hardly better than no findings at all, and intuitions can be strongly influenced by individual preferences and by the limitations of one's own range of experience. In both cases, our approach to people lacks any systematic, empirically grounded understanding of the complexities and constraints of their lives.

Our critical review of literature pertaining to the family also convinced us of the need for holistic studies of family life processes. We became committed to studying families on their own terms, from their own perspective, as a way to understand the important issues and constraints influencing their lives. We believe such an approach assures that nursing interventions take into account the world view of the persons in whose lives they are made.

It is much easier to identify shortcomings than to do something about them. While it is beyond the scope of any one book or study to cover all that one might like to know about families, this book represents an initial attempt to provide the kind of baseline information about family life that is essential to practitioners of any kind who deal with families. We have two distinct purposes in mind. On the one hand, we want to communicate the findings of our studies of families at various points in the life cycle. On the other hand, we hope to convey, by example, a particular way of knowing about families and their members, a way that faithfully represents the world view of those under investigation. Our aim is not to give the reader a prescription for dealing with families but rather to provide baseline data about common family processes and experiences. We view our approach to knowing about and understanding families as relevant and useful to practitioners as well as to researchers.

Since our decision to expand our original thesis advisement group into a research group, our involvement in family research has, quite literally, grown like Topsy. Other faculty and graduate students interested in studying families have joined us, and several graduate students who did their theses in the context of the original group have moved on to new family research projects. Thus we had to agree when, four years after the original "help" sessions, a colleague noted that we had enough data to write a book. Like the group itself, this book is an expression of individual and joint efforts. Some chapters draw heavily on student thesis work. Others are based on data from our ongoing study of socialization into adult family roles. Still others combine information from both sources.

Substantively, the book contains a combination of actual findings and theoretical considerations. The first part serves as a framework for the other five parts. In it we consider the content and quality of much of the family literature currently available to nurses and spell out the theoretical and methodological underpinnings of the research endeavors reported in the following parts. In the last two chapters of the first part we explicate our perspective or rationale for viewing families and the methodological implications of this perspective.

In the second part we begin to present our research findings about families at different stages in the life cycle. We look at dating and courtship and then at married life and parenting. Throughout, we are particularly interested in an individual's movement into new, often added, roles within the family framework. In the final part we return to a discussion of the relationship of the nurse to the family both as a care-giver and as a researcher.

K.A.K.
H.K.G.

Families Across the Life Cycle:
Studies for Nursing

I. Theoretical and Methodological Underpinnings.
Part I provides the framework for the remainder of this book. Any researcher must somehow acknowledge and take into account previous work pertaining to his subject. This we do in Chapter 1 with a selective review of the massive literature on marriage and the family. Yet in Part I we direct our discussion not only to what research has been done but to its relevance and applicability to nursing.

In Chapter 2 we specify the theoretical underpinnings of our various research endeavors. Whether they specify them or not, most researchers make certain assumptions about the nature of man, the social order, and reality. In spite of their highly theoretical nature, our assumptions with regard to these issues have profoundly influenced not only the kinds of research questions we have asked but the specific methodological techniques we have employed. Thus the purpose of Chapter 2 is to state our broad theoretical assumptions and to relate these to our research.

Chapter 2 also considers certain concepts and theoretical formulations pertinent to our investigation of adult family roles. In general, we consider movement into these roles from the perspective of adult socialization. In discussing adult socialization, we use excerpts from actual interviews to illustrate major concepts and ideas. Here again, our aim is to translate abstract formulations into meaningful empirical referents.

Chapter 3 details the methodological consequences of our more theoretical beliefs. This chapter's purpose is to give the reader a fairly complete understanding of the actual process of conducting research. Thus the planning stages of the various investigations reported in the remainder of the book are followed through their data gathering, processing, and analyzing stages.

Taken together, the chapters in this part provide the intellectual and work history of the book. As such, they parallel our own evolution as we moved from looking at what others have done to discussing how we would ideally approach the subject matter and to our actually undertaking the series of research projects reported herein.

1. The Nurse and the Family: Dominant Themes and Perspectives in the Literature. Barbara Bryan Logan

Nursing is at an important crossroads in its developmental history. Past ties to a medical orientation employing the disease model of illness are weakening as the limitations of this model are identified and as a change in orientation from illness to health is advocated. Emphasis is increasingly being placed on prevention of illness. In making these shifts, one of the recognized limitations of nursing has been its orientation toward individuals rather than social networks. Throughout the history of nursing, the nurse-patient relationship has been the primary focus for nursing and nursing education, no matter what the setting. Now pleas for a wider emphasis are being voiced increasingly in the nursing literature and among nursing educators. In particular, these pleas call for a move away from the individual patient approach toward family-centered nursing.

THE FAMILY IN THE TRADITIONAL NURSING CARE OF THE PAST

Certainly, nurses, whatever their specialty, are involved with families, and their use of the family approach is apparent in numerous articles published in the major nursing journals. These articles represent a variety of nursing perspectives. However, whatever the perspective, the articles are highly selective in focus, with primary emphasis on intervention rather than on prevention. Intervention presumes abnormality or dysfunction in some aspect of the family system, and the articles emphasize the role of the nurse in intervening to correct this abnormality or dysfunction. This emphasis is shared by each nursing specialty regardless of its pespective and its particular approach to the family.

Articles written from the obstetrical nursing perspective have centered on recognizing the birth of a child as a family affair. The role of the father in the process has been particularly emphasized [10, 22]. His role has been identified mainly as providing support, and the nurse is reminded that he is a potential

3

ally in the care of his wife. Emphasis is placed on recognizing the supportive nature of the family when complications occur, such as the birth of a premature infant. Nurses are given guidelines on how to assess families' skills and abilities in caring for and becoming involved with premature infants prior to their discharge from the hospital [26]. Articles on pediatric nursing also identify the role of family members, particularly the mother in caring for the sick or disabled child [12, 18]. Yet, although these articles from the obstetrical and the pediatric perspective recognize the importance of the family, their primary focus is the mother-patient or child-patient. Family members are considered only in their advocate or support role in relation to the patient. The model is still that of the individual.

Other articles written from the obstetrical nursing perspective relate to family planning. Nurses are alerted to the techniques, use, and complications of family planning methods. They are, in fact, encouraged to be family planning advocates [8, 23].

The traditional focus of public health nursing on family health is reflected in that perspective's endorsement of family-centered as opposed to individual-centered care. Public health nurses, with their emphasis on home visiting, are alerted to the special needs of certain problem families or multiproblem families. These families are typically members of an ethnic minority such as blacks or from low status occupational groups such as migrant farm workers [3].

Articles written about the family from the medical-surgical nursing perspective teach the nurse to recognize the family's reaction to or adjustment to an individual family member who has a problem. This problem is almost always a disabling disease such as cystic fibrosis or a traumatic condition such as severe burns [5, 7]. The emphasis is either on recognizing that the family as a unit has difficulty accepting or adjusting to these diseases and/or conditions or on alerting the nurse to the fact that the family needs to be mobilized to assist the sick member in coping with that member's physical condition.

Articles written from a psychiatric nursing perspective are similar. Numerous articles highlight families' difficulties accepting and dealing with a family member who has been hospitalized for a psychiatric illness. Many articles emphasize the nurse's role as a family therapist. Psychiatric nursing literature, in particular, has made use of social systems theory and communications theory as frameworks for viewing families primarily from a dysfunctional point of view [13a, 16a].

Some attempt by nurses to cross specialty areas and view the family from a developmental perspective can be seen in the literature. This perspective is apparent in family-related articles dealing with certain stages of the life cycle, particularly adolescence and the middle years. These periods are typically viewed as problematic for the individual; the nurse, therefore, is alerted to potential problems and is given guidelines with which to deal with these problems. For example: "When caring for a middle adult the nurse should tune into the signs of how the person is dealing with increasing his self-esteem by developing more self-awareness, and how he is separating from his parents and children by slowly becoming an independent secure adult. The nurse should also be aware of the implications when a middle adult confronts and reviews his value system and then changes or reinforces it" [9, p. 997]. Again, these articles presume a problem, and a course of action is suggested that the nurse can take to correct or alleviate the problem.

The family is also viewed in nursing literature from a situational perspective; that is, various situations are identified as problematic for families or for society, and the nurse is alerted to these situations as principal targets for primary prevention. An example is widowhood [17]. Potential problems of loneliness, anger, and sadness following the loss of a spouse are highlighted, and the intervening role of the nurse in assisting widowed women to adjust to these problems is emphasized.

A situation often identified as a social problem in which the nurse can successfully intervene is the single-parent family, a family structure deviant from the recognized nuclear family norm consisting of a man, a woman, and their offspring. When dealing with the single-parent family, nurses must remember to evaluate the unique emotional and economic needs of its members in the context of their joint resources and culture [16]. Usually the term *single-parent family* is synonymous with *mother-headed family*. Although single-parent father-headed families do not appear to be as deviant as single-parent mother-headed families, nurses are encouraged to recognize the problems of both families and to intervene similarly [1]. Moreover, adolescent unwed mothers are identified as particularly problem-prone and in need of helpful intervention.

Regardless of the specialty from whose perspective it is written, nursing literature depicts the contrast between the individual and the family or social network approach and the dilemma nurses face in an effort to shift from the former to the latter. Although many articles seem to use a family-centered approach, they typically view the family as a support system or as a resource for an individual member of the family who is defined as "ill." This more or less individual approach is reflected in a majority of the articles on the role of the family in caring for or coping with a physically ill, handicapped, or emotionally disturbed member.

Moreover, most nursing literature is not only directed toward intervention using an individual approach but is also highly prescriptive; that is, a particular method of intervention is prescribed to correct what is presumed to be diseased or dysfunctional about the individual family member or his relationship to other family members.

There are several reasons why the family has been thus neglected in nursing literature. The historical ties between nursing and the medical model have fostered an emphasis on disease or abnormality and its diagnosis and treatment. This emphasis has in turn fostered a problem-oriented approach to health care, exacerbated by the difficulty one encounters when attempting to define normalcy. Added to these reasons is the fact that family theory developed outside the nursing profession.

The historical ties between nursing and the medical model have caused nurses to view health care from a disease model. Nurses are expected to attend first to matters related to the disease process. A convalescing patient who is doing well provides few data considered important enough to chart. Nurses are rewarded for identifying what is going wrong with a patient rather than what is going right; so it is no wonder they approach patients from a disease perspective instead of from a health perspective. It is no wonder they concern themselves most with diagnosis and treatment.

In the process of diagnosing and treating a patient, medical professionals collect data from the patient in order to confirm a diagnosis and to formulate a plan of treatment. Diseases and their proper treatments are defined in medical texts, and nurses are expected to memorize these as a part of their education. Individuals are identified as possessors of a particular disease, and the shift to family health care has not changed this focus entirely. For example, although considerable attention is directed to the family in psychiatric nursing, the family as a whole is now often viewed as the problem. Thus it has replaced the individual as the diseased entity in need of correction and intervention.

Diagnosis and treatment have traditionally been in the physician's domain, and the reluctance of nurses to enter this domain is reflected in the nursing profession's approach to data collection from individuals and from families. We are tentative in our data collection procedures, and our language is characterized by statements such as "it appears to me" or "it seems to me." This tentativeness based on fear of intruding upon the physician's domain has restricted nurses to certain categories of data collection and prevented them from breaking away entirely from the medical model and clearly identifying what is uniquely a nursing function both clinically and theoretically. This pattern is evident in the nursing profession's approach to families. Acting in keeping with the medical model and being attuned to problems, the nurse typically casts families in certain molds and acts toward them accordingly. For example, when he or she encounters a one-parent family, he or she usually assumes that that parent is a woman and that her children are maladjusted because they lack a father figure and the mother lacks male companionship. He or she expects these problems no matter what the family's circumstances.

This problem focus is compounded by the fact that the nurse encounters individuals or families as the expert. He or she begins with his or her own expectations based on his or her knowledge of signs and symptoms of disease, which can be physical or emotional, and he or she sets out to confirm these expectations with the patient or family. The emphasis is not on the patient's or family's description, identification, and report of what they perceive to be wrong but on validation of his or her own definitions.

The disease or problem approach is not unique to nursing; it tends to be characteristic of the entire health care field. One possible explanation for its prevalance is simply the ease with which one focuses on abnormal behavior. Second, problem families or dysfunctional families are more easily identified than are families that are functioning well. Well-functioning families are of little interest to the health care professional; studies of normal functioning are rare. Yet we professionals proceed as if we know what it is for families or individuals to be normal when we have seldom if ever investigated what constitutes normalcy and have reached no agreement on a broad definition of normalcy. We have no valid yardstick by which to measure normalcy, and our definition of normal behavior, derived as it is from the disease model, is "that which is not diseased" or "that which is not abnormal."

How is it possible to free ourselves from this focus? One way is to build a body of knowledge based on normal behavior. So far, such efforts by the nursing profession have been based on theoretical frameworks that originate from disciplines outside nursing, and thus problems have arisen when applying these points of view to the study of families from a nursing perspective. Some of these frameworks—institutional, structural-functional, psychoanalytic, developmental, social systems, and communications—and their limitations are discussed below. In addition, alternative approaches to the study of the family are proposed.

FRAMEWORKS USED TO STUDY THE FAMILY

The *institutional approach* originated in anthropology and sociology and is perhaps the first conceptual framework developed to study the family. Its central focus is the origin and evolution of the family institution over time [24]. Its analysis of family organizations and institutions in different societies permits cross-cultural generalizations about families. Its emphasis on the institutional aspects of marriage and the family allows us to look at family organizations, family patterns, and family norms. As a result, the institutional approach provided nursing professionals with a useful method for analyzing the family as one of society's primary institutions. But such a broad framework is somewhat limited in its usefulness since nurses typically focus on individual families in depth. This approach, however, does allow nurses to view marriage and the family as institutions that serve societal needs, and it alerts nurses to the fact that these institutions may differ across cultures.

The *structural-functional approach* is closely related to the institutional approach. This framework allows us to view the family as a social system whose parts are bound together by interaction and interdependence. Within this framework, attention is focused on the internal dynamics of the family system as well as on relationships between the family and other social systems [21]. The structure in question is the makeup of the family and the position of individual members such as husband-father, and wife-mother. Utilizing this framework, nurses can assess families by exploring, for example, the composition of the family, the relationships of family members to one another, and the functions or activities assumed within the family and by whom. Nurses can also investigate child rearing practices, economic provisions, and role functions within the family. Parsons and Bales [20] have typed the female role in modern Western society as specializing in expressive functions and the male role, instrumental functions. Instrumental functions refer primarily to economic provision and decision making while expressive functions refer to the socioemotional aspects of family life.

7. Themes in the Literature

Expressive functions and instrumental functions are perhaps the most widely used of the structural-functional concepts. Their use is apparent in articles that examine the role of the working wife and the problems that can be anticipated when wives function in a male domain and perform instrumental functions defined as belonging to the male role. The rigid distinction between male and female roles is of course changing in our modern society, but these conventional role definitions still occur in nursing literature and in the behavior of men and women.

Generally, the structural-functional approach to family analysis is concerned with how families are organized and how they operate. Other concepts belonging to this framework that have been used by nurses to determine family organization are the nuclear family (mother and father and their children), the extended family (nuclear family plus other relatives living with and incorporated into the family structure), decision making, and power.

The *developmental approach* views the family as a unit of interacting personalities and is concerned with the life cycle or the stages of development through which the family and its members pass. Within this framework attempts are made to account for changes in patterns of interaction over the family's life span. Thus the focus is on the longitudinal career of the family [14]. Much of the developmental rationale is embodied in the concept of developmental tasks, defined as "a task which arises at, on or about a certain period in the life of an individual, successful achievement of which leads to his happiness and to success with later tasks, while failure leads to unhappiness in the individual, disapproval by society and difficulty with later tasks" [13, p. 2].

Duvall has been a major advocate of and contributor to the developmental approach. Her popular textbook entitled *Family Development* [9a], the first book-length report on the subject, has been used widely by public health nurses, but the concept of developmental tasks has been used by nurses in many specialties. Duvall outlines expectations for individuals or families at different stages during the life cycle.

Developmental tasks can be defined in a number of ways. Dickelmann, for example, applies this concept to the emotional assessment of the "middle adult": "The tasks of the middle adult are different from those of the young or older adult . . . the emotional tasks of the middle adult are often overlooked or misunderstood. . . . During the middle years adults can turn from being other-oriented to being self-oriented" [9, p. 997]. Dickelmann outlines four criteria by which nurses can assess middle adults' achievement of developmental tasks. These are: (1) increasing self-esteem by developing more self-awareness; (2) separating from parents and children by slowly becoming a more independent and secure adult; (3) reviewing personal values by confronting an existing value system and either changing or reinforcing that system; (4) initiating plans for the future by recognizing the aging process and planning for it. Dickelmann explains that although the methods middle adults use to accomplish these tasks differ, each method may greatly affect physical and emotional health and may determine adaptive or maladaptive coping.

Adaptive coping produces a healthy adult; maladaptive coping produces one who is diseased. Dickelmann's article utilizes the developmental approach to describe what should be expected at a particular stage of the life span. It focuses on the individual and is prescriptive in that it alerts the nurse as to what to expect of individuals at a particular stage and suggests how he or she can intervene.

The *psychoanalytic approach* focuses on the role of the family in shaping the personality of the child. It gives priority to inborn instincts, emphasizing the biological core of man and diminishing the role of society. It also dramatizes the first year of life at the expense of later social participation. Freud, the originator of the psychoanalytic framework, conceived the family as the instrument for disciplining the child's biologically fixed instinctual urges. He tended to isolate parent-child relations from the totality of family experience. The psychoanalytic framework also tends to divorce the internal processes of mind from the social environment. It places emphasis on the motivations of the individual as they relate to the emotions of love and hate, pleasure and pain, and sex. Freud's formulations of unconscious motivation point out the possibility that individuals may have a wide range of responses or behavior of which they are unaware. The psychoanalytic framework has been used in many studies of marriage and the family vis-à-vis nursing in a variety of ways. In fact, the individual approach to health care is grounded in the psycho-analytic assumption that man himself is the cause of whatever happens to him in life and that if he is to change, the changes must occur within him. As nursing shifts its focus from the individual to the family, the family instead of the individual is viewed as the diseased entity, which must change itself to "recover."

The *social systems approach* views the family as a set of interacting inter-dependent individuals. It takes a view opposite that of the psychoanalytic framework since it considers the family system to be interacting with and interdependent on many outside systems. This view is based on the definition of a social system as "a set of components interacting with each other and a boundary which possesses the property of filtering both the kind and rate of flow of inputs and outputs to and from the system" [2, p. 14]. Key concepts in the definition are components, interaction, and boundary. The components represent the individuals and their differentiated positions within the family system. Their interaction patterns are indicative of their relation and connection to one another. Their boundary can be thought of as an invisible "semi-permeable membrane," which is either physical (when it applies to the household) or psychological (when it represents divisions between generations and the sexes). It performs a filtering function by regulating the flow of exchanges among individuals within the system and between the family system and outside systems. The systems approach has contributed notably to the field of psychiatry and was introduced into family therapy by therapists at the Mental Health Institute in Palo Alto, California [19]. Assumptions implicit in this framework are: (1) the individual is an open system responsive to others within the larger family system; (2) change in one person within the system will produce change in others within the system; and (3) the family tends to maintain homeostasis and will resist change in any individual within the family system. The extensive use of the social systems framework by nurses for viewing the family is evident in nursing literature [11].

The *communications approach* borrows many concepts and constructs from the social systems framework. In fact, the two are often used interchangeably. The underlying premise of the communications perspective is that all behavior has meaning and that verbal and nonverbal communication is the means by which one learns about the family system. The focus in communications theory is metacommunication, or communication about a communication. Communication is broken down into different components. Watzlawick, Beavin, and Jackson [27] identified three different aspects of communication: *syntactics*, the problem of transmitting information; *semantics*, the meaning of communication; and *pragmatics*, the behavioral aspects of communication, including the content and context of the message.

Jackson [15] identified two components of communication: the *report* component, which relates to the content of the message being communicated, and the *command* component, which defines the nature of the relationship between two parties. Jackson believes that every message contains both types of information.

Watzlawick, Jackson, Bateson, and Satir are the major theorists associated with the communications approach. Their work represents an effort to understand and describe family patterns in both functional and dysfunctional families. They have developed a number of concepts that are particularly useful in working with disturbed families. An example is the concept of the double bind, a faulty communication pattern identified as a major factor in the cause of schizophrenia. Psychiatric nurses also use this concept in describing psychopathology and in assessing dysfunctional families. Communications theory, whether stated explicitly or not, is utilized in many nursing specialties in which nurses advocate clear communication in every relationship in which they are involved. It is particularly useful when emphasis is placed on understanding relationships between individual family members, between the family and outside systems, and between the family and the nurse.

THE SYMBOLIC INTERACTION ALTERNATIVE

Communications theory and the other theoretical frameworks outlined are useful to the nurse in studying and understanding the family because they provide concepts that the nurse can use in family assessment. They are, however, limited in that they emphasize one particular area of family life. Communications theory, for example, advocates very important communication aspects of the family system, but it ignores other, equally important aspects of family life. Similarly, psychoanalytic theory places emphasis on the individual with little regard for the connection between that individual and other social networks. It also ignores the important ways in which these social networks influence the individual. Institutional and structural-functional frameworks, on the other hand, are rather broad and general and therefore do not provide a comprehensive picture of all aspects of family life. A social systems framework is more directly applicable to nursing practice since it emphasizes interactions both within the family and between the family and outside systems.

Except for the social systems and the communications frameworks, nurses typically learn about these theoretical approaches in a beginning sociology or social psychology course. They also typically forget the content of these courses except for a few key concepts that are applicable in nursing practice and can be utilized in a descriptive way. Without additional courses about or study of these frameworks, most nurses' knowledge of them is incomplete. This lack of knowledge is one reason why these frameworks seldom appear in nursing literature. Another reason is that by themselves the approaches are not applicable to what nurses do. A third reason is that they contain assumptions and formulations that may not be applicable to families from a nursing perspective.

Another theoretical approach to family study, *symbolic interaction*, which is discussed in detail in Chapter 2, bases its approach to the family on the premise that family members are the experts about their family life and that consequently family studies must begin with family members' understanding of their situation. This approach evolved from the interactional framework, which originated in sociology and social psychology. It is based on the assumption that man must be studied on his own level, that the most fruitful approach to man's social behavior is through an analysis of the society in which human beings are both actors and reactors [25]. This approach strives to interpret family phenomena in terms of internal processes, role playing, status, relations, communication problems, stress reactions, and decision making. Thus, the symbolic interaction approach utilizes concepts from a variety of frameworks and addresses itself to problems related to relationships between the person and the society, to socialization and personality organization. This framework has produced a number of studies on marital or parental role expectations, perceptions, evaluations, and performances [6]. It is also the framework that guides the studies reported in this book.

The symbolic interaction approach allows us to study and analyze the family in a new and different way, essentially from a nonpathological perspective. We believe that the family comprises a network of individuals interdependently related to one another through performance of complementary roles. How families interact with one another in performing these roles can be observed by nurses in a variety of settings. These observations can then provide baseline data from which nurses can develop theories about various aspects of family life. We also believe that the family is not isolated but is embedded in a variety of other social systems, which exert external influences in addition to those exerted internally within the family. Nurses can also observe how families cope with these external influences and then incorporate these observations into the body of knowledge compiled on families from a nursing perspective. We further believe that the individual cannot be understood completely in isolation from his family and other social networks of which he is an integral part. When building a knowledge base about families, nurses must know a family's position in society and the effects of that position on family interaction and function, as defined by family members. We believe that family members are the experts on their own family life and that we can learn about their family patterns only by direct observation and by listening to what they tell us about the meaning of their behavior.

Thus we approach our studies of the family not as experts seeking to validate certain preconceived ideologies but with an open mind to elicit from families their definitions of their everyday life experiences. For example, instead of assuming that families have problems with decision making and power, we begin by allowing family members to describe the normal events of their lives, such as how the partners met, how their relationship developed, and how they planned their wedding. Thus the nurse can begin to construct models of family patterns built on normalcy, and his or her orientation to data and data collection will be changed from the disease-presumptive model to a model built on presumption of health.

In the process of studying families as they deal with their day-to-day dilemmas, a large number of concerns have come to the surface. As we interview families, they reach out for help, and at that point nurses can be very helpful. In this type of interaction, the whole nurse-patient relationship is altered; the nurse does not assume problems but allows individuals or families the freedom to define what is painful or difficult for them. Such nursing care is given in response to a real need, and it entails first listening and understanding and then a mutual exploration of possible solutions.

Using this approach, the nurse is constantly generating and modifying his or her theoretical constructs of family processes and in so doing is building family theory. Such theory building relies on the use of observational skills to understand what is going on within families and the use of theoretical constructs to apply the observations to a broader framework. Such a framework depicts our recognition of the complexities of family life as it is lived, and our understanding of the inadequacy with which the existing literature about the family portrays these complexities. Often family life as it is lived is much more complex than the simplistic treatment of family issues in the literature would lead us to expect. In this book our descriptions of some very complex processes may also appear simplistic. Families are in a constant state of change while yet maintaining their own particular equilibrium. Studying families is similar to taking photographs: we have captured some moments of the family life processes, but the total picture of the family is infinitely more complex.

The task of the nursing professional in studying and working with the family is to construct a model focused on health rather than on disease and to conduct research using data from normal family life events rather than from signs and symptoms of disease. Nursing models of the family should recognize that the family is more than a support system to be mobilized when an individual member or patient experiences a crisis and that family members are themselves the experts. Theory construction must begin with the perceptions and perspectives of family members instead of with preexisting abstract assumptions. The ultimate goal is to develop a scientific body of knowledge unique to nursing that will guide further research and provide a base for practice. Such a body of knowledge will bring together a wide range of theories and concepts within the framework of real living human people.

REFERENCES

1. Anstice, E. Helping the motherless family. *Nursing Times* 69:432, 1973.
2. Barrien, K. *General and Social Systems*. New Brunswick, N.J.: Rutgers University Press, 1968.
2a. Bateson, G. Schizophrenic distortion of communication. In C. Whittaker (Ed.), *Psychotherapy of Chronic Schizophrenic Patients*. Boston: Little, Brown, 1958.
3. Bauerfriend, L. Strengthening a discouraged family. *American Journal of Nursing* 75:2198, 1975.
4. Blumer, H. *Symbolic Interactionism*. Englewood Cliffs, N.J.: Prentice-Hall, 1969.
5. Bowden, M., and Feller, I. Family reaction to a severe burn. *American Journal of Nursing* 73:317, 1973.
6. Broderick, C. Beyond the Five Conceptual Frameworks: A Decade of Development in Family Theory. In C. Broderick (Ed.), *A Decade of Family Research and Action 1960–1969*. Minneapolis: National Council on Family Relations, 1971.
7. Burnette, B., and Snider, A. Family adjustment to cystic fibrosis. *American Journal of Nursing* 75:111, 1975.
8. Clarke, J. Family planning nurse. *Nursing Times* 70:1856, 1971.
9. Dickelmann, N. Emotional tasks of the adult. *American Journal of Nursing* 75:997, 1975.
9a. Duvall, E. *Family Development* (rev. ed.). Philadelphia: Lippincott, 1962.
10. Fleming, G. Delivering a happy father. *American Journal of Nursing* 72:949, 1972.
11. Haller, L.L. Family systems theory in psychiatric intervention. *American Journal of Nursing* 74:317, 1973.
12. Hardgrove, C., and Rutledge, A. Parenting during hospitalization. *American Journal of Nursing* 75:830, 1975.
13. Havighurst, R.J. *Human Development and Education*. New York: Longmans, Creon, 1953.
13a. Hazzard, E., and Scheurman, M. Family system therapy: New ways to help families in trouble. *Nursing 76* 6:22, 1976.
14. Hill, R., and Rogers, R. The Developmental Approach. In H.T. Christensen (Ed.), *Handbook of Marriage and the Family*. Chicago: Rand McNally, 1964.
15. Jackson, D. The study of the family. *Family Process* 4:1, 1965.
16. Kaserman, C. The single parent family. *Perspectives in Psychiatric Care* 12:113, 1974.
16a. Lantz, J. Family therapy: Using a transactional approach. *Journal of Psychiatric Nursing and Mental Health Services* 15:17, 1977.
17. Miles, H., and Hays, D. Widowhood. *American Journal of Nursing* 75:280, 1975.
18. Murphy, A., and Pucschal, M. Early intervention with families of newborns with Down's syndrome. *Maternal-Child Nursing* 4:1, 1975.
19. Ohlson, D. Marital and family therapy: Integrative review and critique. *Journal of Marriage and the Family* 38:501, 1970.
20. Parsons, T., and Bales, R. *Family Socialization and Interaction*. Glencoe, Ill.: Free Press, 1955.
21. Pitts, J.R. The Structural-Functional Approach. In H.T. Christensen (Ed.), *Handbook of Marriage and the Family*. Chicago: Rand McNally, 1964.
22. Rubin, R. Babies have fathers too. *American Journal of Nursing* 76:1980, 1971.
22a. Satir, U. *Conjoint Family Therapy*. Palo Alto, Calif.: Science and Behavior Books, 1967.
23. Siegel, E., et al. Family planning: Its rationale. *Nursing Digest* 3:55, 1975.

24. Sirjamaki, J.   The Institutional Approach. In H.T. Christensen (Ed.), *Handbook of Marriage and the Family*. Chicago: Rand McNally, 1964.
25. Stryker, S.   The Interactional and Situational Approaches. In H.T. Christensen (Ed.), *Handbook of Marriage and the Family*. Chicago: Rand McNally, 1964.
26. Warrick, L.H.   Family centered care in the premature nursery. *American Journal of Nursing* 70:2134, 1971.
27. Watzlawick, P., Beavin, J., and Jackson, D.   *The Pragmatics of Human Communication*. New York: Norton, 1967.

2. Our Theoretical Framework for Understanding Adult Family Roles. Kathleen Astin Knafl

The kinds of research questions we have addressed throughout this book and the way in which we have conducted our investigations are related to our beliefs about the nature of man and society. After studying families at all points in the life cycle, we have focused on selected issues and dimensions of family life. In this chapter we explicate the underlying rationale for our particular focus. Our rationale stems from the conceptual framework of symbolic interactionism, a social psychology theory that is consistent with our beliefs about the nature of man and society. In spite of its esoteric label, symbolic interactionism stresses a rather practical, common sense interpretation of human behavior. It is built on three basic premises: (1) Persons act toward things on the basis of the meanings these things have for them; (2) The meaning of such things is derived from the social interactions one has with others; (3) The meanings are handled in and modified through an interpretive process and used by the person in dealing with the things he encounters [2]. In short, symbolic interactionism holds that human beings selectively observe and assess the world through a continuous process of interpretation. This ongoing interpretive process makes it possible for individuals to deliberate and adapt their actions rather than to merely release them as a response to a given stimulus. In this context, social interaction is viewed as a formative process in which individuals formulate their respective conduct through a constant anticipation and interpretation of each other's actions.

Following this theoretical approach, we believe that human beings are not compelled to think or act in certain ways simply because they have certain personality characteristics. Thus we have not based our explanations of human behavior on social or psychic forces. Rather we have attempted to understand and explain human behavior by determining how certain individuals define their environment and construct lines of action in it. In short, our aim has been to uncover and then communicate the world view of the various family members we have been studying.

Whereas Chapter 3 details the methodological implications of symbolic interactionism for our various research designs, this chapter outlines these implications in a general way by comparing our approach to studying family life to that of investigators working from other theoretical orientations. Such a comparison may further clarify the impetus for and the context of our work.

SYMBOLIC INTERACTION THEORY

Symbolic interactionists typically begin their research endeavors by asking: How do these people I am studying define their situation? How do they view themselves and the other participants in this situation? Once these basic questions have been answered, the researcher, using this frame of reference, begins to focus on the actual processes by which specific definitions of the situation emerge and how these definitions change over time. Because of their primary commitment to uncovering the respondents' world view, researchers using this approach usually do not formulate hypotheses before collecting their data. Instead, they begin their investigations with rather broad research questions and objectives in mind. For example, we began our study of movement into adult family roles by asking the following general questions:

1. What are the ongoing processes involved in family formation from engagement through the early years of marriage?
2. What are the similarities and differences in couples with regard to their definition and management of the adult family roles of spouse and parent?
3. What do "normal" couples define as problematic or crisis situations, and how do they deal with situations so defined?

In addition, symbolic interactionists usually compare the respondents' various definitions of a given situation to determine if they differ, ultimately exploring the effects of any such differences on the interaction in the setting. Finally, symbolic interactionists consider the relationship between respondents' views and their actual behavior.

In contrast, investigators who believe that an individual's thoughts and behaviors are a function of certain social or personality forces will begin by specifying a set of variables that they believe are important with regard to their subject matter. In studying divorce, for example, they might compare differential divorce rates among couples from different social classes, religions, ethnic backgrounds, or ages. Such investigators do not concern themselves with the meaning that the variables under the study have for the subjects being investigated. On the contrary, once such investigators have specified what from their viewpoint are important variables, they will set out systematically to measure these and determine whether they are interrelated.

Certainly, there is a place for both approaches. The kinds of surveys the latter researchers are likely to do are useful in describing and comparing certain groups. Such surveys have been important contributions to our general understanding of human behavior and the differences between and among various groups. However, if we are to understand fully the complexities of human behavior, we must understand the meanings individuals attach to various situations and aspects of their lives. To know, for example, that members of one socioeconomic class are more likely than those of another to have their marriages end in divorce is probably of minimal help to the nurse involved in family therapy. Before we nurses can make meaningful assessments and interventions, we must be able to determine how our patients and clients view themselves and their worlds. Thus we have chosen to approach our subject matter using the theoretical framework of symbolic interactionism.

Many studies that have employed the symbolic interactionism framework have dealt with adult socialization, an aspect of sociology that encompasses the processes through which adults acquire the skills, knowledge, attitudes, values, and motivations essential to an adequate performance of their social roles [8]. Interestingly, the bulk of such research has dealt with occupational and deviant life style roles. Thus, although by definition adult socialization encompasses the study of adult family roles, these roles have seldom been the subject of research.

Although symbolic interactionists studying adult socialization have contributed greatly to our understanding of the processes involved in moving into occupations and deviant life styles, there is no way of knowing at present if the issues and concepts recognized as important in such studies can be applied to adult family roles. Yet, since individuals often are moving into occupational and family roles simultaneously, research efforts should integrate the occupational and family aspects of adult socialization. It is important that we understand not only the dynamics of the individual processes but the interrelationships between them. This goal is clearly impossible, however, until movement into adult family roles has been studied as thoroughly and intensively as movement into occupational roles. The studies reported in this volume are a means to this end.

ADULT SOCIALIZATION CONCEPTS

Because the influence of adult socialization concepts on our work is evident in our analysis and interpretation of our own data, a brief discussion of some of the core concepts of adult socialization follows. Most of the specific concepts discussed emanate from research done on occupations. They have been chosen either because they were used in our research or because they are particularly pertinent to understanding family life processes.

Investigations of occupational socialization usually consider recruitment into the occupation and the dynamics and specific outcomes of training to be processes that relate to individual identity formation and change. In other words, how do individuals decide to enter certain occupations and what happens to them once they have so decided? Our concerns are analogous to these. We want to find out how persons decide to move into a new role and what are the consequences of such a decision. Moreover, we are interested in the dynamics of preparing oneself for a new role. When analyzing our data on various adult

17. Our Theoretical Framework

family roles, we uncovered some striking contrasts between occupational and adult family role socialization in relation to these broad areas of role recruitment, preparation, and outcome. In studying variants of spouse and parent roles, we have identified interesting differences in the ways people move into and modify family roles.

The process of recruitment into marriage differs from recruitment into occupational roles. Rarely are advertisements placed for potential partners; nor are the qualifications for the position or the conditions of the contract outlined in advance. Our data from interviews with engaged and cohabiting couples as well as from observations made at singles bars indicate that recruitment is an intricate, often time-consuming, process. Typically, it entails a series of sizing-up maneuvers and subsequent evaluation of first encounters and impressions. The process that moves individuals from the status of casual acquaintances to permanent partners is a subtle one:

It really wasn't like all of a sudden I could take going out with him or I could leave it. We had a real nice time and very good conversations and stuff, but in my mind I didn't have any type of marriage or permanency in mind. I think we both let ourselves go more than we really had..wanted to. I don't think there ever came one point in our relationship where we could say we fell in love because it involved so many things. He just seemed like he would sort of fit into all the little wedges [niches], and I cared too, and it just sort of kept growing, and all of a sudden I looked and there it was.

Of equal if not greater complexity is the process of becoming a parent. Unlike recruitment into either spouse or occupational roles, movement into parenthood may or may not involve the making of an explicit decision. It is similar to marriage, however, in that specific qualifications for the role have little bearing on the decision of whether one enters it. A particularly interesting aspect of recruitment into parenthood is the ambivalence that often accompanies this decision, as the following excerpt from an interview with a new mother indicates.

I'd been ambivalent for years about whether or not I wanted to have children. Then when I got pregnant within six weeks of the decision to have one, I was scared. On the one hand, I have a lot of other things that I want to do with my life; on the other hand, I was relieved that I could get pregnant and excited about it.

Ambivalence seems to be a much less salient issue in deciding to marry or pursue a particular occupation.

Once a person has decided to move into a new role, the issue of preparation for the role becomes important. A closely related issue is that of the outcome or consequences of any preparatory endeavors and the ability to identify and evaluate these. In discussing the process and outcomes of professional socialization, Olesen and Whittaker [6] differentiate between an outer or role performance level and an inner or phenomenological level. While the outer level refers to the acquisition of the minimal skills for certification of professional competency, the inner level has to do with the individual's views of self.

Preparation for role performance in marriage is informal and unspecific. All persons, whether or not they eventually marry, are taught certain skills and attitudes necessary for marriage. Certainly, the universality of this kind of role preparation stands in contrast to occupational training, which tends to be highly focused. Yet few if any institutions are responsible for specifically preparing people for marriage and parenthood.

Related to this lack of specific preparation for adult family roles is the lack of definition regarding the abilities one needs to competently perform various family roles. Although we assume that learning is an essential component of movement into new roles, we know little about what knowledge and skills individuals consider important for marriage and parenthood. Also undefined are the ways in which a person might go about acquiring these skills. Again, we simply assume that the individual will be able to handle whatever tasks and challenges arise. Marital and parenting roles are not unlike those occupations in which on-the-job training is the norm, as the following quotes indicate:

As far as marital roles expectations, I thought a lot about going into it, but not a lot about what my role would be. I hadn't really carefully defined that. But as the marriage progressed we talked about things and how to deal with them, a lot about roles and changing roles.

Actually I thought it would be just great, just holding the baby all the time. I hadn't thought very much about it. I didn't know what it would be to take care of diapers and bottles and formula. That I thought about afterward.

Clearly, the hurdles to be managed for entry into marriage and parenthood are not institutionalized. They are unique for each couple rather than a matter of public record.

Socialization into adult family roles must be seen as a multidimensional process. Recruitment and preparation comprise what Olesen and Whittaker labeled the outer or role performance level when discussing professional socialization. Yet this outer level is only one aspect of the process. Adult socialization can be only partially understood as the acquisition of the knowledge and skills necessary for the performance of a given role. As Olesen and Whittaker stress, the inner phenomenological level is also important. Beyond learning the essential cognitive, technical, and interpersonal skills, the person undergoing professional socialization is expected to develop a sense of commitment to the profession and a new sense of self.

Similarly, persons who enter marriage and parenthood are expected to have a high degree of commitment to these roles. Thus the inner dimension of socialization, the development of new views of self, is relevant to a study of family role development. Development of any identity entails a process "by which an individual embraces the roles as a part of self. . . . a transformation by which the individual finds answers to the question, 'Who am I?' " [3, p.

11]. In the case of occupations, identification with the professional role probably approaches what John Lofland [4] has termed a *pivotal identity*, a role that is central to the person's self-concept and around which other role-connected identities cluster and take meaning. A pivotal identity defines who a person "really is" to himself and to others. McCall and Simmons [5] use the term *hierarchy of identities* or *salience hierarchy* to describe how various role identities are arranged in order of their importance to self. It is reasonable to assume that identities associated with marital roles are particularly important to individuals. Berger and Kellner theorize that "marriage occupies a privileged status among the significant validating relationships for adults in our society. . . . Marriage in our society is a dramatic act in which two strangers come together and redefine themselves" [1, p. 53]. The following quote illustrates the impact that marriage can have on one's sense of self:

I've realized that since I've been married I've become more independent. Basically, I'm a people person, but I'm finding I no longer have this craving to go out and be with someone every minute of the day. I think one of the important things that has happened to me is just the fact that I'm a lot more comfortable being by myself. It's because I did need someone else and now a lot of my deep down emotions are expressed to my husband. So now I just, over the past year, feel more comfortable with myself.

Similarly, becoming a parent can profoundly change how the individual views himself. For example, a new mother noted during an interview:

I have become the epitome of all that I held in disdain. I can stay at home and not read, not write, maybe watch some TV and play with the baby. That consumes my day, and I love it.

In viewing any adult family role, it is particularly important to identify this redefinition process and its significance to the family members.

The importance of family role identities to an individual is likely to vary under certain conditions. Sarbin [7] points out that there is particular value placed on playing out roles that are difficult to achieve. For example, the physician in our society occupies a status position that is highly rewarded. In contrast, family roles are seen as relatively easy to achieve and have fewer tangible rewards associated with them. Moreover, severe negative sanctions may be imposed if one does not operate according to expected standards of role performance. If a person has a number of roles to draw upon, it is likely that no one role will predominate. Instead, such a person's life will be an amalgam of roles, and a wide range of behaviors will be available to that person. But the person who has few roles, such as the traditional housewife, must invest each role with great importance. For this reason, we have examined the importance of adult family roles to the individual family members within the context of a broader societal framework.

Throughout this book there is frequent use of the term *role*. Since the word can mean different things to different investigators, it is important for us to specify our use and meaning of the term. For us, a role is something that is both dynamic and emergent. We do not look upon any of the roles being studied as consisting of well-defined sets of behaviors and expectations. Thus we did not assume a detailed knowledge of the components of these roles.

Neither have we viewed our subjects as either succeeding or failing in the enactment of specific, prescribed roles. Rather, we wanted to learn from our respondents how they saw themselves developing and negotiating—or, in short, making—the roles in question. Specifically, we did not assume a knowledge of relevant variables or key issues; rather, we saw ourselves as engaged in a search for these. We wanted to understand our respondents' from the respondents' viewpoint, discovering what they believed to be the important issues and variables. While we believe we possess certain skills needed to elicit, process, analyze, and communicate data, we were convinced that our respondents, and not we, were the experts in the substantive issues under consideration. Our conception of role is consistent with our theoretical framework of symbolic interactionism. It is a conception that allowed us to focus on our respondents' interpretations and interactions.

Our theoretical and conceptual underpinnings have definite methodological implications. Most generally, they imply a division of labor between ourselves as researchers and our respondents. We wanted our respondents to speak for themselves, on their own terms, about the roles in question. Our first task was to encourage them to speak honestly and candidly. Once we had conducted and transcribed these interviews, it was our further responsibility to systematically process, analyze, and interpret what the respondents had told us so it would accurately reflect what they as a group had revealed. The next chapter presents a more detailed discussion of our overall research design. It, in turn, sets the stage for the presentation of our actual findings, which comprise the remainder of the book.

REFERENCES

1. Berger, P., and Kellner, H. Marriage and the Construction of Reality. In H.P. Dreitzel (Ed.), *Recent Sociology No. 2.* New York: Macmillan, 1970.
2. Blumer, H. *Symbolic Interactionism: Perspective and Method.* Englewood Cliffs, N.J.: Prentice-Hall, 1969.
3. Cogswell, B. Rehabilitation of the paraplegic: Processes of socialization. *Social Inquiry* 37:11, 1967.
4. Lofland, J. *Deviance and Identity.* Englewood Cliffs, N.J.: Prentice-Hall, 1969.
5. McCall, G., and Simmons, J.L. *Identities and Interaction.* New York: Free Press, 1966.
6. Olesen, V., and Whittaker, E. *The Silent Dialogue: A Study of the Social Psychology of Professional Socialization.* San Francisco: Jossey-Bass, 1968.
7. Sarbin, T.B. The Culture of Poverty: Social Identity and Cognitive Outcome. In V. Alle (Ed.), *Psychological Factors in Poverty.* Chicago: Markham, 1970.
8. Sewell, W. Some recent developments in socialization theory and research. *American Academy of Political and Social Science.* 349:163, 1963.

3. Our Research Strategies for Understanding Adult Family Roles.

Kathleen Astin Knafl

$Since$ the studies reported in this book employ similar data gathering and analysis techniques, we may describe our common research methodology in a single chapter. The authors of certain chapters have chosen to report specific details of their project's history, but this chapter serves as a general overview the research approach used throughout this book. Our methodological approach is a function of both the theoretical assumptions outlined in the previous chapter and our overall goal of generating data-based theory.

Our specific conclusions and conceptual formulations have invariably emerged from a thoughtful and systematic consideration of the available data. They are never the product of imposing existing theoretical schemata on a set of data. In carrying out our investigations, we wanted our theories to be faithful to the empirical data and our data to be faithful to our respondents' viewpoints.

Consistent with our aim of learning about various family roles from the view point of the family members themselves, we have used the comparatively unstructured data gathering technique of intensive interviewing. Lofland has aptly described the intensive interview as a "guided conversation." He states: "One such flexible strategy of discovery is termed the 'unstructured interview' or 'intensive interviewing with an interview guide.' Its object is not to elicit choices between alternative answers to pre-formed questions but, rather, to elicit from the interviewee what he considers to be important questions relative to a given topic, his descriptions of some situations being explored. Its object is to carry on a guided conversation and to elicit rich, detailed materials that can be used in qualitative analysis. Its object is to find out what kinds of things are happening, rather than to determine the frequency of predetermined kinds of things that the researcher already believes can happen" [3, p. 76]. His definition coincides perfectly with our purposes.

DATA COLLECTION BY MEANS OF INTENSIVE INTERVIEWING

Following Lofland's lead, our first step prior to data gathering was to develop interview guides (see Appendix). The development of these guides was typically a group undertaking. Several of us would get together to discuss what it was we wanted to know about the specific process under consideration. Issues were thus defined, ordered, and developed into a tentative guide, which was then presented to the entire research group for general feedback and revision. We then pilot-tested our guides by interviewing respondents comparable to those who would be actually studied. Pilot testing of guides included questioning respondents both about the issues outlined on the guide and about the quality of the guide itself. We refined the interview guides based on the feedback from our pilot interviews.

The interview guides provided a checklist of topics for interviewers to cover, but interviewers were not constrained to follow the exact wording and order of the guide. Thus, while we structured our interviews to the extent that we introduced general issues and topics for discussion, we simultaneously encouraged respondents to express themselves in depth and to introduce issues that were not covered in the guides but that they believed were important.

Intensive interviewing requires much concentration by the researcher. When interviewing, we wanted to be able to devote our full attention to our subjects' responses, to hear both what was and was not being said, so that we could effectively probe for additional information. Since notetaking would have distracted our attention from the open-ended questioning process, we asked our respondents prior to the actual interview for permission to tape-record their comments, and we were always allowed to do so. This intensive interviewing strategy, we believe, successfully fulfilled our requirement that our method be flexible enough to elicit our respondents' own views of the role processes under investigation.

Our commitment to symbolic interactionism required that our research take into account the emergent nature of the family roles being studied. In actual practice, this accounting was extremely difficult to achieve. Ideally, we might have wished to follow couples across the entire life span, observing both the development of specific roles and the interplay between and among diverse roles. While we obviously have not attempted to follow our respondents for such a long period of time, we have, whenever possible, interviewed the same respondents a number of times. Specifically, the second and third parts of this book draw heavily on data gathered from couples who were interviewed during their engagement and are currently being followed through their first two years of marriage. These couples have been interviewed jointly at six-month intervals and the partners individually once a year. The fourth part also uses longitudinal data gathered from respondents before and after the birth of their children. The remaining parts of the book are based on a more cross-sectional type of data. The interviews on which the fifth and sixth parts were based were conducted with a wide variety of persons fulfilling the roles in question.

Despite our success in designing flexibility into our studies, our need for longitudinal data with which to study families as they develop has been much harder to fulfill. The ideal of following families across the entire life span is most difficult to achieve. Much of the research reported herein is continuing, as we strive to realize the goal of tracing family life throughout the life cycle. Aware of our limitations, we always have tried to indicate when our conclusions are derived from a cross-sectional sampling of respondents and when they stem from longitudinal data.

RESPONDENT SELECTION AND SAMPLING

We wanted our sampling design, as well as our data gathering techniques, to be consistent with our overall goal of developing a data-based theory of adult family roles. Conventional techniques of probability sampling did not suit this aim. While probability techniques are well suited to determining the distribution and frequency of various attitudes and behaviors among a population based on a sample of that population, they are poorly suited to our stated goal of building a data-based theory.

Building a data-based theory entails discovering what the participants in the situation being studied consider the key issues or variables and discerning the patterns of relationships among these. When describing this kind of theory, Glazer and Strauss state that "the elements of theory that are generated by comparative analysis are, first, conceptual properties; and second, hypotheses or generalized relations among the categories and their properties" [2, p. 35]. This statement implies that respondent selection should proceed with an eye to discovering, expanding, and interrelating the categories of the emerging theory. Sampling proceeds on the basis of theoretical relevance. Glazer and Strauss refer to this alternative approach to probability sampling as theoretical sampling, defined as "the process of data collection for generating theory whereby the analyst jointly collects, codes and analyzes his data and decides what data to collect next and where to find them in order to develop his theory as it emerges" [2, p. 35]. With this approach, data collection, analysis, and sampling are inextricably bound together.

Thus generating theory through a process of ongoing comparative analysis, we analyzed data from every interview in terms of what they told us about the specific role process being investigated. We studied data from specific interviews, seeking to identify the key issues or categories, the components of these issues, and the relations between these issues. We were then able to generate a rudimentary theoretical model of some process. Next we evaluated this emergent model in terms of where it needed refinement and expansion. Theory building and data gathering were complementary efforts. Data would contribute to the ongoing elaboration of an emerging model, while model building guided the search for data.

To summarize, the data on which the chapters of this book are grounded were collected with the intent of uncovering our respondents' views about broad areas of concern. To this end, we conducted intensive interviews, using loosely structured interview guides. Our selection of respondents was based on the criteria of theoretical relevance with regard to emerging theories or models of the role processes being considered.

DATA PROCESSING AND INTERPRETATION

When collecting data for the ultimate goal of building theory, the question of how one processes the information and uses it in constructing theory is critically important. Since all our interviews were tape-recorded, our data took the form of interview transcripts. Individual transcripts were usually twenty to fifty single-spaced typewritten pages. Thus we had to decide how to process and then systematically analyze massive amounts of material.

The processing of data began with the transcription of our first interview tapes. Once transcribed, interviews were checked for accuracy against the original tape. As soon as we had several such transcripts, we began developing coding categories. This step was especially important because these categories became the major components of our emergent theoretical models. In order to develop such coding categories, we read a sample of completed interviews and formulated what we believed to be major conceptual themes in the specific process under consideration. These tentative categories were then applied to a second sample of interviews and revised in order to take into account any data not covered by the initial categories. After assigning a number to each category, we read through our transcripts, numbering respondents' comments to correspond to the appropriate coding category or categories. Much of the data was coded by two project members working independently. They met at intervals to compare their application of the coding categories and resolve any differences. During the course of data coding, we all maintained a running record of our criteria for applying specific coding categories to the data.

After coding all the data, we transferred them to qualitative sort cards by making copies of all coded materials, which were then cut up and pasted onto 5 X 8-inch qualitative sort cards. The numbers on these cards were then punched to correspond to the appropriate coding categories. Once these processing steps had been completed, we were able to consider all the data on a given category as well as look at the relationships between and among categories. Although at first we analyzed our data in an informal, ad hoc way, our final stage of analysis was more thorough and more systematic.

The final interpretation of the data typically began with the analysis of individual coding categories and progressed through the formulation, evaluation, and integration of hypotheses. In order to analyze a specific category, we would begin by separating out all the sort cards that had been coded on the category we were to address. We would then read through all the data on that category, noting its primary characteristics and the other categories to which it appeared to be related. For example, at one point we separated out all our data on the "planning the wedding" category. We then read through all the sort cards pertinent to this category, looking for common themes and ways to integrate all the information. With the planning-the-wedding data, we were struck by the wide variations in the amount and focus of conflict on preparing for this event. In trying to explain this phenomenon, we developed a typology of approaches to wedding planning, which we then related to the level of conflict characterizing the planning.

Since data collection and analysis were occurring at the same time, the data-based theories presented in this book have all been revised and refined many times as new data were incorporated into emergent theories. Our approach to data processing and analysis is a guarantee that our conclusions are firmly grounded in the data and not in the researcher's possibly biased or selective impression of that data.

Once the data were analyzed, we believed it was our further responsibility to communicate them in a manner that would allow the reader to evaluate the conclusions drawn from them. In short, we believe that it is important for the reader to understand the process as well as the outcome of any research endeavor. The purpose of this chapter is to convey such an understanding. With regard to final presentation of our material, we agree with Glazer and Strass when they say: "A sociologist contributes most when he reports what he has observed in such fashion that it rings true to insiders, but also in such a fashion that they themselves would not have written it. That is, most useful sociological accounts are precisely those which insiders recognize as sufficiently inside to be true but not so 'inside' that they reveal only what is already known. . . . The sociologist's obligation is to report honestly but according to his own lights" [1, pp. 8-9]. We have attempted to achieve these goals of faithfully conveying our respondents' views while analytically describing the common underlying processes involved as individuals move into, sustain, and modify a variety of adult family roles.

SUBJECTIVE CONSIDERATIONS

The previous discussion has focused on the more technical aspects of our approach to research. In addition, we would like to consider briefly the more personal or subjective side of our investigative efforts. Specifically, we refer to our own feelings and those of our research subjects about participation in these studies.

We believe there are some very real advantages to group research projects, and we would like to make these explicit to our readers; the advantages are both personal and scientific. Since the research process can be alternately a very rewarding and a very frustrating undertaking, having collaborators with whom we could share our individual experiences was personally comforting and helpful. Throughout, we have collaborated in designing projects. We have shared such tangibles as interview guides, coding categories, and even respondents as well as less tangible leads, insights, and hunches. The ongoing sharing has enhanced the quality of both our individual experiences and our finished product.

Our subjects have indicated that they too have been gratified by their participation in our research. We have been impressed by their willingness to be research subjects and by their continuing cooperation once involved. Such ongoing commitment has been crucial to the success of the longitudinal investigation of engaged couples. Prior to their first interview, all respondents were given a general explanation of the overall project and a consent form outlining the terms of our agreement. Although respondents are free to drop out of the project at any time, our attrition rate for other than those individuals who have moved out of the area has been less than 10 percent. Most respondents have indicated that they enjoyed and looked forward to their interviews. One male respondent explained:

I wouldn't say that you made us think of things, because most of what you asked me I had already thought about. Still, it was interesting saying it all at one time. Kind of like pictures in an album; they are all together and you get to look at them and it's just nice. I think we both felt that way.

As noted in the Preface, the group whose research ifndings are reported herein was begun as a means to advise graduate students who were writing their master's theses. We group members hoped to get theses written and advising done in the most satisfying and positive manner possible. In retrospect, we not only accomplished our original goal but succeeded in carrying out a whole series of research projects in a manner that both we and our subjects considered positive and satisfying.

REFERENCES

1. Glazer, B.G., and Strauss, A. *Awareness of Dying.* Chicago: Aldine, 1965.
2. Glazer, B.G., and Strauss, A. *The Discovery of Grounded Theory: Strategies for Qualitative Research.* Chicago: Aldine, 1967.
3. Lofland, J. *Analyzing Social Settings.* Belmont, Calif.: Wadsworth, 1971.

II. Family Beginnings: Premarital Relationships.

"Family Beginnings" is something of a misnomer in that families do not have clear-cut beginnings or endings. We all have families of origin, and many of us will continue the cycle by marrying and starting families of our own. Thus, although certain ceremonial rites of passage "officially" signal the beginning of a new family, socialization into family roles begins much earlier. During childhood, and especially during adolescence, men and women devote considerable time and energy to trying out different forms of behavior as they interact with one another. This experimentation is part of the overall socialization process preparing young men and women to move into adult family roles.

We have chosen to break into this socialization process at the point when many young adults are actively pursuing and exploring a variety of kinds of relationships with members of the opposite sex. Marrying and beginning a family of one's own is only one possible outcome of the same general kind of behavior. Young men and women often find themselves in situations in which they have ample opportunity to interact with and form impressions of one another. For some, these encounters set in motion a relationship that progresses and eventually leads to marriage. For others, the relationship is similarly pursued but ends in cohabitation rather than marriage. Then again, many such encounters are short-lived. Individuals meet, evaluate one another, and decide not to pursue the relationship any further.

While most of the chapters in this book deal with specific family roles and relationships, the chapters in this part consider some alternative outcomes of male-female interaction. They concern the sometimes implicit, sometimes explicit search for a partner. At one extreme are those individuals for whom the search is an active foray into the world of eligibles for the purpose of finding an appropriate mate. At the other extreme are those individuals who are equally intent on avoiding any hint of a commitment to permanence. Specifically, the chapters in Part II present data on couples who are living together as well as on couples who are preparing to marry in the near future. In addition, they consider the kinds of nonpermanent relationships that typify interaction in singles bars.

Although a separate chapter is devoted to each of these topics, common themes cut across chapter boundaries. These common themes are reflected in our use of the same descriptive model to portray the dynamics of diverse kinds of relationships. While the model was developed in the context of investigating engaged couples, it was found to be an equally useful and valid frame for organizing data dealing with singles bars and cohabitation [1]. The model, illustrated on page 30, divides movement toward marriage into three broad stages: initiating stage, sustaining stage, and mutual commitment stage. While Chapter 6, which is based on data from engaged couples, deals with all three stages, the other chapters in this part consider only selected stages or as-

Developmental stages in the process of becoming engaged.

Sizing-up

Checking-out

Comparative analysis (this date vs. all others)

Strategies for maintaining relationship without getting serious

Making relationship public

The engagement event

Planning the marriage

Projections into the future

Initiating Stage

Sustaining Stage

Mutual Commitment Stage

pects of stages. In either case, we specify what components of the model we are discussing and how, specifically, they apply to our data.

REFERENCE

1. Knafl, K.A., and Grace, H.K. Family Beginnings: The Dynamics of Role Making. In C.R. Kneisl and H.S. Wilson (Eds.), *Current Perspectives in Psychiatric Nursing.* Vol. 1, *Issues and Trends.* St. Louis: Mosby, 1976.

4. Singles Bars and the Permanence Dilemma. *Anne Flickinger*

Any stage of the process of developing an identity as a couple may be problematic for the individuals involved. It is, however, axiomatic that one must first meet members of the opposite sex, for without that contact the process cannot be initiated. For many singles residing in large urban areas, what may initially be most problematic is arranging opportunities to meet others to date. One possible way is by patronizing singles bars, bars that are designed to attract single adults.

Data for the study of social interaction in singles bars were collected between the fall of 1973 and the spring of 1974 in a large midwestern city by observing and interviewing the patrons of several bars. The interviews were of two types: brief ones conducted within the bar setting and intensive ones conducted outside the setting. Intensive interviews followed the format described in Chapter 3. The interviewer, following a flexible interview guide (see Appendix), asked participants a variety of questions designed to elicit their opinions and feelings about bar use, bar norms, interaction in bars and elsewhere, desires for long-term relationships, and ways in which bars might facilitate the establishment of such relationships. In addition, bar management personnel were interviewed to ascertain ways in which they structure the setting to meet the needs of their patrons.

A great deal of data was obtained on a variety of aspects of the singles bar experience. Most germane to the conceptual model presented at the beginning of this part are those facets of male-female interactions that are related to the initiation, maintenance, and termination of encounters. This chapter focuses on the ways in which patrons of singles bars structure their encounters, with particular emphasis on the sizing-up element of the initiating stage of the conceptual model. The impact of the bar setting on the interaction process and how the bar influences the formation of long-term relationships will also be discussed.

Of primary importance in this study was the need to examine the motivations for bar use. The data indicate that there are a number of motives for going to singles bars: (1) to meet new people; (2) to find people to date in the hope either of eventually forming a close relationship or of simply having a casual sexual encounter; (3) to escape loneliness; (4) to be with friends in a convivial atmosphere; (5) to drink in populated surroundings; (6) to avoid boredom; (7) to have an outlet for fun and relaxation; and (8) to get back into circulation following the termination of a relationship. Patrons may use the bars for only one or for several of these reasons, and their motives may vary from night to night. Common to all of the reasons enumerated is a need to structure one's social life and people one's environment. Within this context, the motivations patrons cited most frequently were loneliness and the desire to meet members of the opposite sex. The latter motivation was mentioned at one time or another by all individuals interviewed.

Loneliness as a motivating factor is an important consideration when examining the settings in which singles find each other because it is an affect, an emotion that can influence or color the setting. The way patrons choose to cope with this feeling has a generalized effect on the encounters conducted in a bar. Loneliness is both a fact and a feeling; Lopata defines it as "being dependent upon a social self wishing to be involved in meaningful interaction with others" [3, p. 249]. Some patrons would admit to loneliness as a generalized fact, but they had difficulty personalizing it as an experience, as the interview with N.B., a 27-year-old Australian businessman, demonstrates:

N.B.: *I guess loneliness could be a factor, but I don't think that I feel lonely. It's probably a little bit of both boredom and loneliness, but I wouldn't say it's a deep-seated loneliness; it's more of a spur of the moment thing.*

Int: *Do you think a deep-seated loneliness might be a motivating factor for others?*

N.B.: *Oh, I'm sure.*

This example and several others clearly indicate an inability to admit to being lonely oneself while readily attributing the feeling to others.

A.N., a 27-year-old male law student and part-time employee at Bar Alpha,* was asked why he thought people go to bars:

A.N.: *They're lonely.*

Int: *Is that the only reason?*

A.N.: *I'm sure there are variations on this loneliness thing, but they go there for companionship, like most people don't have herds of people coming to their apartment all the time. Being a single person, you're subject to loneliness. I bet most people who go to bars don't really like it, but they have no alternative; so they go.*

*Bar names have been disguised with Greek letter names to protect their privacy.

34. Family Beginnings: Premarital Relationships

Loneliness as a motivating factor was cited by the majority of patrons, even though it was rarely self-attributed. It is as though the patrons were ashamed to admit experiencing a feeling that few would deny is universally felt at one time or another, as though that admission is indicative of some profound inadequacy. An inability to confront such feelings can then influence the honesty with which individuals relate to each other because it circumscribes and limits what can be shared.

The most frequently cited motivation for going to singles bars was the desire to meet members of the opposite sex, although this reason was usually accompanied by other reasons, such as having fun or meeting new people. Regardless of other intentions, a possible opportunity to interact with members of the opposite sex remains at least a hope. The individuals in bars have been engaged in male-female interaction to some degree for a good portion of their lives, and they have learned how to conduct themselves with members of the opposite sex. They may not be successful all of the time, or, indeed, any of the time, and their relations with their opposites may be characterized by chronic uncertainty. Nonetheless, they have developed ideas and thoughts that direct and guide their behavior. In the bar setting, the problem is substantively the same as it is in the outside world, i.e., how to interact successfully with members of the opposite sex; how to initiate, maintain, and terminate encounters; and, even more fundamentally, how to decide with whom to interact. But in the bar setting, the guidelines individuals have established in other settings may not be valid; individuals may have to modify or even totally restructure their outlook if they are to cope with the process of interacting in a bar. For example, upon entering such a bar, one is immediately accorded the status of an an unattached, available person and thus may reasonably expect to be approached for the purposes of beginning an encounter. One need not accept the advances, but one should be neither surprised nor offended when they occur. With the exception of those persons who are there with dates, any individual who enters the bar is assumed to be interested in interactions with others by virtue of his or her presence. If an individual enters for other reasons, he or she must explain his or her status and not assume clairvoyant powers in the other patrons.

Data analysis indicates that patrons of singles bars use a variety of guidelines when addressing the problem of with whom to interact (sizing-up) and with whom to initiate, maintain, and terminate encounters. Some guidelines closely approximate those used in other social settings and public places; others are unique to the singles bar setting and have evolved because established guidelines were inadequate.

SIZING-UP IN PREPARATION FOR AN ENCOUNTER

Sizing-up an individual in terms of attending to physical, social, and personal characteristics is the first step in the initiating stage of our conceptual model. In the singles bar setting, this process begins before the individual enters the bar. Bars are chosen for a variety of reasons, but of paramount importance is the opportunity to be with people with similar characteristics. Possessed of a notion, varying in degree of concreteness, of what sorts of people they hope to meet, individuals patronize certain bars in order to increase the probability that they will find people who meet their criteria. Individuals choose a bar based on information about what kinds of people go to that bar. Such information is obtained by trial and error and word of mouth. The prospective patron evaluates such variables as age, race, life-style, and socioeconomic status. The following interview with S.S., a 22-year old executive trainee, and P.C., a 26-year-old buyer, illustrates this theme:

P.C.: I can't relate to people going to bars grubbing around and looking like hippies. I'm not going to a place like Bar Iota with everyone looking freaky. I mean I'd walk in, turn around, and walk out.

S.S.: And that's just what we did last week: walked in and walked out again.

A similar attitude was expressed by F.E., a 35-year-old male computer programmer:

There's definitely discrimination by bar management against certain socio-economic classes and groups like the man who just got off a street job. It's pretty much white, middle-class, and rising, but I have to admit those are the bars I'm interested in. It makes me sound biased, and I'm sorry to say that.

As these representative examples indicate, one may immediately increase the odds of meeting someone with desirable characteristics by carefully choosing the bars one patronizes.

The bar setting with its dim lighting, population density, and decibel level, which may approach the threshold of pain, influences the pace at which the initial sizing-up process occurs. A leisurely period of getting acquainted is not perceived as an option, and the decision to approach someone in order to begin an interaction is often made quickly and superficially, even though considerable time may elapse before the encounter is verbally initiated. When patrons were asked what was initially attractive about someone, what characteristic might lead them to begin an encounter, physical appearance was mentioned most often. If an individual decides someone is attractive, he or she may then evaluate that person's behavior and interactions with others. A person who appears to be enjoying himself or herself may be evaluated positively; a person who is treating others in a hostile or demeaning fashion will be evaluated negatively, primarily because the evaluator does not wish to receive similar treatment.

Factors characterized as secondarily attractive, those that might influence the patron to continue an interaction once it has been initiated, were of a less superficial nature, such as intelligence, sense of humor, sincerity, reciprocal interests, honesty, conversational ability, and those traits that loosely come under the rubric of "nice personality." Patrons also consider socioeconomic factors. Although they do look for positive qualifiers, they are more attentive to an absence of negative qualifiers such as self-centeredness, lying, poor sense of humor, dullness, ignorance, and an inability to converse. Again, this assessment often occurs rapidly, and an individual who is unable to project a positive self-image in a short span of time will have difficulty in maintaining encounters. Of course, an individual who is only looking for a casual sexual encounter or a one-night stand will be far less concerned with these factors.

INITIATING ENCOUNTERS

For many individuals, the process of initiating an encounter has been divided into two stages. The first may be seen as a preinitiation stage involving the use of eye contact, sizing-up or checking out of the other, spatial maneuvering and stratagems, and deciding who moves first. The second stage involves the actual initiation of the encounter: choosing an opening gambit, making the move, and waiting for a response. Once an encounter has been set in motion, it must be either maintained or terminated.

Eye contact during the preinitiation stage is a device shared by both sexes and is used to some extent by everyone in the bar setting. Eye contact beyond the brief glance that is characteristic of unfocused interaction is perceived as an indication of potential interest when it is sustained or returned. This device is particularly valued and utilized by women in bars, many of whom are reluctant to begin conversations with men. T.M., a 22-year-old student, when asked how she approaches men whom she finds interesting, replied:

I would probably look at them a lot. I guess I try to get eye contact to make them aware that I'm interested.

All those who were interviewed used eye contact to some extent to indicate interest.

Just as the establishment of eye contact may indicate possible interest, failure to reciprocate may suggest lack of interest. Yet even this seemingly obvious device can be problematic for the patron who must decide whether another's refusal to return eye contact is indicative of disinterest, shyness, or idle curiosity. As P.O., a 28-year-old female social worker, stated:

Sometimes, they'll stare, and if you happen to catch them at it, they'll look away. That's rough because then you don't know if they're staring at you because they want to approach you or because you have a piece of lettuce hanging between your teeth. Maybe staring and then looking at the floor means "I'm shy; you approach me." You can see how confusing it gets.

In spite of some confusion, patrons believe that eye contact is a valuable assessment tool and that sustained and reciprocated eye contact indicates at least some degree of interest.

Patrons also must decide who moves first, who initiates the encounter on a verbal level. Generally, the female will indicate interest or at least will fail to demonstrate obvious hostility; the male is then expected to take the first step in initiating the encounter, and the female is expected to respond to the initiating moves. But this process may be disrupted in two ways: a male may initiate an encounter even though it is clear that further communication is undesirable, or a female may initiate an encounter.

A male may initiate an encounter even though a female has demonstrated disinterest by refusing to exchange glances or return a smile. Such unsolicited encounters were observed on numerous occasions and were referred to by women respondents. But they occur much less frequently than do those begun after waiting for cues that indicate interest.

In a reversal of roles, a female may be the one to initiate an encounter after ascertaining that some degree of interest exists. Among the women interviewed, only one indicated that she routinely initiates encounters. Others could do so only with difficulty because they considered such behavior alien to their natures and somewhat aggressive. The only variable that might cause a woman to act differently is a blood alcohol level sufficiently high to overcome her inhibitions.

Stratagems and spatial maneuvering are two additional facets of encounter initiation that are employed to facilitate interaction. Stratagems are those actions that the patron uses to modify existing circumstances to his advantage. Spatial maneuvering occurs when the patron positions himself or herself so as to more easily begin an encounter.

Numerous examples of spatial maneuvering were observed and reported, such as the importance of where one stands or sits in the bar. Men often choose to stand by the women's washroom because, barring an inordinate bladder capacity, any woman who remains in the bar for any length of time will have to pass that way. Where one sits at the bar, assuming one has a choice, is also a spatial maneuver. G.C., one of the few females who initiates encounters, explained:

> If there was a seat here, and there was a girl here, and then a couple of seats, and a guy here, and he looked interesting, I'd probably plop myself down next to him or leave one space and sit close enough so that a conversation could be struck up.

Both of these examples illustrate that spatial maneuvering, although it may appear casual, is a matter of deliberate choice.

Stratagems are designed to modify circumstances and give patrons an advantage they might not otherwise have. C.K., a 29-year-old airline pilot, stated that he might step on a girl's foot or spill her drink to give himself an opening. He has also used more refined stratagems:

> I don't even care if they're escorted if I can get them away from the guy long enough to meet them. I've been known to tell guys there's a phone call for them to get the guy away. I'd even pay a waiter to tell a guy there's a phone call for him.

Stratagems and spatial maneuvering may or may not be successful, but their use at least gives the patrons an opportunity to manipulate the setting in a way that they hope will be to their advantage. Contrived by definition, many stratagems and spatial maneuvers are designed to appear natural and spontaneous.

Once the individual has decided to initiate an encounter on a verbal level, he or she is faced with the need to find an opening gambit. Males who were interviewed indicated that they have tried a variety of opening gambits; after a trial period, they adopt whatever gambit has been most effective. As C.K. stated when asked how he approaches someone who looks interesting:

C.K.: *Generally, I'll look her right in the eye, walk right up, and say Hi. The straightforward approach is as good as any, and I've tried every kind there is.*

Int: *What other kinds have you used?*

C.K.: *Step on their foot, spill a drink on them, don't you live in my building, don't I know you from somewhere, etc., etc.—every conceivable approach that I've ever heard about or read about or seen. I'm trying to tailor-make something that's uniformly successful for me.*

Patrons use a number of opening gambits, a common element of which is an attempt to project a positive self-image and engage the other person so as to maintain the encounter. Faced with the problem of initiating an interaction, participants use whatever works best for them.

Data from the interviews indicate that men and women attach the same or similar meaning to the processes of encounter initiation. When women were asked how they were approached by men, they were able to identify the techniques used. In fact, it is important that opening gambits be invested with the same meaning by both sexes because such actions are accompanied by certain assumptions. If a male sits next to a female and begins a conversation, he assumes that she will know that he is interested; at the same time, she will assume that his behavior indicates interest. The interest is implied rather than stated, and the importance of this implication lies in its face-saving function. Should the female fail to respond affirmatively, the male has not committed himself; he has only gone through motions that have implied interest but could be interpreted as something else.

Initiation of encounters may be accompanied by problems in any social setting, but it is particularly difficult in singles bars, wherein behavior is circumscribed by noise, crowds, drinking, and an aura of conviviality and superficiality. Many of the ways in which individuals usually meet members of the opposite sex are ineffective in this setting; so patrons must develop new behaviors.

MAINTAINING ENCOUNTERS

Once verbal contact has been established, individuals in a bar setting need to assess their impact on others, i.e., is the other person interested in maintaining the encounter? This stage of the encounter process is fraught with fewer problems than the preceding stage because individuals can use evaluative tools they have employed outside the bar setting. Eye contact is used to maintain as well as to initiate encounters. Again, sustained eye contact is perceived as a sign of interest while its absence is generally thought to be indicative of disinterest or a desire to terminate the encounter. Patrons also attend to other nonverbal cues and to the content and direction of the conversation. When F.O., the social worker, was asked how she could tell if someone was interested in maintaining an encounter, her response entailed a description of nonverbal cues:

This nonverbal stuff you hear about is very important. It's like you're talking to someone and thinking "I wonder if he's interested." Then you see him bending his straw into twenty-thousand shapes, tapping his foot, checking out every chick that walks in, then you have a very good idea that he might be bored and looking for a way to get away.

In this case, eye contact and other nonverbal cues are used to surmise one's probable impact.

Patrons of bars also evaluate the content and direction of the conversation. N.B., a 25-year-old nurse, described such evaluation:

You can tell if they're interested by the reaction and response they give. If they don't want to have anything to do with you, they might be a little curt, or there's no response whatsoever in stimulating the conversation. It's maybe a "yes," "no," "uh-uh" kind of answer. . . .

Other participants mentioned the conversational cues from which one might reasonably infer the degree of interest: paying attention, listening, and eagerness to maintain the conversation. Indication of interest may be inferred from the conversational content, as M.B.'s response demonstrates: "It's easy to tell if they aren't interested because they're talking, talking, talking, and it's all about them."

Data analysis indicates that patrons attend to many cues, both positive and negative, but that they pay more attention to and search more actively for the negative ones, such as lack of eye contact, lack of attention, failure to maintain the conversation, or lack of interest in any real exchange or sharing of information. Patrons integrate the cues they perceive and form them into a gestalt of the general impression they think they are making. Most participants employ this same process in other social settings.

The gesture of men buying women drinks may be used as an opening gambit, but it is more frequently employed to maintain an encounter. The gesture is invested with meaning, and normative behavior is attached to it. Because this gesture is specific to the setting, its meaning and the behavior appropriate to it must be learned. In general, a male offers to buy a female a drink if he is interested in talking to her. If she accepts, she is expected to talk to him for the length of time it takes her to consume the drink. The significance of the gesture and the anticipated response is explained by A.T. (male):

I would say it's expected that she talk to you; that's common courtesy. If she's not interested, she shouldn't accept the drink, and I think most girls probably don't. I normally wouldn't buy a girl a drink unless I had already struck up a conversation with her.

The males asked to describe the response they anticipated from a woman indicated that a minimum response would be a polite thank you but that the norm is to remain until the drink is consumed. Male reactions to violations of this norm ranged from anger and indignation to irritation or resignation but were by no means countenanced.

With two exceptions, women interviewed were aware of the normative aspect of this gesture, both in terms of what it means and what is expected. The response from G.C., a 27-year-old nurse, was representative:

I think they at least expect someone to stick with them for the duration of the drink, if not longer. If they're interested enough to spend a dollar for a drink, they want to talk to you and expect you to stay with them. If I'm turned off by someone from just talking to them, I would probably not accept the drink.

These responses demonstrate the congruence of meaning and expected behavior that is attached to the gesture. As long as both men and women understand its import, the gesture is functional as a means of assessing the desire to maintain an encounter.

In general, maintaining an encounter in a singles bar is far less of a problem than initiating or terminating one. The data suggest that the ease with which encounters can be maintained is the result of the patrons' ability to use behavior guidelines and evaluative tools they have developed outside the bar setting. The maintenance process would be far more difficult if patrons had to learn new ways in which to interact with members of the opposite sex.

TERMINATING ENCOUNTERS

Terminating an encounter in a singles bar setting is a complex process both for the person who wishes to terminate and for the person who has been terminated. When unwilling to maintain an encounter, individuals deal with the situation in various ways. One maneuver is to evince the above-mentioned signs of disinterest in the hope that the other person will take the hint and exit, thus sparing the first person the necessity of using stronger tactics. The response of T.M., a 22-year-old female student, was typical of those given by respondents when asked how they terminate encounters:

Go to the washroom. I'm supposed to meet my friend now across the bar. Hope maybe there's another man you know well enough to say, "Excuse me, I have to go and talk to so-and-so." Also, what I've done a lot when I don't want to talk to someone is to refuse drinks from them. That's a good way to cut off a conversation or any attraction, because it's a kind of currency.

This comment illustrates some of the excuses that are used to achieve an

41. Singles Bars and the Permanence Dilemma

amicable termination of an encounter. It is also an example of the meaning invested in offering to buy a drink and in rejecting the offer with the intention of terminating the encounter.

The attempt to be polite is evident in the response given by J.J., a 32-year-old salesman:

J.J.: I usually say, "It's been nice talking to you" and then walk away. Or I might say, "I see someone I know that I'd like to talk to."

Int: It sounds as though you're polite.

J.J.: Definitely. There's no percentage in being rude. It's just a matter of common courtesy, and I don't want to hurt anyone's feelings.

Most patrons seek to terminate an encounter in as reasonable and relatively painless a fashion as possible. The tactic they choose, however, is highly contingent upon the behavior of the other person, who is expected to accept gracefully the fact that termination is desired. Should the other person be recalcitrant or obtuse, the individual is then compelled to state his or her position more forcefully. Faced with a person who is offensive or obnoxious, patrons may drop all pretense of being nice and, in no uncertain terms, tell the other to go away. But because individuals wish to think of themselves as agreeable, courteous, nice persons, they prefer not to adopt Draconian measures. Having to act in a harsh manner is incongruent with their concept of self. They usually rationalize such rudeness by reminding themselves that they are, after all, in a bar and would not be unkind unless needlessly provoked. When asked about terminating encounters, B.Z., a 25-year-old black entertainer, stated:

I say something like, "Excuse me, I have something else to do," or "It's been nice talking to you." If she's really obnoxious, I just say, "I can't talk to you any more," and walk away. Respect is important, and I'm never rude. Rudeness appalls me unless it's warranted.

Initially, most individuals attempt to exit gracefully, but they will employ harsher measures if the other person fails to realize that his or her attentions or further conversation are not desired.

The other person, the individual being terminated, must cope with rejection that is either stated or implied. The bar setting frequently influences this individual's response. Patrons were asked how they react to rejection in a different social setting such as at a party or on a date, and if they believed rejection was easier to accept in a bar. Most of those interviewed indicated that rejection was less painful in a bar, as the following sample responses illustrate:

It's more painful outside a bar; you have nowhere to turn. In a bar, you're with a group, and you have others to talk to.

42. Family Beginnings: Premarital Relationships

Nobody likes to be rejected, but it's easier in a bar because you can always say, "Ah, what the hell do you know," and walk over to talk to someone else.

It's more painful in an outside situation because I'd feel I'd invested more of myself in another type of situation. [The exchange in] a bar is just false currency.

These replies indicate that rejection outside a bar is more painful because the emotional investment is often greater and immediate alternatives are fewer.

Individuals quickly learn that the way in which they cope with rejection outside a singles bar setting is inappropriate in that setting. The dynamics of bar interaction soon points out the necessity of developing a new way of coping. The singles bar is viewed as a setting with a "shoot-down atmosphere wherein "striking out," i.e., failure to arouse reciprocal interest, is an expectation. Faced with the very real possibility that on numerous if not most occasions interest will not be returned, individuals must learn to deal with rejection in a new way. Bars have been described as unserious behavioral settings [1, 2] in which consequentiality is suspended and what occurs is exempt from "counting"; if this description is accepted, then rejection in a bar does not count for anything. The patrons first must learn to expect that they will be "shot down" more often than not. As P.C. stated:

I guess guys expect to get turned down a lot, and so do girls; you don't expect that everyone you meet is someone you'll talk to for very long.

Then they must learn to regard the rejection as unimportant, as not counting. When respondents were asked how they felt about being "shot down," they replied in this manner:

Chalk it up. No big stuff. I've never met anyone at a bar that I was so entranced with that I've felt dejected by their turning me down or ignoring me.

No big deal. That's the breaks.

You have to go with that premise [not to care] or you'll destroy yourself. It doesn't bother me.

These responses are representative of those given by patrons who expressed their belief that being "shot down" is the rule rather than the exception and that it simply does not matter. One of the respondents quoted above took the process a step further, reaching the conclusion that not only the rejection but the person meting it out does not count.

Patrons must also learn how to behave once rejection has occurred. A patron might respond as D.G., a 31-year-old black laboratory technician, responds:

You're a little discouraged naturally, but you don't throw a tantrum. I just say,

"See you again" or *"Have a nice time"* and go talk to someone else. In a bar you expect to get *"shot down"* and approached.

G.C.'s response was similar:

I just pass it off and go on to someone else.

These two typical responses indicate that rejection or the termination of an encounter is usually handled in a reasonable fashion.

An interview with E.D., a 36-year-old school engineer who has been going to singles bars off and on since his college days, reveals the process by which individuals adapt to the bar setting:

Int: How do you feel if you approach someone to talk and she doesn't seem interested?

E.D.: I handle it much better now that I'm older and have been in the bar scene for awhile. Before I used to force the issue.

Int: What do you mean?

E.D.: When I was younger and someone was trying to "shoot me down," espe-cially if she was tactful about it, I'd keep after her to talk to me. And my feel-ings would be hurt. Now I don't feel particularly hurt, and I go on to someone else. It's almost an expectation that you're gonna get it a lot.

In this instance, the patron used to be hurt and unwilling to accept termina-tion. As he learned that such feelings and actions could be painful and did nothing to facilitate encounters, he changed his way of dealing with the situation.

Because encounters in a bar can proceed rapidly from initiation to termina-tion, a certain amount of maneuvering may be employed to minimize the chances that termination will occur immediately. The checking-out behavior discussed in connection with initiation of encounters is one example of such maneuvering. Maneuvering also occurs when individuals first carefully attend to behavioral cues and then attempt to initiate an encounter only when suc-cess is highly probable. A.N.'s response reflects the general feeling that there is no need to ask for rejection:

Usually, the only girls you end up trying to hustle are the ones that you think will be receptive to it.

Terminating an encounter is a problem both for the individual who by im-plication rejects another and for the individual who by implication is rejected by another. Because in singles bars the probability is high that individuals will be both rejected and rejecting, patrons of such bars respond accordingly. They expect their experiences to conform to certain norms: (1) interest in

another person more often than not will be unreciprocated; (2) lack of interest and/or termination of an encounter will be handled politely, other things
being equal; and (3) termination should be accepted gracefully and not taken
personally. Violation of these norms falls within the purview of unsanctioned
behavior, and little sympathy is accorded to those who fail, for whatever
reason, to follow the norms. As C.K. so trenchantly stated:

*"The meek shall inherit the earth" does not apply on the Street of Broken
Dreams [his sobriquet for one bar area]. You gotta be strong.*

One gains strength by expecting to get "shot down," by accepting it with
equanimity, and by "shooting down" without being rude.
   In conclusion, then, encounters between men and women in a singles bar
setting are a problem for both sexes. Individuals who frequent such bars must
develop ways in which to cope with the initiation, maintenance, and termination of such encounters. Some techniques used in the larger social world are
appropriate or require little modification in this setting. Others are inappropriate; so techniques suitable to the bar setting must be designed. Because the
various behaviors exhibited in the bars are invested with certain meanings,
patrons must learn how to interpret those meanings and integrate them into
their own patterns of behavior.

SCORING, OR CAN YOU EVER FIND A MEANINGFUL RELATIONSHIP IN A BAR?

This section describes the phenomena of "scoring," or having an encounter
whose outcome results in sexual intercourse that same night, and its potential
for developing long-term relationships. Synonymous terms for scoring are
"hustling," "picking up someone," "getting laid," and "getting lucky." The
term *one-night stand* implies a sexual encounter of one night's duration, with
no future encounters, sexual or otherwise, scheduled. For many patrons of
singles bars, *scoring* and *one-night stand* may be equivalent terms.
   Scoring has numerous implications beyond the obvious. For some, it moti-
vates bar use, either exclusively or as often as possible. Problems arise when
scoring is the oucome of an encounter; so patrons of singles bars must
develop ways in which to deal with the possibility and reality of such an outcome. Attitudes and admissions about scoring are frequently specific to men
or to women. The use of bars for scoring is related to the desire for close and/
or long-term interpersonal relationships. Most of the data on this topic were
elicited by asking respondents if they had ever dated anyone they met in a
bar for an extended period of time and if at the time they were interested in
a long-term relationship.
   A large percentage of the men interviewed use bars for scoring although it is
not always the sine qua non for going to a bar. J.S., a 29-year-old social
worker, was asked if he thought people go to singles bars looking for a long-
term relationship:

J.S.: I think a lot of people are [looking for long-term relationships]. I'm a firm believer in relationships.

Int: I've heard that a lot of people come down here to get laid. Do you agree?

J.S.: That's why I'm here tonight.

Int: Are you that candid with the girls you meet?

J.S.: I would have to say so. But I believe in forming relationships even if it's for an hour.

Int: What kind of relationship can you form in an hour?

J.S.: A very superficial one.

Although J.S. once had a "quasi-serious" relationship with a woman he met in a bar, this relationship did not alter his desire for casual sexual encounters, a desire that would undoubtedly circumscribe his encounters with women in bars.

A.T., a 33-year-old salesman who goes to bars several nights a week, was asked if he had met anyone at a bar whom he had dated for any length of time:

A.T.: Not really, unless you want to count two or three dates.

Int: I was thinking of a longer period of time.

A.T.: No, usually just one time. That's part of the idea, too; one shot, you're good for the whole night. You figure you want to run into someone, and you want to get lucky. You're not interested in them personally, just, "come on, let's go."

Int: You know ahead that it's going to be a one-shot thing?

A.T.: Yeah.

A.T. is a regular patron of one bar and uses bars for several reasons. When his motive in going is to score, that motive becomes primary. For the majority of males who were interviewed, "getting laid" was a motivation for bar use at least some of the time; for a few, it was the only motivation.

If a male enters a bar hoping to score, he must be prepared to negotiate. To eliminate what might be a time-consuming process, some men are very forthright in their approach. For example, J.G., a 27-year old salesman, was described by his friends as a "real hustler." He stated that he used to go to bars almost solely for the purpose of "getting laid," and then continued:

J.G.: When I was doing it, I found that there was little success difference in the two approaches I used: "Do you want to go to my house and f---?" or "Do you want to go to my house and listen to records?"

46. Family Beginnings: Premarital Relationships

Int: What was your success rate?

J.G.: About 50 percent, and there wasn't much difference based on what I said.

Both approaches meant the same thing to J.G., but when he used the first, his intentions were clear from the outset.

Barring the use of an approach as bold as the one described above, patrons must know what to expect from an encounter continued outside the bar. Certain meanings are imputed to certain types of behavior. N.B. was asked:

Int: Do you ever go into anything knowing ahead of time that it will be a one-night stand?

N.B.: Quite a few times, I take it as it comes.

Int: Does the girl know?

N.B.: Yes, by the time I leave the bar to go home, she has a good idea. Most girls who go home with a guy can take care of themselves, or maybe they just want to sleep with the guy.

If N.B.'s main interest is a one-night stand, he assumes that a female who goes home with him is more than likely consenting to have sexual relations. This assumption was discussed in more detail by A.N. and A.Y.:

Int: What about someone you just want to go to bed with that night? Is there any way you make that clear?

A.Y.: No. I always assume that if some girl will leave with me, things will work out.

A.N.: You have to assume that if some girl will go to your apartment, you'll probably get lucky.

A.Y.: If a girl says yes, it's a rare girl who doesn't know what you might be thinking. Well, you get some girls who come back and say, "Hey, what are you doing?" One in fifteen maybe.

Like N.B., A.N. and A.Y. expect that any woman who returns to their apartments knows why she has been invited. A woman who has other ideas is considered naive.

C.K.'s tactics are a combination of the implicit and the explicit:

Int: So you've met someone and she comes here or you go to her apartment. Is there any expectation . . . ?

C.K.: Of course! You think you're gonna get f-----!

Int: Is that verbalized or is that an expectation?

47. Singles Bars and the Permanence Dilemma

C.K.: Both. In case there's any doubt, I may bring it up, like "Hey, are we gonna f---?"

Int: What kind of response do you get to that?

C.K.: Yes.

Int: That's what everyone says?

C.K.: Everyone doesn't offer to take me to their apartment. But the ones that are offering, a lot of times, it doesn't need to be said. Obviously, two adult people, they want to f---, that's why you're inviting them back. It's not to look at your etchings.

For these males, being able to predict behavior on the basis of assumptions and expectations simplifies the way in which they deal with situations that arise in the bar. A woman who may think she is going to look at etchings is therefore violating what they anticipate will be normative behavior. Of the eleven men who discussed this issue, eight expected the woman to have consented to sexual intercourse by having agreed to accompany them to an apartment. The other three were less categorical in their response, stating that if a woman consented to go home with them, there was a "good chance" that the encounter would end sexually. As J.J. stated, "If a girl goes home with you, it's understood that you're at least going to try." Obviously, such responses indicate that a large number of men in bars expect an evening that ends in someone's apartment to also end in a sexual encounter even if such an outcome is not expressed verbally. At the very minimum, a woman can expect a pass to be made once she is inside the confines of an apartment.

Data gathered from interviews with women indicate that they give a great deal of thought to the issue of scoring. With two exceptions, all of the women queried about scoring believed that it was a major motivation for many men in bars and that many men expect to "get laid" the night they meet someone. Women must decide what a man means by his invitation to leave the bar and how to deal with his intention. G.C. alluded to these decisions when discussing what sort of behavior is not condoned in bars:

G.C.: . . . guys that are more pushy, they'll keep asking things like "Let's go out for the night" or "Let's go out to breakfast"; pushy guys like that don't score.

Int: Does going out to breakfast have any implications?

G.C.: It depends. Sometimes it means just that, and other times a guy has a lot more on his mind, like he wants to "get laid."

Int: Is that made clear ahead of time?

G.C.: Not always, you have to be watching for it. You have to state your position before you go out to breakfast at times to protect whatever your interests are. If your interests are that, fine.

If a male is not candid in expressing his intentions, a female must try to second-guess him by attending to his behavior. If she suspects that their interests are not parallel, then she must make her position clear before she leaves. Going out to breakfast (getting something to eat after the bar has closed) seems innocent enough, but many men hope to continue the evening beyond the meal; so women must be able to surmise the intent of such an apparently simple invitation. If a woman assumes that a man is interested in a sexual encounter, and his interests coincide with hers, then there is no problem.

When M.B. was asked about this process, she stated that she was reluctant to get picked up by a stranger at the risk of contracting venereal disease or suddenly finding herself in close quarters with someone of marginal stability. She addressed the negotiation process:

I think it's discussed at the bar. I would never leave with a guy unless I made it quite clear that I wasn't going to bed with him. I wouldn't leave with him, get to the door, and then say, "I'm not interested." That's unfair because a lot of guys do expect it; the least you can do is be honest about it.

As these responses indicate, women are aware of the problems attendant upon leaving the bar with someone and of the general expectation among males that to culminate an evening in someone's apartment is to "get laid." Women use this knowledge when dealing with bar encounters.

The data demonstrate that men and women report divergent frequencies of scoring. Males indicate that they are scoring, some with great regularity. Females indicate that they usually do not go home with a man the first night they meet him; on those occasions when they do, they indicate that they attempt to convey clearly their intention not to end up in bed. The incongruity is most probably due to our small sample size. Granting a possible male tendency to exaggerate, it is likely that those women who engage in one-night stands were not among those interviewed.

The opposite of scoring and one-night stands is a desire for a long-term, meaningful relationship that embodies trust, closeness, and sharing, the sort of relationship that adults should have the capacity to develop. Everyone interviewed was either involved in some sort of relationship that they regarded as intimate, actively looking for such a relationship, or at least not actively discouraging one. The desire for a close relationship was not synonymous with desire for marriage by any means, but patrons did verbalize a desire for relationships with meaning and closeness attached to them. B.Z. expressed this desire most graphically when asked if he wanted a meaningful relationship:

B.Z.: Yeah. A long-term relationship is heavy, but it's beautiful, especially if it's good. I went out with this chick for two years, and I was really at peace with myself, knowing that everything was okay.

Int: *Could you share some of your thoughts with me on what kind of relationship you'd like to have?*

B.Z.: *I'd enjoy doing things with someone I love or would like to love, doing crazy things like taking a walk at 4:00 A.M. I want them to share my experiences, and I theirs, to share sadness and joy. I want someone who would understand why I might need to sometimes walk out of a room, someone who understands that we have to have differences, who's able to sit down and argue with me, so that I get something out of it, and don't feel a need to make up. Someone who says, "Your hair's too long; I'll cut it," and then screws it up so I have to go to the barber. Yeah, that's where it's really at, and that's what I want.*

Although B.Z. was more articulate than most respondents, his thoughts were representative of what others perhaps wanted to say but were unable to say so explicitly.

Even though most respondents indicated a desire for a meaningful relationship, most had not dated extensively anyone whom they had met in a bar; nor did they believe that bars facilitate the formation of such relationships. They might hope to find someone with whom to form close ties, but the probability of that occurring was viewed with a jaundiced eye. As G.P. stated:

You just have to try, it's a matter of luck, that's all, just a matter of luck.

When asked if she thought bars facilitated the formation of meaningful relationships, F.O., the female social worker, replied:

I wish I could say yes, since that's one of the reasons I go. But I'm not sure. I think the only thing they do is put a lot of people in the same place, and you're on your own from there.

F.O.'s response was typical of those who assessed the impact of singles bars from a fairly neutral stance, i.e., bars neither promote nor hinder; they simply provide a setting in which individuals are placed in proximity to other individuals.

Thus the paradox: individuals who desire serious relationships are going to bars; while this purpose may not be uppermost in their minds at all times, it is an important motivation that rarely reaches fruition. Furthermore, even though most individuals are mildly to severely cynical about the likelihood of a bar encounter developing into a serious relationship, they continue to go to bars. Their failure to establish such relationships relates to two factors: the way people in bars evaluate each other, particularly the men's evaluation of women, and the unserious nature of the bar setting itself, which is not quite like any other.

Men were not asked directly what thoughts they harbored about women who patronize singles bars, but several offered their opinions during the course of the interviews. The harshest opinions were rendered by A.Y. and A.N. while discussing the fact that although women are more sexually liberated of late, they are less inclined than men to admit that they go to bars to meet men:

A.Y.: That's the key to a successful bar, providing the girls with a cover, some reason other than what they're really going for. You get a girl that's even semiclassy. . . . I think that girls that go to bars are low-lifes, almost without exception.

A.N.: He's being more than candid now; he's being flippant.

A.Y.: No! Do you disagree with that statement? With rare exception, the girls that go to bars are not classy. Why don't you date more of the girls that you meet at bars?

A.N.: Well, that's a good. . . .

A.Y.: The girls that I've wound up dating I have not met at bars. By my definition, you meet a lower class of girl at a bar.

At other times during the interview, A.Y. and A.N. were both pejorative and scathing when speculating and commenting on the intelligence and moral character of women who frequent bars. These are the attitudes of one man (A.Y.) who uses bars exclusively to arrange casual sexual encounters and another man (A.N.) who has accumulated so many telephone numbers that he no longer recalls to which women they belong.

E.D. was slightly less caustic:

You can get any girl to mess around, at least any one that you meet in a bar. I don't think there's much difference between girls and guys down here. What does it hurt, if it doesn't hurt anyone?

Even though he stated that men and women go to bars for the same reasons, his negative evaluation of the women is implicit because his assessment of unescorted females in bars was extremely demeaning.

A.A., a 32-year-old physician, was asked about extended relationships with women met in a bar:

A.A.: Do you mean going out more than two times? Anything that's lasting? Never more than twice. That's all.

Int: Why is that?

A.A.: Because of the kind of women you usually meet in these places. Twice is enough.

Although A.A. does not go to bars solely in search of casual sexual encounters, such encounters are an important motivation. He is a self-proclaimed chauvinist and "proud of it"; so his response was hardly unexpected.

When M.K. and D.W., the managers at Bar Alpha, were discussing the rarity of unescorted females in bars, they also noted the general opinion of women who patronize bars. As M.K. stated:

M.K.: Even my girl won't come in alone, and she knows everybody here.

Int: Why is that?

M.K.: Old attitudes. There's a lot of people who still think that any girl you meet in a bar, you don't want to have a relationship with, anything lasting. She's cheap if you meet her in a bar.

Men who offered unsolicited testimony about women who patronize bars generally made remarks of a derogatory nature. They concluded that either she was a very lonely person driven to bars out of desperation, of borderline intelligence, or very likely to be an "easy make." This is not to say that all men who go to bars share these views of the women. Nevertheless, there are men who do feel this way, and women have to deal with them. Clearly, such attitudes automatically preclude any thoughts of a long-term relationship simply because they devalue the woman. Yet none of the women interviewed demonstrated any awareness that their mere presence in a bar would stereotype them in this fashion.

Some of the men who did not voice negative opinions about women in bars commented on the way in which meeting someone in a bar could qualify the relationship. When L.F., a 28-year-old executive, stated that even his "heavy relationships" had been superficial, I asked if he thought beginning them in a bar had anything to do with this superficiality:

L.F.: I think there's a certain stigma attached to meeting someone in a bar. I think a girl is really miffed by that idea.

Int: How about you?

L.F.: Yeah, I'm affected by it too. It's a paradox. People are going to find someone. But even if they do meet a nice girl, they'll keep in the back of their mind that they met her in a bar.

Only one female, T.M., commented on the caliber of people in singles bars, whom she described as "generalized and nondescript in their interests." She was also the only female who stated categorically that she had never met anyone at a bar whom she cared to see for more than one night. This information was unsolicited; none of the other women made any sweeping generalizations about men in bars that even remotely approached the comments made by the men.

The character of the bar setting also militates against the formation of relationships for some patrons. For example, D.G., who initially stated that where one meets a person is unimportant, replied as follows when asked if he thought bars facilitated the establishment of serious relationships:

D.G.: *No, they don't. This might sound hypocritical, but bars tend to inspire transient relationships, those in passing.*

Int: *Why?*

D.G.: *The basic reason is that bars, as opposed to being introduced by friends or at a party, tend to inspire transient relationships between strangers, and you have an "I don't care" attitude. Like if you meet a girl at a bar who is a complete stranger, it's easier to say 'f--- you' than if she was introduced by friends. Just the fact that it's a public place and you're meeting a stranger has a lot to do with your reaction and the kind of relationship you establish.*

The fact that individuals meet in a bar setting, which is defined as unserious, clearly influences the way in which they relate to one another. When introduced by friends, they are more accountable for their behavior; they feel constrained to create a favorable impression. In a bar, they are accountable to no one. L.F., for example, defined the bar setting as an unreal and artificial environment. Because the setting is one in which behavior is exempt from counting, patrons are allowed a wider latitude of behavior, and they are rarely held accountable for their behavior. Obviously, it is difficult to begin a serious relationship in a setting that is not itself serious.

The majority of patrons felt that singles bars do not facilitate the formation of long-term, meaningful relationships but merely provide a locale wherein a large number of people can by their presence be open for an encounter. The nature and direction of the encounter is assessed once contact is made. One cannot assume unequivocally that every man in a bar wants to "get laid," that every woman is looking for a potential husband, or that every person has lurking under layers of the subconscious an immediate desire to get involved in a serious relationship. People go to bars for different reasons at different times; their motivations may vary from night to night. As a result, patrons need to be able to assess accurately the motives of those with whom they are interacting and then to schedule second encounters with those whose interests are parallel.

The fact that so few long-term relationships are established between men and women who meet in a singles bar suggests that the setting itself and the way encounters are conducted within it are important variables. If the setting is unserious, if what occurs there does not count, if consequentiality can be suspended, then any incipient relationship may also be denied significance. People have a tendency to function in terms of polarities; so it is very difficult to say that negative factors do not count while positive ones do; it is more a case of saying that everything counts or nothing does. Thus, in an attempt to cope with the rejection they experience in bars, patrons rationalize what is potentially painful by discounting both the rejection and the individual meting it out. They may then discount everything that goes on in a bar, including relationships that may be potentially meaningful.

The whole aura of the bars also inhibits the formation of relationships. Bars are dim, loud, and crowded; spirits are flowing freely; and sizing-up occurs quickly and superficially. People frequently make rapid, gut-level judgments about others, and a desire to initiate an encounter is often based on physical attractiveness and little else. Individuals with a great deal to offer in a relationship may be entirely overlooked if they are unattractive or unable to convey their positive characteristics in less than 4 minutes.

The data on male-female interaction in singles bars suggest that many patrons consider themselves to be engaged in game playing. Undeniably, much of the behavior has implicit meaning attached to it, and the patrons need to unravel the meaning in order to make a response. But on another level the interaction strikes an observer as markedly adolescent and partially attributable to game playing. Spilling a drink on someone in order to find a reason to interact or fumbling around only to deliver a remarkably jejune comment as an opener are behaviors that seem more appropriate to a junior high school gymnasium where boys and girls are in the beginning stages of learning how to relate to each other. We may conclude from the data that most of the participants are seeking a close relationship in whatever terms they choose to define it. However, they are looking for it in an unserious setting in which much of the interaction is characterized by ruse and guile. The patrons of singles bars simply do not seem to be very honest with others or themselves. Those interviewed stated that they were looking for dates and potential relationships in bars, yet they conceded that such relationships seldom begin in bars. They acted as if they were ashamed they had gone to a bar to seek a relationship, as if admitting to being lonely and to actively wanting and looking for someone to go out with were somehow distasteful and faintly disreputable. Consequently, any relationship they formed in a bar, however tenuous, was characterized by a basic dishonesty in confronting their real feelings and taking the risk to share them. Why individuals are unable or unwilling to be more honest with themselves and others is a topic for further research.

This study of singles bars indicates that such places are needed and that, until some social wizard discovers a better setting, they are likely to remain with us. It has been suggested that bars meet many of the social needs of their patrons, who may lack other resources. Yet many of these patrons have stated that bars do not facilitate the establishment of long-term relationships. Since the possibility of establishing such relationships is a primary motivation for many who patronize these bars, that failure looms large indeed. The owner of Bar Gamma boasted that over five hundred marriages have resulted from meetings in his bar. When we consider that this bar has been around for over 15 years and that millions have passed through the portals, these statistics are hardly encouraging.

REFERENCES

1. Cavan, S. *Liquor License.* Chicago: Aldine Press, 1962.
2. Goffman, E. *Behavior in Public Places.* Glencoe, Ill.: Free Press, 1963.
3. Lopata, H. Loneliness: Forms and components. *Social Problems* 17:249, 1969.

5. Without Benefit of Clergy: Cohabitation as a Noninstitutionalized Marital Role. Jeanie Snodgrass Almo

Popular literature leads us to believe that attitudes toward marriage and family relationships are changing and that couples are attempting to redefine and reestablish their roles and interrelationships. This chapter explores one alternative life-style in this movement toward a redefinition of marriage.

In-depth interviews were conducted with eleven unmarried couples who were living together. They were interviewed together and individually in their places of residence. The individuals ranged in age from 21 to 35 , with a mean age of 26. They had known their respective partners an average of three years and had lived together an average of seventeen months. They were highly educated and middle class; only two persons had less than three years of college, and seven persons had done graduate study beyond the baccalaureate level. Five of the twenty-two respondents had experienced divorce or separation in their families of origin, and five had been previously married for an average of four years and then divorced; two respondents had children by their first marriages.

Communication was each couple's primary need and concern; it characterized each couple's relationship and influenced all the other issues that affected the noninstitutionalized dyad. Because the relationship was not institutional in nature, each couple's negotiations with each other and with others were concentrated on such issues as how to present themselves and define their relationship to others. A couple's ability to communicate with each other was a major factor contributing to the continuation of the relationship.

Communication, in the form of a continuous conversation, is described by Berger and Kellner [1] as the method used to support unstable dyads. These unmarried couples placed greater emphasis on communication than that expected of married couples. The partners had not only the problem of keeping their relationship going but also the problem of defining their relationship to society in acceptable terms.

Marriage in our society has been both a means of social control and an organized form of psychological and social protection and approval for the adult. As such, the institution of marriage offers a set of rules to guide decision making, a framework for creation of a family, and a mechanism to meet adult needs. Berger and Kellner state that marriage is one of the few formalized constructs of our society that provides persons with a taken-for-granted image of a heterosexual dyad and urges them to step into taken-for-granted roles. In other words, marriage is a ready-made world into which persons merely step. If intense communication is needed in this ready-made world of traditional marriages, it is no surprise that such communication is essential for couples engaged in a noninstitutionalized relationship in which roles and images are not ready-made.

Unlike traditionally married couples, living-together-unmarried couples experience no ceremonial rites of passage that signal the beginning of the "official" marital unit. Their relationship may to an extent parallel that of other couples whose relationship develops according to the stages outlined in Chapter 6. Cohabiting couples experience the initiating and sustaining stages in much the same way as couples whose relationships progress to traditional marriage. But cohabiting couples' movement into the next stage, mutual commitment, although apparent, is not formalized by the external social event of the wedding ceremony. Instead, living-together-unmarried couples adopt an alternative, socially nonsanctioned life-style.

NEGOTIATION AND COLLECTIVE BARGAINING

When a couple's status changes from dating to living together, new negotiations are imperative. There is need to define the relationship and its meaning; to define the boundaries of the relationship and who is to be included and excluded from these boundaries; to define what are the appropriate roles for the individuals in the relationship; to determine how decisions are to be made, how activities of daily living are to he handled, how communication lines will be constructed, and how to present themselves as individuals and as a unit to the larger society; and to identify the future direction of the relationship. Negotiation and bargaining occur at all levels of the relationship.

Negotiations fall naturally into two categories: interpersonal negotiations between partners and negotiations with others, conducted both individually and as a unit. Because the couple's status is neither formally established nor recognized by social sanctions and rules, many issues that might be easily settled by traditional marital agreements must be defined by the partners themselves. They must decide how they will describe their relationship and their own status in it to significant others such as parents, colleagues, friends, landlords, and health services agencies. Questions such as to whom should the mailman deliver the mail and in whose name should the telephone be listed become issues to resolve. Other issues to be negotiated include how partners will refer to each other in order to convey the nature of their relationship to outsiders and whether their socializing patterns as single persons will remain the same or change to reflect their new status. At the heart of many of these issues is the question of what exactly is their new status — single, married, or other? Technical issues normally settled by a legal marriage ceremony, such as property rights, financial responsibilities, and joint ownership, must be negotiated and resolved by the couple.

Personal issues, such as how long do they plan to stay together, for what reasons would they part, what is the nature and depth of their commitment to each other and to the relationship, and in what direction would the relationship go if in the future it were to change, must be either settled or understood by mutual agreement to be open-ended and unresolvable at that time.

Parents

For many of the couples in the study, one of the first major issues to be mutually resolved was what to tell their respective parents about their living arrangements, or whether to tell their parents at all. When one couple was asked how they each told their parents they were living together, the male partner explained:

I never really came right out and told them. When they came over, there were always two pillows on the bed, and a couple of times she [mother] would find her [the female partner's] underwear around the room. So . . . it's like I know and she knows but we're going to pretend as if neither of us knows. . . . Finally, she said, "I know what you're doing but I don't approve", still she accepts us pretty well. But still she won't come over to dinner here because that's an act of approval.

When asked how the couple agreed to answer the telephone given these circumstances, the man stated:

I'm not the one that answers all the time. I used to do it in the other place, but it just got to be such a hassle! How much did they know? When could we stop playing the game? It was a bad issue . . . I never really made a decision to tell them. . . . I just stopped picking up her things or the extra pillow when my mother came over. I just stopped covering up. It was easier to let them just come upon it. . . . I took the easier way out.

Another woman described how she handled the issue of who would answer the telephone in a different way:

For one thing, I have two phone lines. I can answer either, but he can answer only one. If I'm not home, no one answers the other.

Couples who sensed parental resistance to living together solved the problem of parental reaction by not talking explicitly about the relationship, an evasion about which they and their parents mutually agreed. In contrast, several other couples encountered little or no resistance to the news that they were living together. When asked how their parents had come to know they were living together one couple replied:

He: Just gradually, they assimilated it. It wasn't that big a deal. Anybody in my family could do anything they wanted; my parents will never comment. My father did have occasion to comment [about] my sister who has been living with a man for about a year; he said that she should get married if they were going to continue to live together. That was all they said. . . . I just told them that if they wanted to get a hold of me, call me at her place. There was no big problem.

She: I just told them that he was living with me. We went home shortly after that . . . we were staying at their house, and we just told them we wanted a room together. I had had someone stay there before, and there had been all this stuff about staying together and sleeping in the same room; so we had already been through that. So they never questioned it; they expected it.

This couple's parents had had to deal previously with the topic of sleeping together and living together. In the woman's case she herself and in the man's case a sibling had established a precedent that the couple could then follow.

Most couples informed their parents about their living together gradually, often by default, or when they just decided to "quit covering up." Others have continued for more than a year's time to prevent their parents from knowing about their joint residency. They have installed two phones or asked their partners to leave when their parents came to visit. However, most couples have in some way, either by direct notification or by permitting their parents gradual awareness, let it be known that they are living together as a couple. In all but four cases, this knowledge has been a point of contention and difficulty in the parent-couple relationship.

Landlords and Others

In most cases, the couples eventually sought new quarters where they could be together in their own mutually chosen apartment or house. They therefore had to present themselves to a prospective landlord either as a couple or furtively as an individual, with whom the other partner would then move in.

Most couples stated that acquiring an apartment was no problem as long as they could prove they had jobs and could pay the rent. Several couples lived in apartments leased by one party only. In three instances, the male partner moved into an apartment already inhabited by his mate. Among those couples who did look for their own apartments together, several decided it would be easier to present themselves as married to avoid potential confrontation. One man stated:

When you go apartment hunting, you have to describe your husband or wife; so you play a little game with the people. This particular man thinks we're married . . . she wasn't here when the lease was signed . . . our names are on the mailbox separately, though. One landlord asked us how long we had been married, and we said we weren't. He just said okay. It was acceptable to him. But here, he thought we were married; we just never corrected him.

One couple had not acknowledged that they were living in the same apartment. However, the couple seemed to have reached an understanding with the mailman, even though they had never openly admitted their situation to him. The man stated:

The lease is in her name, it's really her apartment . . . my name isn't on the mailbox, but the mailman knows I'm here. . . .

Although couples often do not explicitly define their relationships, others quickly become attuned to the nature of the association.

Another couple expressed their difficulty in trying to present themselves honestly and described how they chose to deal with it. The man explained:

In one building we told the guy we weren't married and we didn't get the apartment. So when we looked here, we told him we were. It's such a hassle, having to put my name only on the mailbox, instead of her own name, too. Why can't she have her own name? It really isn't fair. . . . People from work had to be told if anyone called there checking to see if Mrs. M. worked there, to tell them yes. It's just really such a hassle. It makes you feel like you're doing something wrong.

One couple thought that their being an unmarried, interracial couple limited them to certain neighborhoods and forced them into higher rent districts, which were considered more "hip" areas in which to live. They chose a certain neighborhood, in spite of the greater cost, because they thought the area was more open and knew there would be no problem. They expressed some bitterness that they had to pay in so many ways for the "privilege" of living together.

The couples cited other difficult situations with which they had to deal. When one woman was rushed to the hospital during a miscarriage, her partner had difficulty describing his relationship to her. Hospital personnel would not accept him in the role of "next of kin." Several persons remarked about the difficulty they experienced when doing simple activities such as buying furniture together and being compelled to sign "Mr. and Mrs." to the bill of sale because the salesman insisted that they *both* must sign. In a social structure in which marriage is regarded as the only legitimate way to pursue an ongoing heterosexual relationship, even the most mundane business transactions become difficult for a cohabiting couple to manage.

Employers and Colleagues

Several respondents experienced much pressure in their places of employment on occasions when they had to decide how to describe their relationship or living arrangements. Those who chose not to acknowledge their living together status left themselves open to uncomfortable interactions with colleagues. For example, one woman executive stated:

In my office there are about seven men who are all married. They say to all the single girls, "Do you have a date for this weekend?" I don't think it's any of their business . . . it puts me in a funny position . . . I feel kind of torn. I guess their assumptions really bother me; they say, "Look, she's however old she is and still single and probably sits home every night by herself and waits for the phone to ring." This is really uncomfortable because I'm one of the executives, too; but because I'm a single woman they feel they can ask me, whereas no one would ask one of the male executives personal information!

Being single and living with a man created some uncomfortable moments for this woman in her professional relationships. Her partner also had experienced some discomfort at work relative to their living together, but his discomfort was not as great:

Someone did ask me once if I was married. My boss wanted me to get married. He told me he would give me a raise if I got married. . . . Companies prefer married men because they think they're more stable. . . .

Both men and women who live together without being married experience difficulties at work. In many instances, individuals handled this difficulty by avoiding discussing with whom they lived or by lying and stating that they lived alone or with a "roommate." One man stated that although people where he worked were very conservative, his boss thought it was "neat" that he lived unmarried with a woman:

For him, it's a point in my favor; to live with a girl is acceptable, like a game; you've got all the good things without the responsibility.

In this instance, the man gained status in his colleague's eyes. Yet women who participate in such relationships are often automatically demeaned.

Employed couples had to decide how to describe their partners on legal papers such as insurance policies or those forms that request whom to notify in case of emergency. Most respondents did not stipulate their partners but avoided the issue by listing their fathers, brothers, or some other relative.

Many respondents were somewhat concerned about this omission because in the case of an emergency the person actually closest to them might not be informed and might not be considered beneficiary of jointly purchased property or joint savings, unless specific alternate arrangements had been made.

One experience caused a particular problem for one couple. When the woman's mother died and her partner wanted to take time off from work to be with her and her family, he had to fill out forms requesting the time. To be eligible, he had to be a member of the immediate family. So he "just lied and wrote down mother-in-law" because that relationship was what he felt he had, and he was not going to let bureaucratic procedures keep him away.

Many couples met with neutral reactions when they described their relationships to colleagues; for them, the telling was uneventful. The factors that seemed to influence these reactions were the work environment, the outlook of other employees, and the role model expected within the profession. For many respondents, their living arrangements made no difference at work. For some, however, these arrangements made all the difference in the world, both at work and in their social lives. One woman, a teacher, experienced great difficulty in deciding how to handle the situation vis-à-vis her colleagues. Her response was:

I've lied; I've just flatly lied! They say, "Are you living alone?" I say, "Yes." I'm just not sure if it's the interracial part or our living together; I think it's difficult to separate [these points]. If we were just living together, would I still lie? I don't know; I possibly still would. Mostly because the people that I teach with would be against it. I'm sure I fear rejection from them, a kind of social stick-out. Always in the back of my mind is: "Would I be rejected or accepted outside of school in accordance with the way I live?" Some of the teachers are outwardly sociable and say, "Let's go out for a drink," or something, but I keep pretty much to myself out of fear that if they knew, would I be accepted. It's like a wall. So I'm sure the relationship has some effect on my relationships to school and other people.

Certainly, fear of being cut off socially and its attendant need to hide a living together arrangement places additional strain on a couple's relationship.

One factor that greatly influenced whether couples could describe their relationship to others was their own acceptance of it and the confidence with which they presented themselves. It appeared that many of the couples who chose not to describe their living situation did so out of fear of problems, and not because they had actually experienced such problems.

Labeling

As the O'Neills [3] pointed out, society does not provide a sanctioned title for a couple living outside the legal marriage contract. With a marriage ceremony comes the titles Mr. and Mrs. But what titles are appropriate when two persons are living together? Institutions carry labels, but cohabitation has not become a recognized institution. Cohabiting couples must decide what title to give to themselves and their relationship.

Couples gave elaborate descriptions when asked how they described their relationships to others and what terms they used when referring to each other. Many couples expressed the quandary in these ways:

> There's no term that's adequate. I've heard people describe each other, even their husband, as "roommate" or "partner." I just think there's no proper term.

> There is no word to connote the relationship we have, "roommate" or "boyfriend" connotes other things. It's not a big deal, but it's a constant small irritation.

> We live together with the feeling of permanence, but there's just no way to describe that to anybody, even friends.

Several couples use labels, but indicated that they were dissatisfied with the choices available, as seen in the following example:

> Mostly we say roommates . . . I wouldn't use either the label "girlfriend" or "wife." I have used "girlfriend" in the past simply because of lack of anything else. I wouldn't use the term "girlfriend" in the company of anyone who knew me; if they knew me, they would know what she means to me . . . it's just not a very descriptive term. It's also a pejorative term to the feminist movement. I would say "friend," "roommate," "lover" — all of those terms apply. I think "wife" is also a pejorative term and implies possession.

The response evoked by the frustration of not having a proper term to use was often anger. One man expressed this anger by saying:

> The term "girlfriend" seems like such an adolescent term. If it's someone that I'm close to, I say "the girl I live with." Nothing fits right. After I've had to use some improper term, I feel so angry, more than anything. I feel like, "Cut the crap, dammit, why can't I say it!" I feel especially weird with the people I work with. You want to say what's true, what's there. . . . She's more than my girlfriend and my roommate; put the two together and someone figure it out!

For one woman, the lack of a term and the difficulty describing the relationship led to her avoiding discussion of it with others, which in turn led to difficulties described by her partner:

> It bothers me; I feel cheated. When she denies our relationship to people she works with or others, I feel cheated! It pisses me off! It's as if she's ashamed or something!

It was apparent that the lack of a proper term to describe the relationship and the members in it was a bone of contention for all persons. For some it was mildly irritating; for others it proved to be a source of interpersonal problems. All persons expressed the need for a means to better describe the relationship, and all expressed disappointment that no term available to them implied the depth or quality of their feelings. The noninstitutionalized nature of the living together relationship is readily apparent in the paucity of terms available to describe the relationship and its participants.

Friends and Social Life

Couples also have to deal with their friends and peers. Most couples stated that their friends were very accepting, with some very happy for them and others neutral. In only a few instances did friends respond negatively to cohabitation, and even then they asked only why the couple had not gotten married. Such responses came mainly from persons who were married and were encouraging their friends to be likewise. Most individuals replied that their cohabitation seemed to be accepted and accompanied by no specific fanfare, a circumstance which they partly attributed to the fact that their "moving in together" happened gradually without an identifiable event, in contrast to a traditional wedding, which is planned in advance in most instances and during which some ceremony is shared with friends. Many couples had friends or relatives who were also living together; so cohabitation was an accepted state among most of their peers.

Most couples socialized primarily with other couples rather than with individuals, unlike when they were "single." The couples indicated that they socialized with married, dating, and living together couples equally. All felt that there were really no distinctions among the various categories. The differences that were mentioned related to couples who lived in the suburbs rather than in the city and thus had different life-styles and to couples who had children and thus were not as free to socialize as couples without children. Life-style and availability, not marital state, determined their circle of friends.

Having neither the official status of "single" or "married," cohabiting individuals must decide how to present themselves and their social availability to outsiders. If the fact that a person is cohabiting is not common knowledge at his or her place of employment, how can it be made known that he or she is "not available" or is "available on a limited basis"? Or if a person decides to continue dating members of the opposite sex, how can he or she best communicate that decision to the present partner? One woman, in describing how she handled the question of socializing with other men, stated:

Some fellows where I work are asking me out, but I don't want to go out with anyone else. I just tell them I'm married.

65. *Cohabitation as a Marital Role*

Her partner also expressed his desire to date no one else. However, he handled the situation this way:

There are some girls at work that I find myself attracted to, but I don't feel I could handle that right now. So I let them know in a nice way that I'm free to be their friend, but only in a brotherly sort of way. It's really hard. I usually end up telling them about her as a way of explaining.

Obviously, the handling of usual social relationships and expected roles for singles in our society becomes complicated for those living together.

One couple had decided after much debate to continue dating outside their relationship. However, this decision caused some difficulties between them. They expressed their arrangement thus:

He: When I see someone outside of our relationship, I don't necessarily explain my living arrangements to her. I feel it's necessary to explain before you get on such intimate terms that there will obviously be a conflict of interest.

She: At first you didn't tell people, and I felt you were denying me. I didn't feel it was fair to them or to me.

He: Anybody who had reason to know knew!

She: I have a lot of strong feminist feelings, and one of them is that there is a traditional double standard, with women programmed to be misled. I'm very sensitive on the subject. So I was very strong from the beginning that everything should be made very explicit to everyone concerned.

The questions then arose: what is the difference between married men and women and men and women who are living together? How is this difference expressed to unknowing suitors? The couples had not resolved these questions clearly for themselves or for others.

COMMUNICATION BETWEEN PARTNERS

The couples interviewed had to decide not only how they would present themselves to society but how they would approach each other. Communication between the two partners was the network through which all other decisions and negotiations proceeded. The quality of this communication determined the success with which the couples made decisions on a number of sensitive issues, such as sexual aspects of the relationship, the degree of their mutual commitment, fidelity, the meaning of their relationship, whether to stay together or part, and whether to marry. They also had to agree on their joint and individual socializing patterns and settle issues related to daily household upkeep and finances. In describing their relationship and its meaning, the couples spoke in terms of how well they communicated, of what issues they could and could not discuss. In general, they used ease of communication as a barometer of how well the relationship was faring.

Meaning of the Relationship

No couple described the status of their relationship as "officially engaged." Most individuals considered their agreement to be somewhere between "no specific agreement as to the permanence or meaning of the relationship" and an "agreement to stay together as long as things are good." Only two couples indicated that they definitely planned to separate in the near future. When asked what they meant by "no specific agreement as to the permanence of the relationship," many couples stated that although they had never made any verbal agreements, they had reached implicit understandings about what they expected from the relationship in regard to such issues as fidelity, openness, and how long they would be together. Many couples, however, were discussing such issues openly for the first time during the interview. Several respondents were reluctant to describe the permanence, stating, "I don't think in terms of tomorrow or long-term anything." Many stated that they live from day to day; if things go well, they will stay together. The couples who "probably" or "possibly" would be married in the future made that decision contingent upon their ability to "work some things out first." Those who planned to stay together indefinitely also reported that their staying together would depend on their ability to come to definitely agree on specific issues and to "make things workable." Most couples considered open discussion of the meaning of the relationship to be unnecessary or unwise. Many alluded to implicit "understandings" about the bases of their relationships and were reluctant to make those understandings explicit.

Commitment, Sex, and Fidelity

Couples had difficulty identifying the point at which commitment to the relationship began; whether it was before living together, at the time of moving in together, or a product of the living together experience. One woman admitted that when she stopped contributing to the rent on her old apartment and began to share the rent with her partner, she became frightened about the "decision" she had just made, questioning whether she was ready for such a commitment. One man acknowledged that he had never before felt deep commitments to anything or anyone but that the relationship with his partner helped him to talk and to feel "released" and able to be more open about who he was and how he felt about love and life in general. As a result, he felt deeply committed to her and their relationship and to his own self-growth.

Most couples felt that they had made a strong commitment when they decided to live together and that even if this commitment was never made explicit, they could feel secure in their definite agreement to be together in a deep relationship before the joint residency. Only one couple indicated that such an understanding had been vague; this couple now planned to separate.

For some couples, commitment meant sexual exclusiveness. Although one couple had not explicitly agreed on sexual exclusiveness, they felt it was understood. The woman stated:

I feel free enough that if I wanted to see other men, I probably would move out. I wouldn't do it in this situation. It's not part of my understanding and I know it's not part of his. . . . In this way I think we are both here to be with each other. That's understood.

For others, sexual exclusiveness was not an assumption. When sexual fidelity was part of a couple's commitment, it was openly discussed and agreed upon. When outside sexual relationships were to be allowed, they also were discussed and understood, although not always mutually agreed to. Some couples, however, had agreed that commitment should not be discussed in terms of sexual exclusiveness and some partners were reluctant to discuss openly their feelings about outside encounters. All couples, including those who granted the possibility of outside relationships, agreed that commitment meant that their relationships were structured around each other.

Several respondents expressed the belief that if two people were really committed to each other, there was no need to get married, that a legal certificate did not change the degree of their commitment. One man felt, however, that living together enabled him to avoid the more "in-depth," "life-long" commitment of marriage, which he had made once, unsuccessfully. Among the couples interviewed, the feeling of being committed to a relationship was contingent upon a feeling that the relationship had some mutual, if unspoken, understanding of permanence and included a certain degree of planning for the future together, similar to the phenomenon of mutual commitment described in Chapter 6.

Many individuals were generally unclear about the nature of their commitments, which were based on unspoken and vague mutual agreements to "be together as long as things are good." Some of the respondents' statements revealed conflicts:

I can't make that kind of life-long commitment again, so why get married?

If I've already made the commitment, what's the need to get married?

What a commitment meant to many individuals was unclear in their own minds. But although their commitment was often unclear and unspoken, all but two of the twenty-two participants expressed strong feelings of commitment to their respective relationships and partners.

The sexual aspect of their relationship was a major area of negotiation for these couples. Only two couples described their sexual relationships as very good and satisfying; one couple said they had no specific problems; and

the other eight couples described their sexual relationships as ranging
from mildly troubled to irreparably damaged. The reasons cited for the
difficulties included guilt about living together, personal unresolved sexual
hang-ups, decreased desire and withdrawal from their partners when depressed or angry about something in the relationship, erratic hours kept
by one or both partners, and a difference in the level of need and desire
of the partners. All but two of the couples stated that the frequency and
quality of their sexual encounters had diminished over the time they had
lived together. All agreed that their sexual relationship reflected their overall relationship, especially when problems arose.

Communication played a major part in negotiations about sex. For most
couples, sex was a difficult subject to broach and was usually avoided
until it had become an obvious problem and had created tension that
generalized to other aspects of the relationship. When this subject was
brought up by one partner, both parties seemed to feel that attempts to
resolve the problems through discussion had for the most part been unsuccessful. This lack of success was attributed to difficulty in talking about
sex openly and to differing opinions on how to go about resolving the
conflicts. In several instances, one partner did not feel the need to change
his or her sexual habits while the other partner (who often desired an increase
in intensity and frequency of love making) not only felt a need for change
but defined the disparity as a problem the couple definitely wished to
alter. The need for change itself became a problem because it was not
felt as intensely by both persons. It seems that change, like communication
is more difficult when only one person feels the need for it.

Like Macklin [2], we observed that sex was a part of the total relationship, not a major reason for living together, and not a major factor keeping
the couple together. In many instances, couples stayed together in spite
of unsatisfactory sexual relationships. They were able to resolve sexual
problems to the extent that they were able to communicate about it. All
respondents indicated that their ability to talk about their sexual problems
was the key factor controlling satisfactory physical adjustment. If such
problems could not be discussed, they could not be dealt with. For this
reason, some of the couples had sought out professionals to help them
learn to communicate better.

Because living together is a socially and culturally undefined state, the
matter of what constitutes fidelity had to be defined by each couple. Was
their relationship to be a sexually closed dyad or one open to the inclusion of others by one or both parties? Was their arrangement to be formal
and binding, reached and agreed to openly by both partners? Or was it
understood that each person was free to do as he or she pleased? Or was
their arrangement something both persons agreed silently not to open up
for discussion, instead acting independently and secretly in whatever way
they saw fit?

The two couples who had discussed their arrangement the most were
the two who, after a great deal of painful debate, tears, and anger, had

agreed, or conceded, to allow each partner to see others independently both for dating and for sex. One woman described her and her partner's decision as follows:

I didn't want to have outside sexual relationships, and he did; so we fought about it, and then I guess I changed my mind . . . to the point where I agreed it was a big difficulty. . . . It has taken about 11 months out of the 13 to reach the agreement. When we first started discussing going out with other people, the double standard always made it easier for men to go out and not women. One of the points I made was that when a couple goes out with each other, they usually wind up at the woman's apartment. But where do I go? So he said come here. But I can't do that! It really has been a bone of contention as far as I'm concerned. I still really don't want to go out with other people. And although I do agree that I have no right to demand that he stay home with only me, I don't like his going out.

Although this couple had spent a great deal of their time together negotiating the decision to see other people, the woman's dissatisfaction remained. It was partly this dissatisfaction that later led to this couple's separation.

For most couples, seeing "outside others" was a taboo topic not open for discussion. Most persons stated that they had at one time or another during their present relationship seen someone else, but that the action had not been openly discussed between the partners. Two couples had not talked with each other about outside dating prior to the interview, and they indicated that they did not wish to broach that topic during the joint interview. In interviews, each of these four individuals stated that he or she would not share information about outside encounters with his or her partner. These respondents also indicated that they did not wish to know about corresponding activities by their partners. The couples remained silent on this issue by mutual agreement. One couple stated that they had agreed that to set limits on outside friendships was unnatural and unhealthy and that no one had the right to monitor someone else's relationships. The woman described their resolution this way:

We used to have long arguments about what would constitute being unfaithful, and we agreed that we each would have outside relationships, too; we never really agreed on how far the other person could go without our getting concerned. Any relationship that you start with someone is an open-ended one; you never know what may happen, but you can't forbid it or prevent it. I think a lot of couples are living together and are committed to each other but are ideologically committed to a nonmonogamous relationship and really feel obliged to go out and start something up. It gets to be very strange because they get into relationships that aren't really emotionally involved for them but [that] people feel obligated to get into; then there's jealousy. One of the reasons I thought we should get

married was that our relationship has been very monogamous, although
not exclusive, and just very much centered on each other. I don't think
we want it to remain exclusive; we think it's important to have friends
outside of either sex. I feel that just being close to people is a very wonder-
ful thing, and I don't want to cut that off. . . .

This couple continued to discuss this problem after their marriage. They indicated that during five years of negotiation, commitment had come to mean that their relationship was structured around each other but not to the exclusion of other important friends. At the time of the interviews, their relationship did not include any outside sexual partners.

Two couples who were not seeing others stated individually that they had thought about it. Fear of hurting the partner was cited by each of the four persons as the major reason he or she decided not to see others. Each felt an outside relationship would be too traumatic to the present relationship and would be potential cause for its termination. Each felt that he or she could not keep hidden from the respective partner information about seeing someone else because their relationship was, as far as he or she was concerned, very open and honest; not telling the partner would change the underlying concept of their relationship.

Communication, it its many forms, was the theme underlying all other issues. When couples were asked to describe their relationships, they mentioned their ability or inability to communicate well with their partners as the major indicator of the success of the relationship. When discussing their ability to solve problems together, to make joint decisions, to describe their own growth and personal goals within the relationship, all emphasized the need for a more honest discussion of needs and expectations. They thought that better communication would enable them to stay together and to enjoy the relationship to the fullest possible degree. Communication was their major problem; other problems revolved around it. Other relational difficulties seemed to be symptoms of more general communication difficulties.

REFERENCES

1. Berger, P., and Kellner, H. Marriage and the Construction of Reality. In H.P. Dreitzel, (Ed.) *Recent Sociology, No. 2.* New York: Macmillan, 1970.
2. Macklin, E.D. Heterosexual cohabitation among unmarried college students. *The Family Coordinator* 463, 1972.
3. O'Neill, N., and O'Neill, G. *Open Marriage: A New Life Style for Couples.* New York: M. Evans, 1972.

6. Relationships in Process: Forming a Couple Identity. Beverly J. Bernstein, Donna M. Dixon, and Kathleen Astin Knafl

Individuals date for many reasons. While some are earnestly seeking a permanent partner, others date simply for the fun and companionship that dating can provide and have no real interest in developing a long-term relationship. Dating outcomes vary as well. For the couples who later marry, the first date is also a first step toward marriage. For other couples at the opposite extreme, the relationship terminates after this first encounter. This chapter focuses on those dating relationships that develop into permanent commitments. In the course of becoming committed to a life together, couples move through stages. Our description and interpretation of these stages are built on a model first presented in an article by Knafl and Grace [2] (illustrated, p. 30). This model divides couple relationships into three broad stages: the initiating stage, the sustaining stage, and the mutual commitment stage. Drawing on respondents' descriptions of the progress of their respective relationships from their first meetings through their engagements, this chapter expands and further refines the original model.

Our data are drawn from sixty interviews with twenty engaged couples who were interviewed both individually and jointly during the course of their engagements. The twenty couples were selected on the basis of their availability and willingness to be interviewed. In general, the individuals were in the middle or upper class. All had had some college, and 65 percent (thirteen) of both the men and the women had earned a college degree. The individuals came from Protestant, Roman Catholic, and Jewish backgrounds, and in all but three cases partners had the same religious affiliation. The mean age of the male respondents was 25 at the time of the first interview. The mean age of the females at this time was 24. Except in three cases in which the man was five or six years older than his fiancée, partners' ages were within three years of each other.

While respondents did not have to be "officially" engaged in terms of a

73

formal wedding announcement or engagement ring, we interviewed only those couples who were explicitly planning to marry. Three of the forty respondents had been married previously. In each case, partners were interviewed together within six months of their planned wedding date. Approximately two to three weeks after this joint interview, we conducted an individual interview with each partner. While joint interviews concentrated on the development of the couple's relationship, individual ones focused on individual dating histories and family backgrounds. The length of these couples' relationships and engagements varied. Approximately half the couples had been dating for over one year when they became engaged. The engagements ranged from three months to two years, with the majority of couples being engaged for one year or less before their marriage.

When reading over the interviews for the first time, we were struck by the obvious diversity of the couples' experiences. We were confronted with both rapidly and gradually developing relationships, high- and low-conflict situations, and a multitude of rationales for the decision to marry. Individual as well as couple differences abounded. Respondents described widely varying family backgrounds and experiences. Some were well established in their occupations while others were still seeking fields of endeavor. Some respondents were experiencing their first serious heterosexual relationships. Other respondents had dated extensively. Some had been engaged previously, and three had been married before. Only after numerous independent analyses of both the intact interview transcripts and the coded data did we begin to discern issues and themes that characterized the relationships of all couples despite their individual uniqueness and diversity. We recognize the existence and the importance of this myriad of individual differences, but in this chapter we have chosen to concentrate on what the couples' relationships had in common.

As two individuals move from being casual acquaintances to marriage partners, quantitative and qualitative changes in their relationship take place. These changes ultimately contribute to the formation of a couple identity. In her article on the transition to marriage, Rapoport [3] points to forming a couple identity as one of the tasks of the engagement period. The individuals develop a sense of we-ness, a feeling of being a functioning unit, as their relationship evolves. Thus they are able to describe what kind of a couple they are and to discuss their own and their partner's individual qualities. It is important to note that couple identity neither supersedes nor replaces individual identity. It is a component of individual identity, not a substitute for it. In our analysis of the developmental stages of couple relationships, we pay particular attention to qualitative and quantitative changes that contribute to the formation of this sense of couple identity. Berger and Kellner [1] discuss such a process in the context of marital relationships. We find that it begins during the engagement period.

Of course, relationships do not develop in a vacuum. While partners may ultimately spend very large amounts of time and energy on one another, they never completely exclude the outside world. Various significant others usually influence the course and nature of the couple's relationship. In this chapter we take these important external influences into account. Finally, relationships develop at varying rates. Rate of development is an important issue in both the initiating and sustaining stages of the relationship. In this chapter we consider a variety of factors that influence the rate at which a relationship develops.

THE INITIATING STAGE

The initiating stage of a couple's relationship begins with the first encounter. During this stage the partners see each other irregularly. On their first few interactions they form initial impressions of each other, and on subsequent dates they attempt to validate these initial impressions and further expand their knowledge of each other.

First encounters of the twenty couples interviewed ranged from casual social interactions to actual dates. Whatever their form, these encounters provided the partners with an opportunity to assess each other's physical, social, and personality characteristics. This sizing-up process varied according to the type and number of characteristics evaluated. Some respondents described this process only in terms of physical appearances. For instance, one man was initially attracted to his fiancée, whom he met in a singles bar, because she looked "real lively and sexy." He continued to discuss his initial impression by describing how her attire complemented the color of her hair. Other respondents considered a variety of personal and social attributes when initially assessing their partners. For example, one man stated:

Well, the very first thing I noticed on our very first date was [that] we thought along the same wavelengths. By that I mean many, many things were in common. We felt the same way about many things. Some things about her personality just appealed to me. Because when we described each other, or described ourselves to each other, I should say, I could see an awful lot in her that made her attractive. She was a very intelligent girl, quite attractive, and she seemed to pay attention to the same things I paid attention to.

In contrast to the previously quoted respondent, this individual's favorable first impression was predicated on personality characteristics rather than on physical appearance. He was highly analytical and explicit in pinpointing initial likes and dislikes.

Couples' initial reactions to each other varied. Some couples were strongly drawn to one another at their first meeting; others were almost as strongly repelled. Most were neither strongly attracted nor repelled. The following quotes illustrate the diversity of these initial reactions:

Well, when I came over and we were deciding what movie to go to, I told her that I'd like to see this, and she told me she had already seen it. She didn't mind seeing it again if I hadn't seen it. I knew she wasn't domineering right off the bat.

75. Forming a Couple Identity

He just seemed like a real honest, down-to-earth, nice person. He was genuinely interested in what you had to say. He wasn't really trying to show off,
to impress you, like a lot of people. He was never pushy, and he didn't
make you feel like you had to put on false airs.

During their first few times together, the couples confirmed and further
refined their initial impressions.

Those couples who initially had evaluated each other negatively did not
begin to date until their original assessments had changed. In these cases,
respondents identified specific incidents leading them to reevaluate their
first impressions of each other.

Once an individual defined someone as a promising dating partner, he or
she began to undertake a rather thorough, systematic assessment of that
person's various attributes and the possible benefits to himself or herself of
continuing the relationship. During this process, the individuals explicitly
considered reasons for maintaining or terminating the relationship. Although
thus begun in the initiating stage, this evaluative process continued through
all stages of the relationship.

Some individuals considered only one or a very limited number of traits
that were particularly important to them. One woman, for example, noted
that after a few dates with her fiancé she was satisfied that he was not an
overly aggressive person. She went on to explain that she was not attracted
to such persons and that it was very important to her to determine that
her fiancé harbored no hidden aggressiveness.

Other respondents described evaluating a wide range of attributes before
deciding that the relationship merited pursuing. The following quote illustrates this kind of broad evaluation:

The first thing I judged a girl by was intelligence. I paid close attention to that—
how they acted or reacted to things, how they reacted toward me. Obviously,
I wasn't interested in a girl that despised me for some reason, and most
girls that I dated more than once were pretty much intelligent girls. They
were either in college or had finished college. For the most part we could
communicate with each other. Personality is a big thing. I worried about how
they reacted toward my friends or, if we were out by ourselves, what things
we had in common. Like, well, let's say we went to a movie and started
talking about it. You could judge a person by his reactions. I wanted attractive girls too. I did have this thing about being seen with girls who were
presentable. I felt that if they had enough pride in their own appearance,
that would mean a lot.

This man had very definite criteria for evaluating his dating partners. In
discussing his image of his fiancee, he was able to state how she measured up
to his expectations with regard to the various qualities he had defined as
important. During this early dating period, all the individuals focused on

verifying the presence of positive qualities and making sure that they would not be surprised by previously undetected negative traits.

When deciding whether to continue a relationship, the individuals also considered the possible benefits to themselves. Simply having someone to date was sometimes an important factor in an individual's decision to continue a relationship. For example, one woman stated that she had decided to continue dating her fiancé because "there was no one else I was interested in, and I had just broken off with another guy and needed someone to date for an interim period." In this case, the fiancé's having filled a social gap in the respondent's life was sufficient incentive to continue dating. In another instance, a man said that he decided to continue dating his partner because "it was hard finding someone to date at school; so I just sort of kept asking her out." Thus even convenience can be considered reason enough to continue dating. While certain couples stated that their dating continued because they were strongly attracted to each other, others cited more pragmatic reasons.

Our data revealed several interesting differences in the reasons men and women cited for deciding to continue relationships. The majority of the men interviewed stated that they had continued to date their fiancées because the women bolstered their self-images. As the following quote illustrates, men regarded ego boosting as an important reward of the dating relationship:

She took more interest in me than other girls did. She liked to do the things I did when she came down to school. I was 19 and she was 16 when we started dating. I was a big college man to her, and there was a great degree of respect and trust in her attitude toward me that was very good for my ego.

In addition, men were favorably impressed if their partners allowed them to establish specific dating patterns.

Women, on the other hand, considered those relationships rewarding enough to pursue that did not impose unreasonable or unattainable demands on them. In other words, if a woman was able to fulfill the man's expectations comfortably, she was also willing to continue the relationship at this point. But this initial pattern of male control often changed as the relationship progressed. For the twenty couples studied, these first encounters moved the relationship forward either by solidifying an already positive impression or by reversing an initially negative one.

Friends and family entered into the sizing-up stage of the relationship to the extent that their opinions of the individual as a dating partner were taken into account. Half of the couples in the sample had been introduced through friends. In these instances, friends' "approval" of the twosome actually preceded the first date. In other instances, respondents stated that they discussed the person with other people, thus validating their initial impressions by comparing them to someone else's reactions. In several instances, respondents noted that they had continued to date their fiancés in spite of an initially unfavorable impression because friends had encouraged them to do so.

If the respondents lived at home or resided in the same general area as their parents, they usually introduced each other to their families during this stage of the relationship. These meetings were typically brief and casual, as the following quote indicates:

It was just a matter of introducing everyone. It was no big thing. I was always having someone over, and he was just a new person. My parents were kind of indifferent. He was one of my friends, a nice guy, no one special.

Not until the relationship had progressed beyond the initiating stage did parents begin to evaluate the dating partner more critically. Respondents distinguished between these first, casual introductions and later meetings, when prospective in-laws assessed the partner in terms of his or her becoming a family member.

Because the men usually initiated encounters during this stage of the relationship, they assumed an active role in determining the pace of development of the relationship. With few exceptions, women expected their partners to initiate and plan their dates. The men, in turn, considered such behavior to be highly appropriate. The woman's typically more passive role at this point is illustrated in the following quote:

I figured he could make the next move. I was going back to school, and he knew where I was going to be. I knew it was a long distance [between] where he was going to live and where I was going to live, and I was not going to push it. So I wasn't sure if anything would happen. I wasn't going to die if he didn't call, but I thought it would be nice. It was up to him.

While women occasionally slowed the rate of development of the relationship by refusing dates, they rarely attempted to accelerate the pace at this stage.

Initial dating patterns varied considerably. However, as couples progressed to the sustaining stage of their relationship, they began dating regularly and usually frequently. The transition from the initiating to the sustaining stage of the relationship marked a turning point in the couple's relationship. Anselm Strauss defines a turning point, stating that "Anyone who has fallen in love, grown to hate an enemy, or found a friend will quickly recognize that although some of the evolvement was gradual, certain high points, certain events occurred after which we were 'closer' or 'further'. After these events, one is a different person to the other, and he is different to you" [4, p. 63]. Couples identified such specific events or situations that temporarily accelerated the development of their relationship and propelled them to a more intense level of involvement. Although the respondents identified a wide variety of turning points, these fell into three broad categories: (1) separations, (2) extended interactions, and (3) definite actions. In several instances, couples experienced early in their relationship separations that they described as turning points because of the accompanying sense of loss over the absence of the other person. In other cases, extended periods of time together such as weekend trips or going out several days in succession brought about a reevaluation of the meaning of the relationship. In the following quote, a woman discussed the combined effect of extended interaction followed by separation:

He had to leave town for a couple of weeks, a business thing. The week before he left I saw him three times. I started feeling sort of like [we were] a couple. Then that weekend I drove him to the airport. I really missed him while he was gone because I was seeing more of him before he left.

In this case, the separation caused the couple to redefine their relationship in terms of greater seriousness.

Half of the couples reported that their transition to the sustaining stage was the result of one partner's taking a definite action to move the relationship forward. These definite actions included such conduct as "getting pinned" or terminating other dating relationships. The men initiated such actions, and when the women responded positively, the transition to the next stage was complete. Whatever their form, these turning points marked the boundary between the initiating and sustaining stages of the relationship.

THE SUSTAINING STAGE

The beginning of a couple's relationship serves as a testing ground for compatibility. When individuals consistently enjoy each other's company, they begin to think in terms of a lasting relationship.

The sustaining stage is a series of small steps that moves couples from a fun-oriented dating relationship to a commitment to permanence. These steps, which are both gradual and abrupt, contribute to the eventual development of a couple identity. Associated with these developments is an increasing amount of interaction between partners. Encounters become consistent and predictable, and individuals terminate other dating relationships. The increased frequency of interaction contributes to a deeper level of mutual understanding. In the process of establishing satisfying rules and role behaviors for their relationship, the couple becomes a workable unit.

At this stage, however, couples are not overtly aware of the guidelines they need to function successfully. In fact, this stage is predominantly a pleasurable, fun-oriented time for couples. Initially, the partners are uncertain of the future of the relationship, but with increasing involvement, they become more comfortable and secure. Dating is for fun and companionship, a time to enjoy each other's company.

Soon after beginning to date steadily, thirteen of the couples interviewed confronted the issue of dating others. Sometimes they decided to terminate other relationships in favor of the developing one. The men ceased to ask other women for dates, and the women stopped accepting dates from other men. This exclusiveness symbolized the importance of the developing relationship, freed the partners to concentrate on maintaining the relationship, and allowed them to pursue actively getting to know one another. One man who realized his new partner's dilemma over a past boyfriend waited for her to resolve her problem before he began to ask her out on a regular basis. This couple explained this phenomenon thus:

He: I didn't want to make things more complicated for her before she went home to see her ex-fiancé [to break up], to make her decision more difficult. But when she came back things just kind of blossomed. . . . It was a little more resolved in her mind. And I thought, I think she's ready now.

She: Then he really started to move in.

Once past relationships were resolved, the new relationship could move forward.

The process of establishing an interpersonal relationship became more complex as couples entered the sustaining stage. On first dates, conversation usually centered on basic data gathering about the person and his or her social world. Once this initial information was obtained, the individuals sought to understand each other's less obvious characteristics. Initially, individuals looked for gross disqualifiers and outstanding attributes in assessing their partners. In addition, they drew on their assessments of past relationships or the relationships of others to help them identify less obvious qualities. Such comparative analysis then permitted a more explicit checking-out process. A woman described her comparative process as follows:

Other people that I have gone out with were really closed, and you'd practically have to drag out of them how they were feeling about things. J. would say: "Come on, let's stop right here and talk about it. I sense that something is bothering you." I don't remember ever playing any dating games with him. The flirtatiousness was never there as much. [Laugh]

By validating early initial and later impressions and/or comparing this partner to others dated, each person began to construct a complete picture of his or her partner. Individuals were especially concerned with comparing their current partner's treatment of them to that of others they had known and dated.

The couples studied saw each other regularly, dated exclusively, and learned more about each other as the sustaining stage continued. A new orientation and a new element was added to their lives as they became part of each other's daily round of activities. Being together was enjoyable; so leisure activities were planned and carried out together. Their individual lives took on a new "we" orientation. The couples described themselves as "serious" and "involved" during this stage. In addition, their friends and family also regarded the pair as a couple pursuing a "serious" relationship.

During either the initiating or the sustaining stage, each partner introduced the other to respective friends. Dating patterns emerged that included going to parties or spending time with other couples. Friends who initially were identified with one partner became identified with both. A woman explained how this process gradually occurs:

My Mom is very interested in my friends and N.'s friends—our friends. In one instance, N. has a friend who's married—they are both of our friends now, but they are from dental school so I distinguish them as N.'s.

Consistent with the emerging "we" orientation of the sustaining stage, this couple began to share the same network of friends.

Meeting each other's family usually required special arrangements if the respondents had met at college. Parents recognized the significance of these meetings and offered their impressions of the person. As dating continued, family activities included this new individual. With the exception of one man, all of the respondents stated that they "got along" with their prospective in-laws and did not anticipate serious problems with them after marriage.

Up to this point, the evolving relationship has been described as a predominantly fun-oriented time. Most couples also perceived this stage as a romantic time. They identified and communicated feelings of love for each other. For example, one woman stated:

I'm very sentimental about things. Like I said I wanted to wait until Valentine's Day to even say "I love you" to him. Both of us are like that.

This woman enhanced the meaning of expressing love by waiting for an appropriately romantic holiday. Being in love was synonymous with "being serious" or "going steady" for many couples. Feelings of dependency, close friendship, and attraction were described as components of this romantic feeling.

Respondents had difficulty defining or describing their sense of being in love. For some, it was a unique sensation. One man described his feelings in this way:

It was just something different. I felt I wanted to be with her. I had a fantastic time with her. I just loved being with her, little things about her. And finally one day I just said it.

Maintaining an active relationship requires forward movement. Verbalizing love was one of the many small steps on the way to eventual marriage.

The sustaining stage was not invariably the time when couples fell in love. For some, love was associated with a strong attraction in the initiating stage. Those couples who fell in love later associated this feeling with wanting that person for a permanent partner. For example, a woman said:

I think I purposely tried not to use the word love because I felt like I'm not

81. Forming a Couple Identity

*really sure what it means. I didn't want to demean the value in terms of love
by calling this great emotion of attraction that I was having for P.; I didn't
want to call that love.*

Respondents not only voiced differing ideas about what love was but also
distinguished different levels of intensity of being in love. Often they noted
that their present feelings of love for each other were much stronger than they
had been when they initially admitted such feelings to each other. This
gradually increasing intensity of feeling was another component of the emerging couple identity.

As individuals began to think of each other as possible marriage partners,
they worked to make their relationship uniformly satisfying. The establishment of consistent dating patterns in the sustaining stage gave couples the
opportunity to construct mutually satisfying guidelines for their relationship. During the course of their interactions, they negotiated personal rules
or norms for governing the various aspects of their relationship. Typically
such rules emerged from situations in which decisions had to be made or
conflicts resolved. Once instituted, these norms provided guidelines for
subsequent decision making and conflict resolution.

Usually both partners participated in this negotiation process as disagreements surfaced. Often disagreements concerned behavior. One couple discussed conduct at parties. They held different opinions about the amount
of time to be spent together or apart while socializing with others. Discussion
resolved the issue and led to the establishment of unwritten rules to which both
partners agreed. These rules then guided the couple's arguments or discussions
about other issues. Rules were more obvious for couples with many conflicts.
One man who identified numerous areas of disagreement with his fiancée
stated:

*. . . like an unwritten law. You can fight all you want to but just don't walk
out. We'll slam doors and walk out of the room but you can't walk out of
the house.*

Other rules, such as discussing an issue immediately or not ending a date
angry at each other, became standard ways of resolving disputes. Because
couples wanted to continue dating, they were willing to invest much time in
devising mutually acceptable patterns of behavior suited to their relationship.

When defining role behaviors, the respondents often identified their partners' objectionable personality characteristics. Stubbornness, aggressiveness,
and a volatile temper were among the traits mentioned. Those couples who
explicitly confronted these initial points of conflict reported that the amount
of strain they placed on the relationship usually decreased after each partner
explained his or her feelings about them.

Role behaviors defined by one partner as expected of the other caused
problems for some couples. When interviewed individually a woman noted:

Another thing we disagree about is his schooling or his lack of it. He could do
a lot better than with his current job. He wouldn't have to have a degree,
just some training in one field or another that he's happy with. If I get preg-
nant, he wouldn't be able to support a wife and child. He'd be much happier
in something else.

After spending much time discussing this issue, the couple finally decided
that the man would look for a new and better job immediately after the
honeymoon and that the woman would stop hassling him about the issue.
In this case, the conflict was dealt with by temporarily tabling the issue.

Areas of conflict varied greatly from couple to couple. Yet all couples
reported that during the course of dating they were faced with various
situations requiring a negotiation process. In short, all couples attempted to
coordinate their individual preferences and behaviors.

In addition to having to negotiate problems pertinent to the quality of
their interpersonal relationship, the couples also had to deal with problems
external to their relationship. These problems usually involved either a relationship one or both partners had with some other person or a work or
school situation. In one instance, the man reported that all his fiancée wanted
to talk about was the clashes she was having with some of her friends. Families were a source of stress at this stage if they had reservations about the
seriousness of the couple's relationship or the desirability of the chosen
partner.

Resolution of both internal and external problems helped each person to
know and understand the other better. External conflicts, however, took on
an added dimension if one person focused on them to such an extent that he
or she neglected or offended his or her partner. Establishing rules for behavior
and working through problems can further strengthen a relationship and a
sense of couple identity. As the individuals studied began to think of one another as future spouses, they willingly attempted to establish guidelines and
solve both interpersonal and external problems.

Occasionally, individuals moved through the various stages of their relationship at different paces. For example, the man may be seriously considering
permanence while the woman is still in the beginning stage of validating her
initial impressions. Special constraints appear when the relationship develops
at a different pace for each partner. Progression through the sustaining stage
of the relationship varied from several weeks to several years for the couples
interviewed. Each partner's level of commitment to the relationship influenced the rate of progress through this stage. Eleven couples maintained
similar levels of commitment throughout the course of their relationship,
moving through the various stages of development at somewhat the same
pace. These couples typically described this progression as a gradual, almost
imperceptible progression. One couple explained:

He: It was sort of an understanding. It just came about. I didn't have to ask her
'cause she knew I wanted to and I knew she wanted to.

83. Forming a Couple Identity

She: I guess a year and a half ago we started talking about it [getting married] but just didn't know when.

The progression to mutual commitment was perceived, in these instances, as the natural, expected outcome of the relationship.

The other nine couples indicated that the partners moved through this stage of the relationship at discrepant rates, creating an obstacle that had to be surmounted before further progress could occur. Discrepant pacing can be a source of stress for both partners, as one woman reported:

Int: When did you begin to feel that you were in love?

She: December sometime. Probably before but I didn't want to admit it. He kept saying to me he loved me, but I said I wasn't ready. He had asked me to get engaged, and I still said no but I said sometime. And he kept saying, "Well if you think you are, why not now." And I said "No, I want to wait till I'm ready. If you can't wait for me I guess you'll have to go." I was afraid if I was pushed into it, I would regret it.

This woman's fiancé stopped pressuring her and passively waited until she conveyed that she was "ready," but discrepant pacing imposed a strain on the relationship.

One woman placed time limits on when she expected a similar commitment from her partner. She described her thinking:

Last winter when it was so cold, I was getting more and more up-tight about us. See, I had told myself, not him, that if we weren't planning to marry by June, I'd leave. I told myself that before I ever moved out here with him last August.

If this respondent's passive strategy of waiting had proved ineffective, she had anticipated undertaking an active maneuver. Her fiancé described their relationship as stressed by "an underlying tension to marry" despite the woman's passive strategy.

Turning points were identified by each couple as especially important events in their developing relationship. Within the sustaining stage, turning points influenced the rate at which the relationship developed. For example, one couple's saying "I love you" served to move the relationship forward at a temporarily increased rate:

She: I think we both knew our feelings were pretty strong, but until he said it, I don't think either one of us had it solidified in our minds. And that just catalyzed the whole thing.

He: Yeah, then we knew we were stuck.

Expressing love for one another symbolized the importance of the relationship for each partner. When it accelerates the pace of the relationship, it can be viewed as a turning point.

Two couples experienced negative turning points. In one case, one partner wanted to marry and the other was adamantly against it; as a result, they separated for one year. In the other case, the woman could not deal with some of her partner's personality traits and broke off the relationship for two weeks. Dating was reestablished when rules were successfully negotiated to govern the development of the relationship from that point. For each couple, the sense of loss that both experienced during the separation constituted a turning point in the relationship.

Turning points also occurred when discrepant pacing was resolved. The relationship could then move forward at the same rate for both partners. Nine couples stated that sometime during the relationship one person had been behind the other concerning the degree of commitment. For six of these couples, discrepant pacing influenced the decision to marry. In these instances, the person more committed either actively or passively attempted to solve the problem. One couple noted:

He: She prodded me a little bit: "Do you want to get married now?" The very last month [before engagement] she started threatening me that we'd better be engaged by her birthday.

She: If I wasn't engaged by my birthday, I was just going to go out and start having a good time again.

We found both women and men who admitted wanting to marry before their partner did. When this issue was resolved, the couples moved into the mutual commitment stage of their relationships.

Couples reported increasing sexual intimacy consistent with the overall progression of their relationship. For some, this aspect of the relationship developed quickly, and they engaged in premarital sex relatively early in the relationship. Other couples reported a more gradually developing sexual relationship and did not anticipate engaging in intercourse until after marriage. Regardless of the rate at which the sexual aspect of the relationship developed, all couples viewed sex as a dynamic and evolving component of their life together. Whether or not they experienced intercourse prior to marriage, all respondents anticipated that marriage would enhance this aspect of the relationship.

Couples who had had sexual intercourse viewed it as a natural act that both symbolized and advanced the more general progression of their relationship. In the following example, a woman places the movement toward sexual intimacy within the context of the wider, developing relationship:

We got to the point where we developed a really good, just a really open, sincere, warm relationship, and I think that was possible because we were together all of the time. . . . I remember sometimes he used to say, "I'm going to keep you here one night," and I said "Oh no you're not" and so one night he did

[Chuckle]. And that started everything. . . . We started dating seriously at the end of August, and I think in November we started getting close physically. At that time we had already planned on getting married.

Couples who became sexually intimate early in their relationship redefined the meaning of the sex act as their relationship progressed. A man described this progression:

There's more of a feeling involved with sex now than there was when I first met her. When I first met her, I guess it was just to have sex. Now there's more love involved.

Clearly, their growing commitment to one another made their sexual relationship a more meaningful experience for this couple.

As couples progressed through the sustaining stage of their relationships, the level of sexual intimacy invariably increased. Even those couples who postponed coitus until after the wedding developed a more serious sexual involvement during the sustaining stage. This greater involvement is apparent in one woman's statement:

We haven't encountered the whole sexual act, shall we say. We're waiting for it, eventually [Laugh]. Let me say it is very difficult at this point. It's getting harder and harder.

Couples decided to postpone intercourse until after marriage for a variety of philosophical and practical reasons. Several couples cited religious convictions as the reason they had mutually agreed to postpone having premarital sexual relationships. Both partners living at home was a definite barrier to the development of sexual intimacy, as was the lack of a safe, reliable form of birth control.

In spite of marked differences in how far their sexual relationships had progressed, all of the couples interviewed had similar feelings about the importance and place of sex in their relationship. Sex was regarded as one of the many elements necessary to the development of a satisfying, adult heterosexual relationship. Respondents viewed sexual relationships as an important component of their couple identity, but one no more important than such other factors as open communication, sharing, and trust.

THE MUTUAL COMMITMENT STAGE

During the sustaining stage of their relationship, individuals actively and often systematically evaluate each other as possible marriage partners. This evaluation occurs in the context of regular dating and gives the individuals an opportunity to find out if they can negotiate mutually satisfying patterns of interaction. When the couples studied moved into the mutual commitment stage of their relationships, they explicitly decided to marry and communicated this decision to their families and friends. Informing others of their plans to marry propelled them to actually set the date for their weddings.

The engagement event may or may not include the traditional pattern of the male making a formal proposal. For those couples whose relationship had developed gradually over an extended time span, engagement was viewed as the next logical step. As the following quote illustrates, some couples hesitated to take this next step because of certain external constraints impinging on their lives:

He: I'd say within the last couple of years, maybe two and a half years; [it was] along into the relationship that we seriously started thinking that we should marry.

She: It really couldn't have been before because we were so young when we met and . . . being still in school. I finished high school in three years and college in three years, but I think I was always rushing to get through with school so that we could get married sooner.

Six couples noted that one partner was more eager than the other to marry. In these instances, the less eager member of the pair was quick to cite external factors as the reason for the hesitancy. One man noted:

One big thing was I had a lot of financial responsibilities, and I just didn't want to make any final commitments to her until I knew where we were going. I didn't want to start our marriage out with owing debts and this type of thing — starting out on the wrong foot.

Thus the actual timing of the engagement or formal decision to marry was often a function of both external factors and the nature of the couple's relationship. Partners who disagreed on this issue did so because they had different ideas about various outside factors. By this stage, the couples had reached a mutual understanding regarding the meaning and seriousness of their relationship. Disagreements pertaining to the marriage date emerged from discrepant definitions of external factors. In short, some individuals were obviously more concerned than their prospective partners that they marry only when the circumstances were exactly right. Usually, this appropriateness meant that both had completed their education and that they could function as a financially independent unit. In these instances, the more anxious partner was always at least partially successful in advancing the wedding date, a finding that is hardly surprising since by this point in the relationship the couple has agreed to the idea, if not the actual timing, of marriage.

Public announcement of the decision to marry also varied. While some couples immediately communicated their intentions to family and friends, others preferred to wait. A woman described her reasons for waiting:

I think in the beginning, when we first became engaged, I had to have a little

time to get used to it. I felt sure enough of him and us that we got engaged
and at first it took a little time to get used to it before we had all the relatives
and everybody descending on us. So we didn't tell anybody right away, and it
took a couple of months before I really felt like a couple. You know, like you
see your parents and they are "a couple" together, and I didn't feel like that
immediately because I didn't expect to be engaged. But now, I feel like half
of a pair. You know, really solidly a pair. We are a couple.

By waiting to announce their plans to marry, this couple had time to further so-
lidify their relationship and sense of being a couple unit. The authors of the next
chapter, on planning the wedding, point out that couples who immediately
announce their engagement and begin wedding preparations move into a
"developmental moratorium" in terms of the ongoing development of their
relationship. Those couples interviewed who instead chose to keep their
engagement a "secret" had added time to focus on their relationship before
getting caught up in the work of planning the wedding.

On the other hand, some couples reported that their perception of themselves as a couple unit was reinforced when they told their families of their
plans to marry. While some respondents indicated that one or both parents
had criticized their choice of a spouse, others reported that their parents
reacted enthusiastically when told the decision. One woman described an
especially enthusiastic reaction to the formal announcement:

We decided to come back and tell our parents. We walked back into the house
with these grins on our faces. My mother knew. She could guess from the
looks on our faces. It was funny with his mother. We walked into his house.
I had met her casually. We walked in and he says, "Mom, I'd like you to meet
your daughter-in-law." Her face just dropped and she said, "Now or future?"
He said, "In the future." Then she got all excited and started yelling and
screaming. We hadn't seen such emotion from his mother. Well, then the word
got out. His mother had to tell everyone.

Family reactions such as this reinforced both the couple's decision and their
sense of identity as a couple unit.

Mutual commitment brings about certain changes in male and female roles.
Changes in patterns of control are apparent. In the initiating stage, the men
essentially control the amount of couple interaction. As hypothesized by
Knafl and Grace [2], women, as they became more comfortable and secure
in the relationship, assert themselves to fulfill their needs. In response to this
behavior, men assume a more passive, conforming stance. The men interviewed reacted in various ways to their partner's increased assertiveness.
Some viewed their partner's demands as a new-found source of friction between them. Others were pleased with the change and its impact on the
relationship. The following quotes illustrate these two reactions:

A week later she had the ring on her finger, and we were telling everybody. And

I started talking to her friends, and she got very upset. On the way back she said, "This is the night we announced our engagement to the world. You didn't pay any attention to me. You just paid attention to my friends." At that point I could see the one problem we were going to have is that she demands attention.

She is more assertive now. The relationship is much more that of equals, rather than in the beginning, where it was — like I had my say in just about everything because she thought that my opinion was so high. We're much more equal as far as the attitude toward things, and, you know, the amount of give and take in the relationship.

During the mutual commitment stage, role negotiation continued to be the means by which the couples made decisions and resolved conflicts.

This stage has not been examined in as great a depth as the other stages. The reason is that planning a wedding forces a couple to spend time negotiating with others. The couple becomes so involved in this process that the quantity and quality of their interaction changes. Therefore, Chapter 7, which discusses the events involved in preparing for a wedding, describes what, for most couples, transpires during the mutual commitment stage.

Individuals progress through various stages in the process of developing a serious relationship. They adapt or change their personality attributes and role behaviors as a result of interacting with each other. Our data — the descriptions of the experiences and interactions of twenty couples studied as their relationships progressed — reveal the developmental process involved in the formation of a couple identity. Within their new, socially defined relationship, individuals adopted different role behaviors, learned about the likes and dislikes of their partner, and were able to anticipate certain responses or behavior patterns of their partner. Further research and data analysis could correlate the importance of development of a working couple identity to adjustment in beginning marriage roles.

REFERENCES

1. Berger, P., and Kellner, H.   Marriage and the Construction of Reality. In H.P. Dreitzel (Ed.), *Recent Sociology No. 2*. New York: Macmillan, 1970.
2. Knafl, K.A., and Grace, H.K.   Family Beginnings: The Dynamics of Role Making. In C.R. Kneisl and H.S. Wilson, (Eds.), *Current Perspectives in Psychiatric Nursing*. St. Louis: Mosby, 1976.
3. Rapoport, R.   The transition from engagement to marriage. *Acta Sociologica* 8:36, 1964.
4. Strauss, A.   *Mirrors and Masks: The Search for Identity*. Glencoe, Ill.: The Free Press, 1959.

7. Staging a Status Passage: The Wedding Event. Kathleen Astin Knafl and Helen K. Grace

Planning a wedding may seem an unlikely topic for a nursing textbook. Its inclusion, however, stems from our commitment, outlined in Chapter 3, to studying people on their own terms from their own perspectives.
This commitment has produced some surprising findings. Some of our initial
hunches regarding important issues and variables have been radically altered
after seeing the data. On the other hand, issues we never anticipated have
emerged as crucial from our subjects' point of view. This chapter reports the
dynamics of one such issue.

As we began to analyze the data on engaged couples, we discovered that
the individuals interviewed had not used the engagement period as an opportunity to prepare for married life. This unanticipated finding was associated
with a second and equally unanticipated discovery. The couples clearly had
invested more time and energy in planning and carrying out their wedding
than in negotiating the guidelines by which they would lead their lives after
the wedding.

Few studies have considered the dynamics of the engagement period and
the events surrounding the wedding ceremony, reception, and honeymoon.
The research available has emphasized the function of the engagement period
as a special time set aside for readying oneself for married life. For example,
Rapoport [1], who views marriage as a critical role transition, has identified a
series of developmental tasks that she believes couples must accomplish in
order to successfully manage the transition. She assumes that such matters as
establishing a couple identity and negotiating mutually agreeable arrangements regarding sex, family planning, friends, families, decision making, and
work are important matters that should be dealt with explicitly during the
engagement.

In view of Rapoport's work, the responses of the couples interviewed to
questions touching on the priorities and focal concerns of their engagement

are especially intriguing. Usually their interest in anything but their weddings as planned and executed is minimal. In fact, once the planning begins, the couples often slip into a developmental moratorium with regard to their relationship. Preparing for married life in terms of negotiating or resolving specific issues that are usually encountered by married couples receives little attention compared to the concentrated efforts directed at wedding planning.

Without exception, the twenty couples interviewed encountered problems when planning and executing the event. This chapter concentrates on the issues that arose during the wedding planning period. The distinct planning styles the couples followed in preparing for their weddings are described and interpreted in terms of how they either minimized conflict or contributed to its escalation.

The decision to marry and the subsequent involvement in wedding planning typically necessitates a qualitative change in the nature of a couple's relationship. When questioned about their courtships, the individuals usually responded enthusiastically, describing essentially carefree times characterized by numerous shared, pleasurable experiences. On the contrary, when questioned about their wedding plans, they characteristically responded in another tone of voice, and focused on the amount of work and the problems involved. The following interview excerpt illustrates this qualitative shift in the nature of a couple's relationship. When asked about their courtship, both partners noted: "As long as we were together we had fun." However, when questioned about their wedding plans, they admitted:

She: We've had disagreements; the biggest one has been about the wedding and about who pays for what and how many guests each person is allotted.

He: It got to the point where I was fed up already. And there was this whole mix-up with invitations. I was fed up; I was to the point of calling off the ceremony and just having a small wedding.

The wedding is a tangible piece of work that the couple undertakes. To successfully stage this event, they must negotiate and implement a number of decisions. They have to integrate their views about the type of wedding each would prefer, what their parents and peers expect, and the financial and more mundane constraints of their situation. While weddings are supposedly happy events, the actual staging process may be fraught with innumerable tensions and strains.

INTERPERSONAL AND EXTERNAL CONFLICT

All couples reported conflicts in the early stages of wedding planning. These initial conflicts occurred between partners and/or between the couple and various significant others. They revolved around establishing the broad dimensions of the wedding and the reception. As the couples explored their ideas and preferences with each other and with their families, they inevitably encountered differences of opinion that easily led to conflict. Yet, although all couples reported some initial conflicts, only half indicated that the entire planning period was conflict-laden. Some couples were able to resolve initial conflicts and plan their weddings in an atmosphere comparatively free of strife while others became involved in protracted, multiple conflicts.

Although the small sample size precludes any kind of sophisticated statistical analyses of the correlates of conflict in this situation, a comparative analysis of the twenty cases demonstrated some interesting differences between the high- and low-conflict couples in terms of how they went about planning their weddings. These data reveal important insights into how individuals go about structuring and negotiating their relationships and the consequences of their actions in this situation. Couples differed in the extent to which they worked together in preparing for their weddings as well as in the extent to which family members were included in the planning and decision making. In general, the couples interviewed experienced less conflict to the degree that they either individually or as a couple defined wedding planning as a negotiable process and were thus open to compromise.

Half of the couples decided to share the work of wedding planning and were in essential agreement about the type of wedding they preferred. However, even partners who agreed about the kind of wedding they wanted and who were comfortable working together were not always able to proceed free of conflict. Conflicts arose when various significant others with whom the couple came in contact had ideas about the wedding that differed from their own. Faced with a host of seemingly unresolvable and incompatible expectations, some couples decided to focus on their own preferences. Often, however, the engaged pair had great difficulty in actually implementing such a decision. Efforts to ignore the demands of significant others did not always eliminate such demands. At times it even increased the ardor with which the demands were made. One respondent described the situation in the following way:

A big thing with the wedding is when are we going to have it. And, if you don't think of yourself first, you're up a creek. You can't have it this day because of Aunt Mary; you can't have it some other day because of Uncle Jack. . . . But you know, it's your wedding and if they can't make it, it's their loss, but still we keep getting screamed at.

In short, a couple's efforts to discount others' expectations in favor of their own can be all but impossible.

The decision, as one man stated, "to stick to our guns" was characterized by comparatively intense and continuous conflict with various significant others throughout the course of the preparations. The three couples who attempted to pursue their own preferences with minimal compromise to the opposing demands of others all described the planning process as an overwhelming hassle.

Planning for the wedding was especially difficult for those couples whose families used them as vehicles for communicating differences of opinion. One man described such a situation:

She defends her parents; I defend mine; and we've had some really heavy arguments.

These couples found themselves in the situation of arguing with one another about something on which they essentially agreed. They were caught up in a situation of simultaneously justifying their viewpoint as a couple to their individual families and their families' conflicting points of view to each other.

A slightly different situation occurred when the two sets of parents agreed about the kind of wedding they envisioned but their view was contrary to what the couple desired. The conflict in these cases took on a "them against us" quality and was both less complicated and less pervasive than the conflict that ensued when the respective parents disagreed. A woman described this situation:

George and I agreed on what we wanted, but it took a lot of hassles explaining it to our parents. They finally agreed with us, but there were more hassles, and we ended up having to do more of the planning ourselves.

Couples who stood firm in their preferences discovered that their families' willingness to provide help diminished. Whether the couple was facing united or divided family opposition, their wedding plans were fraught with conflict.

A notably less conflict-laden situation ensued when couples explicitly decided that the wedding was for their parents as well as for themselves and that the nature of the event was therefore negotiable. Five couples planned from this point of view. These couples reported a general willingness to compromise on the part of all those involved, with a consequent diminution in both the amount and the intensity of conflict associated with planning their weddings. Couples in this category described wedding planning as a series of compromises between themselves and their parents. These couples reported that the bulk of the compromises were made by the parents. As a result, these weddings more closely approximated the couples', as opposed to the parents', ideal. For example, one woman discussed her mother's reaction to plans for a nontraditional wedding in the following way:

She really tried to be tolerant. She's not really pleased, but she sort of tried to be tolerant.

This planning style, in contrast to the uncompromising style, was characterized by comparatively little conflict.

The ten couples just described emphasized working through wedding plans together. In doing so, some experienced a great deal of conflict with family members while others encountered minimal conflicts. They considered themselves to be jointly responsible for the event and reported that the decisions related to it were arrived at mutually. Moreover, the actual tasks involved were either shared or equitably divided; neither partner dominated the planning or staging process. The amount of conflict the couples encountered in planning was a function of their orientation to the various significant others with whom they had to deal. Couples who acknowledged that the wedding was for their families as well as for themselves were willing to compromise at least some of their own preferences in order to accommodate those of their families. Low levels of conflict accompanied this orientation. On the other hand, an unwillingness to take into account at least some of the family members' preferences that deviated from those of the couple resulted in intense and lingering conflicts over the nature of the event.

Couples who did not work out their wedding plans together fell into three distinct categories. In some cases, one partner dominated the planning, the other being only marginally involved. Four of the couples interviewed followed this pattern. Three couples followed another style whereby they relinquished most of the responsibility for planning to the woman's mother. Finally, three other couples who initially decided to work together in staging their weddings found that they had serious disagreements about the kind of event it should be. In each of these three categories, the amount of conflict associated with wedding planning varied.

In the four instances in which one partner dominated the wedding planning, the pattern was for the woman and her mother to work together and the man to be only marginally involved. Half of these couples reported high conflict in planning their weddings and half reported low conflict. Conflict, when it was present, occurred between the mother-daughter pair and various others. One woman explained:

With the wedding, my Mom and I planned it. But then his mother — no one asked her opinion, so I really thought she had no right to say a word — but every time she talked to me she'd say how she hated yellow and how the wedding color should be blue.

The outside opposition encountered by the woman and her mother in planning was analogous to that encountered by couples who worked together on the event. The woman and her mother, rather than the couple, worked together and negotiated their plans with various others. When the women and their mothers were allowed to plan the wedding alone, they worked together with relatively little conflict, drawing on negotiation patterns they had developed over the years. As the following dialogue illustrates, these women and their mothers worked through their differences even in spite of great discrepancies in their ideas about the preferred wedding:

Int: What kinds of plans have you been making for the wedding?

She: It started out to be a few people for cocktails and it's now two hundred people for a sit down evening reception. But what would happen is my mother would come to me with a tear in her voice asking, "Would it be all right if. . . ," and I'd think, "Well, that's just one small concession." Well, the concessions added up, the the next thing I knew I had this giant wedding. I'm an only daughter, and she's looked forward to this since I was 1 or 2.

Again, the women and their mothers drew on long-established patterns of working with one another, patterns that the couples who worked together in planning had to develop and test in the actual course of the preparations.

Three couples virtually relinquished all responsibility for planning to the woman's mother. In such cases, the planning process was essentially conflict-free. One woman explained such a situation:

This is really mother's party. We've been down several times and made major decisions, but the rest has been hers. We got into an argument over some small things about the reception and she said, "Don't you understand? The reception is our chance to say thank you to all the people who have been so nice to you." After that I let her have her way because that made sense.

The pattern was for either the couple or the woman to negotiate a general outline of plans with the woman's mother, who then assumed the bulk of planning responsibility.

Finally, three couples who initially had decided to plan together for this event subsequently found themselves at odds with one another over the kind of wedding they preferred. The conflict in these cases occurred between partners and not between the couple and various significant others. In one such case, the disagreement stemmed more from differing orientations toward planning in general than from the specifics involved. The man explained the couple's differences:

I think she is worrying too much about the wedding. She's afraid things aren't going to go smoothly. She is much more of a pessimist than I am. I'm the optimist, and I just keep trying to tell her that whatever happens will happen; we'll have a good time.

This man's fiancée interpreted his optimistic outlook as disinterest. She responded with regret:

It's a very exciting time in your life, and it's too bad that I have to do it alone.

This couple's wedding planning was characterized by a failure to understand each other's point of view and a resulting sense of mutual disappointment.

Two couples had protracted conflicts about the character of the wedding. One couple recounted in detail the arguments they had been having concerning the size of the wedding, its date and time of day, the reception size and seating arrangements, the number of attendants, the color scheme, the flower arrangements, and the invitations. This couple never mentioned a point of agreement or one positive aspect of wedding planning. In fact, at the end of the interview, when asked if they would like to say anything else, the man answered that "the sooner the wedding is over the better off we will all be." The second couple who reported a high level of interpersonal conflict over wedding preparations indicated that their disagreement centered on one issue, the color of the woman's dress. This couple addressed their difference of opinion in the following dialogue:

· *He: Let me say this. We've both had relations with other people, but we reached an understanding as a couple that we would wait, and I felt that there was a certain amount of symbolism involved which was appropriate due to our particular situation.*

She: I rejected the symbolism because it's all a bunch of garbage. I told him I was not going to wear white, and he got terribly upset about it.

Whereas the former couple's disagreements involved wedding planning specifics, the latter couple's conflicts touched on issues pertinent to the quality and meaning of their relationship. The latter couple filed for divorce within three months of getting married. Clearly, they were expressing some of their rather serious incompatibilities through the wedding dress issue.

ASSESSING THE BYPRODUCTS OF CONFLICT

Planning for a wedding is a complicated, often traumatic, undertaking that assumes a variety of forms. The couples interviewed dealt differently with each other and the significant others involved in the wedding planning process. Their various planning styles elicited different levels of conflict attendant on the process. Since we intend to periodically interview these couples during their first two years of marriage, we will have ample time and opportunity to systematically explore current speculations and tentative ideas about the immediate and long-range significance of the wedding event for the couple involved.

Clearly, the process leading to the "happy event" can be less than happy itself. The degree to which couples appreciated the time interval between their decision to marry on a specific date and the actual event varied greatly among the several planning styles described. Those couples who fell into the low-conflict categories, particularly those who had relinquished all or part of the responsibility of wedding preparations to someone else, were more likely than couples in the high-conflict categories to perceive this as a time to be savored and enjoyed.

Some couples regarded this time interval as an opportunity to work together, to learn to negotiate decisions both with each other and with various family members and friends. Others regarded wedding planning as "woman's work," possibly making a first, implicit move in the direction of a fairly conventional definition of marital roles. For these individuals, the wedding was not so much a beginning opportunity to negotiate and forge new roles for themselves as it was a chance to take on what they perceived as appropriate roles.

Planning the wedding can become something of a testing ground for a couple's ability to assume or negotiate a workable, satisfying relationship. If this is indeed the case, then all the work, frustration, and stress that is typically incumbent on wedding planning would seem to serve a useful purpose. The problem is that even if a couple discovers or begins to suspect in the course of planning that a workable, satisfying relationship is not likely, they will discover that calling off a wedding is extremely difficult at best, once arrangements are well under way. One woman expressed this dilemma in the following manner:

You know, there are things about Jeff that are upsetting me more and more. It's close to the wedding, and I am getting nervous. I keep preparing for the wedding, but maybe in reality I'm not supposed to marry him. When I am by myself, I wonder if I am making the right decision.

It is difficult for individuals to sort out whether their doubts are byproducts of the stresses engendered by planning or last-minute jitters, or are indicative of more serious problems in the relationship. Our data indicate that most couples are willing to give the relationship the benefit of the doubt and to assume that the quality of their lives and their relationship will improve once the honeymoon is over.

REFERENCE

1. Rapoport, R.   The transition from engagement to marriage. *Acta Sociologica* 8:36, 1964.

III. Family Beginnings: Marital Interaction.

Entering marriage did not precipitate problems for the couples interviewed for Part III. The couples consistently said that they were ready emotionally to marry. Setting up a household with another person and coordinating personal habits and preferences constitute most of the initial adjustments to marriage. Establishing marital relationships that will function effectively requires designing or expanding open communication patterns and mutually acceptable rules to guide daily living. Dating provides a foundation from which to build. The chapters in this part each deal in some way with the further development of these communication patterns and rules.

Chapter 8 addresses the issues particular to the first year of marriage. Chapter 9 illustrates that couples who live together before they marry have already established certain rules and communication patterns for daily routine by the time the wedding ceremony takes place. Our data indicate that these couples did not find marriage much different from living together. Chapter 10 examines the black wife's premarital expectations and adjustments to marriage. She must adjust not only to her new spouse but to a new view of herself as well.

Negotiation is an integral part of marital interaction. Chapter 11 delineates four negotiation patterns present in troubled marriages that result in divorce. The interaction processes of these couples reflect the problems inherent in their relationships.

Two persons who decide to marry construct for themselves the type of world in which they wish to live. Each marriage situation, then, is unique. The interaction patterns the couples define for themselves determine the character of their marital relationship.

8. The First Year of Marriage: Adjustments and Negotiations. Norma Link Curley and Karen Skerrett

As suggested in the preceding chapter, couples who are agonizing over wedding preparations typically look forward to an improvement in the quality of their lives and their relationship once this event is behind them. In the Chapters 8 and 9 we explore what actually occurs during early marriage. In so doing we concentrate on what couples identify as the major adjustments of married life and how they, individually and as a couple, deal with these. Each chapter focuses on a different group of young marrieds. The present chapter is based on interviews with fifteen couples who had not lived together before getting married. In Chapter 9 we consider data from a sample of couples who had cohabited before marrying. While the two chapters do not entail formal comparisons of these two groups, we do, on occasion, point out interesting or striking differences between them.

Data for this chapter come from intensive interviews with fifteen couples. All respondents had been raised in the Midwest and were between 20 and 30 years old. All had completed college, and many held advanced degrees. Not surprisingly, the majority of these couples had met in college and had dated one another for several years. Most couples were interviewed once three to six months after marrying and again after approximately a year. The interview and data processing techniques employed conform to those described in Chapter 3. After a brief discussion of the honeymoon period and initial adjustments, the chapter focuses on the major marital adjustment issues encountered by the respondents.

INITIAL ADJUSTMENTS

The honeymoon was the first topic addressed during the three-month interviews. All of the couples except one took a trip after the wedding. All of them considered the honeymoon to be important for recuperation from the strain of the wedding before facing jobs, apartments, and marriage. They expressed a sense of disbelief at being married and a new sense of strangeness about each other. Most couples described the honeymoon as a time to be alone to get to know each other in a new way. For them, it was a relaxed, fun time, like a vacation. They did not begin to feel the strain and adjustment of marriage until after they got home. One woman said:

We needed a vacation. It was very restful. We were so tired after the wedding. Mostly it was just relaxing. We had the most delightful week's vacation doing what we wanted to do.

One man said:

It was just another vacation, with a little added twist.

For other couples, the honeymoon was a more stressful time. The partners quickly realize that they are having to spend all their time with someone who does little things to annoy them. The ambivalence that was expressed many times later was apparent in these statements by one couple during their first interview:

He: I enjoyed it; we got to know each other better than before.

She: But during the first days of marriage there is a nervous strain; you are not used to no privacy. That is wearing. Some say it is a special time with lights around it, but I didn't see any lights. It's a special time because you are so close to someone. But it wasn't what people led me to expect it to be by describing it. It's more fun now because we aren't so self-conscious. I can see how a delayed honeymoon would be fun. If you are somewhere special, you'd enjoy it because you know the person you are with so much more.

The man spoke for the couple who did not take a honeymoon:

I will offer this piece of advice to those who haven't married yet. We made a very bad mistake by not getting away; we realize now. After you are married, you can call it a honeymoon, you can call it an escape, anything, but for your own peace of mind, get away from your family.

The interviews reflect the very great adjustments and negotiations that occur during the first year of marriage. The ambivalence couples feel is striking. It stems from their having conflicting feelings simultaneously. The newlyweds are happy to be married and very much in love, but at the same time they experience many problems that require continual negotiations.

Feelings of affection and concern were expressed immediately by every couple. They felt closer than they could have imagined before the wedding. One woman said:

Suddenly looking back, you find you care more than before, and it surprises you because you think you loved him as much as possible then.

A man said:

I knew we'd get along, but I didn't expect we'd get along as well as we do. What bothers me is a small percent; 2 percent bothers me, and 98 percent is okay.

But during the interviews that 2 percent sometimes comes across as 98 percent. The conflict arises from the stress that accompanies the passage from being single individuals to being married couples. This passage is a most difficult and complicated process, for two individuals from different backgrounds with two separate identities must establish an identity as a couple while maintaining separate identities and growing as individuals [1]. Other studies have found the first stage of marriage to be characterized by adaptation and conflicts [3, 7, 8].

Our data allowed us to identify seven aspects of the adjustment process. We found that couples had to: (1) regard themselves and each other in new ways; (2) define what marriage is for them; (3) maintain their own identities within the relationship; (4) negotiate a division of labor; (5) manage conflict; (6) establish a sexual relationship; and (7) redefine relationships with friends and family members. In addition to identifying these aspects of marital adjustment, couples also evaluate their progress toward achieving marital adjustment. The remainder of the chapter discusses the seven areas of adjustment listed above. It concludes with a description of couples' views of the extent to which they have attained satisfactory adjustments in these areas.

Although in this chapter each of these aspects is explored separately, they are experienced simultaneously, as integral elements of a complex and dynamic process. Although this adjustment process is more pronounced and intense during the first year of marriage, the issues it addresses are never completely resolved. At different stages of family life and individual growth, old issues have to be readdressed. However, by the end of the first year, the intensity of the adjustment process lessens, the couples having defined a basic style of relating that serves as a framework within which future redefinitions take place.

REGARDING SELF AND EACH OTHER IN NEW WAYS

Every couple interviewed mentioned at least a few annoying personal habits or ways of doing things that either were noticed for the first time or took on new significance early in the marriage. One woman described the experience:

[Before marriage] things bothered me but I knew he would be leaving in a little while and they wouldn't bother me any more. . . .[Now] you notice something and then it happens again and is reinforced. Suddenly you are aware.

Several other individuals also described this heightened awareness that came from being with each other day in and day out and noticing the other and experiencing him or her in different ways. One man commented:

It is just the perception of the other person, how they are feeling; or if something is bothering them, the other person knows pretty quick. We can help each other out.

Partners may learn new things about each other or experience previously known characteristics more intensely. What is learned may or may not cause problems. One woman said:

We started to notice things two or three weeks after the wedding. I started to get upset about minor things. J. said, "The biggest problem now is adjustment, nothing really major, [you] just need to understand it and get used to it." I thought it was really true. Now we usually say what bothers us, and it helps a lot.

Every couple mentioned that they had to solve minor problems such as where to squeeze the toothpaste, how to find a comfortable temperature in the house, and when to have the radio on at night or in the morning. The most difficult problem seemed to be learning to sleep with another person. One couple vividly described what they had experienced:

He: The bed is four inches too short; so I sleep diagonally and crowd her. And I got four teeth pulled last week, and she hasn't slept very well; she's afraid she will hit me in the night. I don't sleep with reckless abandon like I used to because one fell swoop of my arm and I could maim her.

She: We pretty much adjusted that, but the first weeks it was hard finding a comfortable spot.

He: We had a lot of adjusting. Finally we ended up changing sides of the bed; it seemed to work out much better. It was kind of funny; I slept on my left side and she on her right. We ended up bumping butts all night long.

She: We decided it was better to face each other; so we switched sides.

The couples also learned more about their respective personality characteristics. Sometimes this new information elicited problems; sometimes it did not. When problems occurred, they were apt to be mentioned. Most couples had difficulty verbalizing positive development, but what bothered them surfaced easily. The knowledge was particularly difficult for one man to handle. He and his partner stated:

He: I think she's a different person now. I'm aggravated in some ways that I married this person and now a couple of months later she is different.

She: I think girls do it. When trying to get someone, they do a lot of things. It's *kind of a game, but I really didn't know I was playing. Before I was trying to please him. Now I'm more relaxed and not constantly asking how do you want this to be done.*

This new awareness process included the individuals' learning new things about themselves or regarding themselves in new ways as a result of an intimate, close relationship in which they see themselves through another's eyes and hear themselves in new situations. One couple explained:

He: The only thing I can think of is when I was by myself I didn't realize I was just plain lazy.

She: I am still a little spoiled, but I realize it doesn't accomplish anything to be that way. When I felt frustrated, I'd just let loose and stomp around. I used to do it with my parents. They accepted it. My mother just ignored it.

He: One thing I notice about myself is how organized I am and [how I] can't stand anything out of place. One thing I learned about myself is that I put things on her but not on myself. For example, one week she spent all her household money on Christmas presents. I was really mad, but then I noticed how I spend more money than I should sometimes but don't get mad at myself.

When interviewed three months after marriage, the couples were just beginning to verbalize these new awarenesses to each other and to discuss the implications for their own identity and the development of the relationship. They related to each other more in individual terms than in couple or relationship terms. For example, the pronoun "I" was used more frequently than "we," whereas in later interviews the opposite occurred.

There was a noticeable difference in the feeling tone of the eight- and twelve-month interviews. By the twelfth month, the feelings were more relaxed; loving expressions occurred more often than unhappy and stressful ones. Adjustments were being made, and the partners were getting along better. They had learned more about each other than they had ever dreamed possible. They began to relate more in relationship and couple terms and to talk to each other instead of to the interviewer. The relaxation process occurred during daily interaction, and the difference it made in the individuals was the subject of comments by one or both partners. One woman commented that she helped her husband to:

. . . loosen up, let go, even use a few bad words. Everyone at work tells him he is more conscientious and demands more now. I help him stand up for himself.

One man said:

We are getting to know each other better and getting a personality as a couple, but not that much has changed. We kind of accept each other's likes and

105. *The First Year of Marriage: Adjustments*

dislikes and just go our way. . . . It's just that now more than ever I know that sometimes she says things she doesn't mean, and every once in a while I'll explode and say things I don't mean. We look at it for what it is. It isn't that serious any more. We don't have any real serious fights.

DEFINING WHAT MARRIAGE IS FOR THE COUPLE

Each couple's next major step in the adjustment process was to define marriage for themselves. Initially, the couples began to notice small differences between being single and being married. They then had to consider more overtly what marriage meant to them and to further negotiate and more fully define their own relationship. In the early interviews, they tended to discuss the institution of marriage rather than what the marriage meant to them personally. The latter they began to discuss in the later interviews.

The couples began to feel what it was to be independent, on their own away from their parents. One partner commented:

If we want to go out, we go. If we don't want to be bothered, we say no. We can do whatever we want; we aren't tied down to a specific time. One of the nicest things is I don't have to drive you home at 12:00 P.M. and drive all the way back home.

However, the recognition of independence in this sense is limited by an awareness of dependence, of having to consider the other person and responsibilities when planning activities and daily living. One couple explained:

She: You can't pick up and go whenever you feel like going out. There's someone to worry about more than yourself. You have to really want to share your time and pleasures with another person. I had to alter my thinking, saying: I can't sit in the library for four hours. When you're married there's always something to do in the house.

He: You don't want to go out and leave your wife at home. You feel funny going bowling with the guys. I do my ice skating while she's teaching Hebrew school, so I don't feel so guilty. Saturday when I sent you with the girls, I felt funny staying here and washing the dishes.

She: And I felt funny leaving him home with all the work that had to be done in the house.

Frequently accompanying this discussion was the realization of how much more they needed to do both as a couple and individually to develop and maintain the relationship. For example, one couple described their awareness of their differences and their efforts to adjust:

He: I like to read and I can't read in the same room with the television. So I go in the bedroom, and M. comes in and bothers me. I'll just be getting involved, and she comes in and shoots the concentration.

She: After a whole day of not being around D., I like to at least have him in the same room.

He: We talked about it and adjusted. Last week four commercials went by before she came in.

She: I'll get used to having him around; as I get more things to do, I'll not have to bother him.

He: Then I'll probably cry that you aren't paying attention to me. In the beginning I tried to understand why M. was doing this. I try to relate that I want to be alone, then I thought I was being selfish. I'm a loner in a way; sometimes I want to be by myself, read and do things alone. But when I go out, I like M. to be with me.

Not until the eight- to twelve-month interviews did couples talk at any length about the personal meaning of marriage. All couples mentioned feeling closer now than ever before. For example, one partner commented:

[The marriage] seems fuller now. I don't know how to describe it; it just seems like there is more to it than before.

Another couple described an increase in confidence in each other and in the relationship.

Most couples mentioned the companionship and friendship of marriage. As the following quotes illustrate, they had someone with whom to share their lives:

Now I've found someone I'd like to live the rest of my life with; it makes me very happy.

Someone that's your best friend and everything else combined. I like the companionship. I always hated being alone.

It's living a life together, and doing things for each other and helping each other out when it's needed, planning together, doing things together.

All the couples were asked how living together (as they imagined it) would compare with being married. Every couple mentioned the security and responsibility to work things out in marriage. The following statement is representative:

Marriage is a more secure and enjoyable relationship than just living together. If you only share mutual attraction with no bonds, when things upset you, you just leave. Now you care about the relationship and work at it more.

Every couple also believed that the hardest part of being husband and wife was two individuals' having to learn to live together. One partner commented:

First and foremost you have to learn to live with each other. Everything else is insignificant.

Another summarized:

Really, to be perfectly frank about it, I feel that your ideals change after marriage because you come to the realization that marriage is just a piece of paper. You're brought up to believe that you get married and all of a sudden you develop responsibility. Being married and what have you, if you didn't have responsibility before you got married, you certainly won't have it during marriage. And I believe that most of my ideals of a wife, husband, father, were false. Basically an ideal husband or wife is a companion, lover, and a friend. It can't be any more, it can't be any less, because if there is a change after marriage in the person, then the person you married is not the person you knew before.

An interesting comment by four couples concerned how much reading about divorce or the divorces of couples they knew bothered them. One woman said:

The Tribune will have something about divorced women. You read that, and it's like the feeling I have. I can't imagine ever not having [that feeling], and you begin to wonder every once in awhile, how can this feeling which seems so natural ever leave you.

MAINTAINING SEPARATE IDENTITIES

All the couples agreed it was good to maintain individual hobbies or activities in order to relieve the intensity of intimacy and to maintain individuality. However, such individuality was advocated with ambivalence, for the issue offered the partners an opportunity to ventilate their negative feelings about what they had given up for marriage. All couples expressed such feelings despite their desire to be married and their happiness. One couple's conflicting feelings are apparent in the following dialogue:

He: It's curtailed my bridge game; I miss the bridge a little. But I still participate in the sports with my friends. You give up something for other things anyway. She gets jealous of my sports sometimes.

She: I want him to be with me. . . . [I'd] rather do things together, but if it works out not to do things together, it's okay.

He: We try to plan things so we do them together. I don't really want to leave her, and I'll kill her if she wants to leave me.

She: And I realize it's not fair to expect him to be with me all the time.

One couple told of a number of fights about her being late from a teachers' outing to which she had gone every Friday night before marriage. The man commented:

One night I came home on a Friday; she wasn't home; this upset me. I knew how long she had been there. It was reaching the point that I was going up and get her. You could have called me and let me know when you were coming home.

Another man said:

It's been a hard change for S. I remember the day she yelled out, "I'm still an individual and you know I still have my own friends and things like that!"

After a year had elapsed, a few had the courage to mention that they sometimes think about what it would be like to be single again. One partner admitted:

There are times it would be nice to be cut loose. Every once in awhile I would like to be free, not free but more in a position to do what I want. Once in awhile I think: what if I hadn't gotten married; I could do that.

The couples realized other differences between being married and being single. The men felt an increased sense of responsibility, and the women were aware of their increased workload. Because of this workload, the women thought marriage was more of an adjustment for them. One woman stated her case:

I talked with friends who just got married a couple of weeks ago. We all felt it was a bigger change for the girls because the guys didn't have to do anything they didn't do before, no cooking or cleaning.

The men argued that their increased responsibility is equal to the women's workload. The men's attitude is apparent in the following dialogue:

He: I feel more responsible.

She: I don't have that feeling.

He: Because I pay the bills.

Other comments recorded at three to six months addressed whether marriage was as couples had expected it to be. One couple stated:

He: We don't behave any differently from unmarried people, basically just living together like two roommates in the apartment, but I think we're a little closer.

109. The First Year of Marriage: Adjustments

She: Before I was married I thought married people are like one person, but now I think everybody is different.

One man offered his definition of marriage:

I never considered marriage as different from what it is, a convenience. . . . It's a piece of paper. . . . Marriage is a subconscious and conscious effort between two individuals whether the law or anybody says you must stay together. If this subconscious or conscious effort breaks down, there is no marriage. So there really was no difference when I got married and when I wasn't married. I'm really strange about that. I don't believe in marriage licenses and rabbis and divorces and what have you. I mean it's passé. It's a convenience, really.

NEGOTIATING A DIVISION OF LABOR

Thus far, we have been discussing relationship definitions. Division of labor is another phase of this process and a part of marital adjustment. Our prediction that role definitions are more traditional among couples who had not lived together was supported by our interview data. All couples agreed that housework was basically the wife's role. All planned to have children in two to five years. The wife would work until after the birth of the children, then stay home to do the housework and the majority of child raising. No individual in this group thought it was good for a mother to work before her children are in school; all individuals thought that if she went to work afterward, her work should be confined to school hours. All the husbands had apparently agreed before marriage to help with housework while their wives worked. After they were married, the degree to which they followed through on this promise varied.

They had little discussion about how the daily work would get done. Instead, the individuals had stated their preference or beliefs about how the work should get done and had then settled into a daily routine. Whoever was unhappy with this routine broached the subject of roles for further discussion.

Several husbands did next to nothing to help with the housework. For one wife this failure to help was a major source of conflict while other wives expected to do most of the housekeeping anyway. Whether or not it was a major issue, all the wives mentioned this failure of the husband to help after marriage.

One couple shared the work; in fact, for them there was a reversal of sorts — he expected more from her around the house. Before marriage they had discussed the importance of not getting in ruts, keeping things spontaneous, and sharing the work equally. The man outlined that couple's concept of roles:

We both read Open Marriage *[5]; that's the type we strive for. Not have set roles; if something has to be done, both do it. If no one feels like cooking, no one does it. Neither is classified in one role. Also to try not to get in a routine.*

110. Family Beginnings: Marital Interaction

We catch ourselves now sometimes falling into a rut. I know some say there are things a wife should do all the time, but she shouldn't let me fall into that. It's not right for something to be your role for the rest of your life.

One man did help with the housework. His wife cooked, laundered clothes, and cleaned the kitchen while he did the remainder of the cleaning. He said:

I told her definitely her job is laundry. Before we got married, that was the first specification. . . . We both clean the house; there is no arrangement.

Two men were not working; one was in school, and the other had not found a job. Their wives were working, so the husbands did the majority of the housework. What work the men did not complete, the women helped them accomplish in the evening and on Saturday. Both couples planned to continue this sharing when the man began working. We had predicted prior to our study that such sharing would continue since the men already knew what needed to be done and how to do it. Nevertheless, these men had difficulty accepting this role reversal. One man explained:

At first I didn't like the idea of her working and my staying home. But she told me I look cute in an apron.

Another man commented:

We made an agreement: whoever it's easier for at the time will do it. It works out better than saying you are supposed to do this all the time.

Although these men agreed to do the major portion of the housework, their wives still had to keep after them to get it done. One man described his situation:

Temporarily it's working out. It's not all on my back or hers. It really wasn't decided I'll do this and that. She just said you do this and that.

Several couples mentioned the influence on their marriage of their families' way of doing things. One woman reported:

My mom said to me a long time ago, it was not the woman's place to vacuum, wash the floor, or do the walls. That's his job.

One woman's anger at having to do all the work came from her family-generated feeling that weekends were special. She did not want to do household tasks on weekends; so she tried to complete them during the week despite her husband's being unavailable to help. Since his family did household chores on Saturday mornings, he felt compelled to continue the pattern in his own marriage. One couple summarized the influences they felt in deciding that the woman should do most of the housework:

He: Some things of the role are from society or parents. Others are a necessity because I can't do them, so M. gets the pressure of the relationship. You can classify what she does as the wife's job, but you can also generalize it and say there are things to do, and it's not the wife's role always, but it has to be done, and she is there to do it. The husband could do it, but it isn't defined as the man's role.

She: Not biologically, but by society.

He: Society, necessity, or pressures of marriage or relationship. She is capable and does it if he is not going to do it.

She: Most of it is worked out by what is working in the relationship.

One couple's more equal distribution of tasks is reflected in this statement:

When there are two people living in a house and both work and there is a mess, to stand around and walk past and say why don't you clean up the mess is ridiculous. I mean we both clean the house.

The negotiations that accompanied interactions involving even the most mundane tasks helped define a couple's relationship. One man's failure to help his wife implied to her a lack of consideration:

It seems what is to be done is so obvious. It makes me mad, like a personal insult, yet I know it's not. I guess I've read too many romantic novels. Because I expect things; wouldn't it be nice if he did this or that? Then he doesn't do it, and I get mad.

Another man interpreted his wife's leaving pudding to be prepared as an example of her taking advantage of him:

Then I laid down the law; a favor is one thing, but being a slave is another. I began to think this is the way it is supposed to be; you just can't lie down and serve as a doormat either.

Handling financial matters and paying the bills was another aspect of role negotiation. Again the interactions defined the relationship. One man said:

Seems like I took over the money to make sure all the bills got paid and there was enough money in the checking account. I told M. she could sign my name if she had to. The way she handles it, I don't trust her.

Another man said:

We had a couple of arguments before the wedding about buying silver, but I came out on top. If nothing else it taught her to let me manage the money.

Most couples, however, acknowledged equality regarding money matters. They believed it was important that they both know about family financial matters in case something happened to one of them. In these cases, no matter who paid bills or made initial decisions about money, all major decisions were made jointly. None of the couples had major difficulty deciding how money should be spent.

The man paid the bills, bought insurance, and handled financial transactions for the majority of couples. These roles seemed to be quite important to the men. They were defensive of their territory. The other couples handled these matters together or divided the work. One woman paid bills and handled daily financial matters while her husband handled insurance and investments. Another couple paid bills together, but, since he was home, he handled most daily financial matters. Another man who had his own business handled all matters pertaining to the business, but his wife handled household finances. They made all financial decisions jointly. The remaining couples either had separate accounts or planned to get them so that each had his or her own money.

In summary, the ideal division of labor was discussed before marriage. After marriage, tasks were done according to either likes-dislikes, traditional division, or equality while the wife worked. Only if one partner was unhappy with the division was it discussed further. All agreed basically that the wife's responsibility was housework and the husband's was breadwinning. But to get the family on a more secure financial basis and to give the wife an opportunity to use her education before having children, the wife worked, and as a result the couples frequently shared or tried to share household tasks. Who handled daily finances was decided differently by each couple, but they all seemed to make major financial decisions jointly. Although task division was basically traditional, attempts at equality were referred to frequently. The women seemed to have much say about these arrangements. Several studies of white, middle-class, well-educated, suburban couples report the same finding [2, 4, 6].

CONFLICT MANAGEMENT

Each couple worked out a method of handling disagreements that was effective for them and agreeable to both. The overall process of conflict management, however, was the same for all couples. First, over a period of time during which the couples had several disagreements, they became aware of how conflict occurred and which features they liked and did not like about their and their partners' reactions to it. Then they talked about the conflict. Again they argued and again talked about it. Over time either one or both partners changed their individual conflict patterns to accommodate the other.

Every couple mentioned the need and desirability to be open and to discuss differences. But such openness was easier for some individuals than for others. Two initial patterns commonly developed. The first was a pattern whereby one partner, usually the woman, would broach a problem and the other partner would either fail to react or not want to talk about it. As a result, the partner who initiated the disagreement would be frustrated. One couple described such a situation:

She: In the beginning it was a problem; he wouldn't fight with me. I wanted a good fight every now and then, a good argument. And somehow we always ended up laughing.

He: She starts yelling, and I start laughing.

She: And I start laughing at him because he's laughing at me, and that's how it went. But it's better now; you've been giving me more reaction lately, and I haven't been getting so upset either.

The second was a pattern whereby one partner vented anger immediately while the other let his or her anger build up and then unleashed these feelings all at once. One man described this discrepancy:

Sometimes it's hard to talk about it because I know she's upset about something, but trying to find out what it is is difficult. I know I've done something; I want to know what, not have someone sulking. Or she won't say anything for several days then get really mad at a small incident. Then it comes out.

Many individuals used their parents' styles of handling disagreements as a reference point. If they liked the style, they imitated it; if they disliked it, they tried to be different. One partner commented:

My parents had the attitude that if you don't like something, you don't say anything. We don't agree, and I really try to be more open. I'm doing better, but I still have a way to go.

All the couples planned to wait two to five years to have children. There were two reasons for this decision. The first was the conviction that it was important to get to know each other and to settle down in marriage. The second was the need for the financial security the wife's income could provide. The following comment was typical:

We'd like to get the things we want to get and get to know each other better before we have children.

Two husbands were very reluctant to have children because they were unsure about the responsibility of raising them. One man said:

I'm not against children. You have to put children in a perspective. I think more children are being neglected and abused simply because people who have them are not prepared to have them. I'm too young. I'm not prepared for children. I'm not going to have a child to tie me down. A child is a nuisance, and I'm not prepared to take on responsibility.

All of the women wanted children, so having a family was not a source of conflict for them.

One woman stated that she would work two years in order to clear the couple's debt and accumulate some money before having a child. Her decision was quite agreeable to her spouse. During the last interview, however, she talked about not teaching the next year and having a child. Another woman was pregnant at the eight-month interview. Both these couples were using a rhythm method of birth control. A third couple concluded that they really wanted a child when they observed that they willingly had intercourse at the wrong time of the month. All the other couples were using the pill. For all couples, birth control was a mutual decision made before marriage. All considered it important for both partners to be involved in this decision.

All the couples planned to have two or three children, even the Catholic couples who might have been expected to want large families. An understanding of the need for population control seemed to be universal. The following comment is typical:

I'd like to have a large family, but I'm conscious of the fact there are too many children as it is; so maybe we'll just have two.

ESTABLISHING A SEXUAL RELATIONSHIP

A couple's sexual relationship was a difficult topic to discuss unless the couple had problems, which the majority of couples did not have. One woman had experienced a definite decrease in desire and was consulting a physician for help. Her husband was reported to be very understanding and supportive. Another woman had a back problem that interfered with intercourse. But by the first-year interview her condition and the couple's sexual relationship had improved. Nevertheless, they thought they were lagging behind other couples in working out their sexual relationship.

The sexual lives of most of the couples appeared to take on a pattern. At first couples had sex very frequently, from five to seven times a week at any time of the day or night. Then after one year they began having sex less in the morning because they had to get to work and less at the end of the day because they were tired. The majority had intercourse after work in the evening or on weekends, when they were relaxed. The number of encounters gradually decreased to three or four a week. In all cases, either partner could initiate sex. In fact, the men seemed to enjoy their wives' being aggressive. All partners commented about how they try to get the other in the mood when they want to have sex.

Most couples felt the actual physical act to be not as important as the affection and love associated with intercourse. Several commented that wrestling while touching and teasing was as enjoyable as intercourse. For example, one partner said:

It isn't a primary motive behind marriage. There are times sex has its very special moments, neat and warming. But there are other times just a squeeze of the hand, or a smile, or pat on the fanny, that's more important. You reach a point where the physical side of sex is needed. But I think the emotional side of the needing of the other is more important.

Although most couples were much less specific about the sexual aspect of their relationships, they did comment that the first year was a time when they were adjusting to each other's needs and finding what satisfied the other. After being together one year, the couples were more relaxed and described their sexual relationship as having improved. One partner commented:

Like we mentioned before, we have an unspoken thing because we know when the time is right. This didn't come about overnight; it took awhile. We had to sort of learn about each other, what each expected of the other. Yeah, we know just what works and what doesn't, what we can do and what we can't, what we like and what we don't like.

REDEFINING RELATIONSHIPS WITH FRIENDS AND FAMILY MEMBERS

Every partner said that friendships change with marriage. The following comments are typical:

The friendship is still there as close as it ever was, but the type of relationship is different.

I still talk to my girlfriends and see them a lot. But I don't know why, my relationship with them is a lot different.

With me most of my friends have to go home and make dinner for their husbands and clean the house. One night during the summer the girls I work with had a barbecue because one girl was leaving. That's the only time we've gotten together.

Single people don't like to go out with married people unless they are going with someone. We have a friend who ignores us. We have to bribe him with dinner to get him here. Friendships have gotten a little distant. Part of it is our move; they don't want to drive 30 minutes to come down.

Distance was a common reason for friendship changes. One man said:

One of the major influences on my friendships is the fact that we moved far away from her home, and all our friends live far on the West Side, and we don't go there that often.

116. Family Beginnings: Marital Interaction

On the other hand, several couples had groups of friends they saw before marriage whom they continued to see after marriage. Partners who had best friends nearby continued to see them frequently.

The adjustment to the altered expectations of friends was less stressful than other adjustments. One reason may be that couples knew what to expect, as the following comments illustrate:

I took sociology in college. The teacher said that a wife's friends are dropped after marriage, but my college friends and our husbands get along so I don't feel I've lost friends but gained some.

I don't see some friends as often now. But I experienced that with my girlfriend. When she got married, we hardly ever saw each other. So I was prepared for that.

Their changed relationship with their parents was more of an issue for these couples than it was for those couples who had lived together prior to marriage. This issue was conflict-ridden for most couples and a major problem for one couple. A variety of situations contributed to the nature of the couples' conflict with parents.

A few individuals had gone to school out of town and stayed away. No conflicts developed in these cases because both the individuals and the parents had adjusted earlier to being apart. These individuals thought that their present relationships with their parents were fine but expected that with the arrival of grandchildren their parents would want to see them more often.

Many individuals had parents living in town who initially called them daily and visited frequently. They tolerated this situation for a time, thinking it might be a temporary problem. When it continued, however, they made comments such as "I'm too busy to talk now" or "Yes, we're still in bed. What do you want now?" Or they told their parents that they were calling too often or at the wrong time. These couples tended to ignore their parents' requests that they visit frequently. If the parents' demands continued, the couples intended to let their parents know that their expectations were too high. Usually the couples agreed about how to handle these situations. The partners tried to be understanding about parental problems, which often were experienced by both partners simultaneously. They talked about the problem and supported each other in an effort to encourage setting limits on parents.

Only four individuals thought there were no problems with their parents. The parents were trying very hard not to expect too much or to interfere, and the individuals and their parents agreed on the frequency of calls and visits. One couple had a call system with both sets of parents. If either the couple or the parents received the signal and were too busy or did not want to talk, they either would not return the call or would wait until later to do so. Another couple did not claim to have a serious problem with the parents but disagreed about the way in which they each treated the other's parents.

One couple had a major problem with the wife's parents. They had not approved of the marriage from the beginning, and several arguments had erupted between the couple and the woman's parents while the couple was dating. After the wedding, they did not see her parents very often and were very cool and polite when they did. After she became pregnant, her parents began making reconciliation gestures. The central issue became how much her parents affected her way of acting and how upset her husband became about this influence. She was trying to change, and he was trying to understand, but her parents' influence continued to be a major adjustment issue for them.

Most of the couples who had problems adjusting their relationships with their parents experienced less stress with fewer phone calls and less visiting expected as time passed. Their later interviews reflect their more relaxed feelings.

EVALUATING ONE'S OWN ADJUSTMENT PROCESS

Thus we have examined seven aspects of adjustment reported by the couples interviewed for our study during their first year of marriage. We may also consider how the couples described the amount of stress they experienced and what factors they believed influenced this stress. Two couples thought their adjustment period was minimal. One of the couples had dated for seven years and thus felt that they knew each other quite well before marriage. Their premarital interviews reflected resolutions of relationship issues that were similar to those other couples experienced during the first year of marriage. This couple remarked:

He: There were no major adjustments. We always felt married; we might as well have been married. I have had no attitude changes, and my life-style hasn't changed dramatically.

She: I don't know; I've adjusted to having my own house; that's a big difference because Mom isn't going to come and clean for me. Besides that, no personal adjustments, nothing I've had to give up that I like or do, anything that I hate or wasn't prepared for, nothing really big.

However, all the other couples felt the adjustments more acutely, some more than others. For the majority, the most intense feelings occurred when one partner felt that he or she had been deceived during the premarital relationship about personal characteristics or fulfillment of the relationship and role expectations after marriage.

Individual differences in temperament were the most important determinant of the amount of disappointment and stress the partners experienced. Those who labeled themselves as emotional people expressed themselves more strongly about all issues. Two wives observed:

Things bother him more than me. He lets them bother him while I just accept it.

118. Family Beginnings: Marital Interaction

*D. is a more tolerant person; for various reasons little things don't bother him;
he can procrastinate and I can't.*

The factors that influenced the amount of tension the couples experienced
when adjusting were related to how well prepared the couples were for marriage, especially to how much of an adjustment they had expected to make.
Those who had expected that adjustment would be difficult were surprised
how easy it was while those who had expected that adjustments would be
easy were surprised how hard it was: These two reactions are apparent in
these comments:

*There isn't much of a change really. We more or less knew each other's faults.
I knew what was coming. It's a lot easier than I thought. I wish I could make
more people less afraid of it.*

*He: I might stick my neck out and say it has been a little easier than I thought it
would be in the beginning.*

*She: On the other hand I had the reverse expectation: that it would be easier
than it was.*

Couples felt that the most important preparation they had for marriage
was knowing that their parents had a basically happy marriage. They concluded that they must have learned something from their parents and that
after the adjustments had been made they, too, would be happy. Couples
identified their parents as "the major keys," typically explaining: "My
mother and father got along well. I was never afraid of marriage." Parents
did not appear to overtly prepare their children for the adjustment; in fact,
the little guidance couples actually got from their parents was striking. One
person commented:

*Families are defensive and only show you concrete objective things like insur-
ance, finances, cars, but not about problems that come up.*

Another factor mentioned as influential in decreasing the intensity of the
adjustment was having known each other for a long time before marrying.
One person explained:

*I would say long engagement is a definite advantage. We went through a lot of
problems together.*

A final factor mentioned by most couples was being older or having been
on their own before marriage. Many couples felt they had done everything
they had wanted and were ready to settle down. Even the younger individuals in the group felt that they were at least older and more mature than
many who married out of high school. One person's comment is typical:

It is best at this age; I got kicked around, traveled, went out. When you are

119. The First Year of Marriage: Adjustments

*younger you expect more from life; you are disappointed easier. Now I'm
more settled, mature.*

Several couples mentioned having talked with other newlyweds about the
adjustment they were making. Knowing that adjustment is normal and that
others experience the same tensions made them feel better about themselves
and made the adjustments easier to handle. One person said:

*I have talked to quite a few married friends about their problems and seeing
the way they act with each other and the problems they face and the things
they've shared, and that helped. It made me realize I'm not the only one
having problems.*

One couple was not able to resolve as many problems as the other couples
had resolved because the woman had been hospitalized with a back injury.
This couple felt that most couples had gotten farther in their first year than
they had managed to do. They remarked:

*She: We've come a long way in the past year, but we haven't gone far enough.
I mean there's a lot more experimenting, learning that is yet to come. If we
had accomplished everything in one year, what would we have to look forward to?*

*He: We've only been married a little over a year, and five months of that was
out of service as far as sexual, social, emotional difficulties. I'm not one to
fight with somebody when they're sick; so anything that went on while she
was sick was just passed over. So there were no arguments or any maturing
of the relationship during that period of time.*

Despite a small sample size, our study demonstrated several patterns in
newlywed adaptation. The couples interviewed supported the prediction
that the first year of marriage was a stressful, conflict-ridden time requiring
many adjustments. The first three months were especially difficult. This was
a time during which the couples were just beginning to discuss differences,
make adjustments, and negotiate roles. By the end of the first year, all the
couples were more relaxed when interviewed and were able to report that
differences were being resolved. As predicted, the couples' changed relationships with parents were an important issue.

Age and dependency on parents did not seem to affect the degree of stress
the couples experienced. Individuals who were in their late twenties and who
had lived away from home seemed to feel the stress of marriage as much as
the others. Instead, the degree of stress experienced seemed to be determined
by personality, the agreement between expectation and the reality of marriage, and the duration of the premarital relationship. Those couples who
had known each other the longest, who had discussed their differences and
had expected marital disagreements prior to marriage, reported the least
stress throughout the first year.

As expected, role definitions were found to be essentially traditional despite the fact that equality and less sex-specific division of labor were frequently valued and desired. Some couples were clearly more successful than others in achieving this ideal. Finally, our data indicate that the women interviewed had more input and participated more equally in decision making than previous research has indicated. The following chapter investigates more specifically how the experiences of those couples who had not lived together compared to those of couples who had lived together prior to marriage.

REFERENCES

1. Berger, P., and Kellner, H.   Marriage and the Construction of Reality. In H.P. Dreitzel (Ed.), *Recent Sociology No. 2.* New York: Macmillan, 1970.
2. Giele, J.Z.   Changes in the modern family: Their impact on sex roles. *American Journal of Orthopsychiatry* 41:757, 1971.
3. Goodrich, W., Ryder. R.G., and Rausch, H.L.   Patterns of newlywed marriage. *Journal of Marriage and the Family* 30:389, 1968.
4. Kenkel, W.F.   Influence Differentiation in Family Decision Making. In J. Heiss (Ed.), *Family Roles and Interaction: An Anthology.* Chicago: Rand McNally, 1968.
5. O'Neill, N., and O'Neill, G.   *Open Marriage: A New Life Style for Couples.* New York: M. Evans, 1972.
6. Pfeil, E.   Role expectations when entering into marriage. *Journal of Marriage and the Family* 30:161, 1968.
7. Rausch, H.L., Goodrich, W., and Campbell, J.D.   Adaptation to the first years of marriage. *Psychiatry* 26:368, 1963.
8. Waller, W., and Hill, R.   Becoming a Married Person. In J. Heiss (Ed.), *Family Roles and Interaction: An Anthology.* Chicago: Rand McNally, 1968.

9. Nontraditional Marriage. Karen Skerrett

Among the couples being followed through their first years of marriage, several couples had lived together for varying lengths of time prior to marriage. Despite the fact that alternate marriage forms such as communal living and cohabitation prior to marriage gained notoriety during the late nineteen-sixties and early seventies, very little research has been conducted and published describing these life-styles or the kinds of individuals who opt for something other than the traditional dating-engagement-marriage pattern.

Admittedly, our sample is very small and may not be representative of the phenomenon of living together before marriage for all people. Nevertheless, it became obvious that the rich information supplied by the couples interviewed could be meaningfully pursued with the intent of identifying characteristics that did or did not distinguish these individuals from their more traditional counterparts. These individuals became known as the nontraditional couples, which simply meant that they had lived together prior to getting married.

Most of the published research [1, 4] has examined cohabitation among college students. Since college attendance continues to reflect a minority, somewhat privileged position, the studies admittedly are observing an essentially middle-class phenomenon. These studies provide an image of the couples who when they lived together were good students; not well integrated into college or community life; affluent; in poor communication with parents [4]; and independent, outgoing, and aggressive [1]. Joesting and Joesting [2], who studied antiwar demonstrators, found that those who were living together expressed more liberal views about sex roles. The couples we studied, while all out of college, had much in common with the couples cited in the published studies. They tended to be college-educated and articulate, and to describe themselves as "outgoing" or "aggressive."

Both partners worked in semiskilled or professional occupations, the majority having professional roles. Several men and women were studying for advanced degrees in addition to working. One woman had been married previously and had an 8-year-old daughter who was temporarily living with an aunt while this woman returned to school. The majority of the couples were interviewed once about eight to nine months following marriage. One couple was interviewed twice, at six months and at one and a half years. These interviews constitute the source of information presented in this chapter.

LIVING TOGETHER . . . OR COURTSHIP STYLE?

At the outset we must explore the notion of cohabitation or, as the couples said, "living together." What precisely did the term mean to them? How and why did they decide to set up housekeeping together? What kind of changes in individual life-styles accompanied the living together process? Most importantly, what triggered the decision to marry?

All of the couples we studied were similar to Arafat and Yohurg's [1] college students, for whom the change to living together was a casual process. The couples had dated for periods of several months to over a year, and the cohabitation occurred gradually, typically without any explicit understandings between the pair concerning the significance of the move, its duration, or the rules according to which change would be negotiated. One woman's remarks are typical:

I began staying overnight, then a couple nights, then weekends, then I finally had so many clothes over there that we just figured I might as well move in.

The presence or absence of roommates made little difference. One woman believed that she became invaluable to her partner because her cooking came to be praised and relied upon by his two apartment-mates. For all except one woman, who had lived with several men she had dated, the cohabitation was a first experience for both the men and the women.

Parental attitudes were an important factor in the couples' views on living together. Most sought to avoid offending their parents. For example, one woman said:

I'd recommend living together for everyone — if they could get away with it, that is.

This woman and her partner's living together arrangement, like those of other couples, many of whose parents lived out of town, was never known to either set of parents. The same woman stated:

If our parents had known that we were openly living together before, their attitude would have been different. By the time he came to my parents' attention, and vice versa, we were pretty close to getting married.

No data indicated that these couples had poor relationships with their parents; on the contrary, they seemed to be sensitive to parental values and expectations, and many expressed concern about parental approval.

Parents, then, generally did not represent a problem to be contended with when dealing with the practical, routine matters inherent in setting up housekeeping. For all but one couple, however, living together would have been an issue had the parents lived nearby. The new arrangement was announced to friends gradually and was perceived by them as a positive step.

The changes the couples underwent during the time they lived together were typical of those described by the traditional newlyweds. Most of the couples tried to share household responsibility, but the specifics of work allocation were poorly defined and were seldom overtly negotiated. Setting up housekeeping was thus a trial-and-error process.

Like their implicit decision to live together, the couples' decisions to marry were only a bit more focused and identifiable. The following dialogue typifies the couples' responses when asked why they decided to marry:

She: It's interesting. I'm not sure why we did.

He: I know you badgered me enough. [Laugh]

She: No.

He: Remember? Three sheets to the wind and you say, "By the way, you gonna marry me?" I say, "Yeah, go to sleep."

She: Well, technically, it was for the legal thing, which I've discovered is for shit. And the business of changing your name – that really makes me mad. The biggest thing I think was if we wanted to adopt kids or something.

Int: How about you?

He: Well, I looked at it this way, this girl is not getting any younger.

She: Be serious.

He: I figured I had a choice: I could go for a vacation in Mexico or get married.

She: You probably never thought about it.

He: You're right. Right, I didn't one way or the other. I just got no negative thoughts from it.

Several couples recognized the meaningfulness of formalizing their relationship in a ceremony in front of friends and family, but they did not cite it as a factor in the decision to marry per se. Similarly, while all the couples cited the importance of marriage for raising children, none based their decision to marry on the decision to have a child.

How, then, did cohabitation change after marriage for these couples who had lived together from several months to several years? How did they define marriage and perceive their roles in the relationship? The clear consensus among all couples was that the act of marriage itself made little, if any, difference in their relationships. The marriage event, while felt to be special, caused no specific changes in the living habits of each partner. One couple even believed that the reason their marriage was working was precisely because they did not let being married change the way they related to each other. This couple explained their reasoning:

He: *Immediately, once people get married and get so-called socially acceptable, then each one immediately grabs hold of all the old failure things that go with all of that, and they're doomed from that instant. See, we never stopped being the way we were before.*

She: *Before, you were able to look at the faults of each other without a bond to blame them on, you know. As soon as you get married you must realize this — the faults are the same, regardless. But even I catch myself saying I'll bet if we hadn't gotten married, we wouldn't be so bored or whatever. And then I realized, that's not the truth at all 'cause before there were lots of times when I didn't want to be around you for a day or two or whatever.*

The couples believed that the differences they cited between married and nonmarried life were purely circumstantial. The changes that the couples had experienced in their lives since marriage were attributed to residential moves, jobs, or school rather than to marriage itself.

With one exception, none of the couples "felt married." The one couple said that they felt married because they no longer felt "single and alone." Several couples stated that they "felt married" only around their parents or when they were introduced as Mr. and Mrs. Several women discussed the difficulty they had getting used to a new name. One couple, however, did recognize a difference involving their marital status, which they expressed as follows:

He: *Apart from the fact that marriage is to create children, I think it's consider- ably harder to back out of marriage. Things have to goof up more radically for a marriage to end than [for] two people living together [to part]. The main purpose [of marriage] is to put a stronger buffer on things.*

She: *It's a stabilizer. . . . I mean if society didn't have something like this to kind of regulate people's relationships, there would be a lot more people who would just get in and get out of things sporadically and very temporary.*

He: *The whole point of marriage is not that you're bound forever but that you're basically committed to having a much higher level of aggravation.*

Although this same couple claimed that marriage had made no difference in their relationship, the new status did seem to carry with it altered expecta- tions for role performance. Similar contradictions expressed by several other couples may indicate that whatever changes had occurred in self-other perception were both too new and too subtle to be fully integrated into a couple's working awareness. These contradictions were verbalized by one woman:

When I start thinking of [what influenced me] as a young girl, there are still things in the back of my mind telling me what marriage is supposed to be. When I start thinking I should be doing this, or should be doing that, and I take seriously what it entails . . . that's when the whole thing gets me down. But when I act myself just as I've always acted toward B. or toward anyone else, I feel honest and face no problems at all.

Thus it may be that, for this woman at least, the expectations of behaving differently when married were still somewhat intangible and had not been translated into actual behavioral differences in her relating to her husband.

All the couples recommended living together, clearly relating its benefits to marriage and subsequent adjustment. Their perspectives, however, must be borne in mind: all the couples did marry; so their views on the value of living together are spoken from the context of an ongoing marital relationship. The couples referred to such values as "knowing what the other person is like 24-hours a day, not just 10" or "working out your disagreements and finding out if you're sexually compatible." These comments lend credence to Montgomery's [3] suggestion that living together represents an alternate form of courtship rather than a parallel to traditional marriage. The fact that several couples concluded that their experience of living together probably increased their chances for a successful marriage makes the living together experience more a preparation for marriage than a true alternative to marriage. Like the couples Montgomery studied, the couples we interviewed regarded living together as a temporary part of a permanent relationship despite the fact that this commitment was not clearly articulated prior to the decision to live together. Looking back, all the couples tended to view their living together arrangement as "probably permanent." The kind of marriage relationship that stems from living together is similar to that that develops between couples who did not live together. One woman's definition of marriage reflected the attitudes of the majority of nontraditional couples:

It's a lot of work, hard work. Having to compromise on so many things you're used to doing your own way. You've got to work all that out and try to respect the other person's way of looking at things. It's consolidating two points of view after you've pretty much done things your own way and think your way is right.

This definition of marriage is certainly neither unique nor radical; nor is it a view that stems from or is contingent upon having lived with someone. What, then, is unique about the married lives of these nontraditional couples? Their uniqueness rests in the character of their negotiations, which are examined below as they relate to interpersonal and external rules.

NEGOTIATING INTERPERSONAL RULES

All couples routinely interact according to a myriad of rules, not all of which they are aware of. Some obvious examples of rules are: "You do the cooking; I manage the money" or "We should have an active social life." Other rules are much less explicit: "I am dominant; you are submissive" or "I can't cry." These kinds of rules are frequently communicated in very subtle ways through body language or through the use of conflicting and simultaneous messages. Such sets of rules lend structure to a relationship and give meaning to self, others, and the world.

The study of traditional couples in Chapter 8 indicated that during the first year of marriage a great deal of energy is directed at establishing rules that govern the character of the relationship: new rules are made and old ones are modified. In this chapter we consider whether this process is any different for individuals who have already experienced living with another person. What rules govern the behavior of nontraditional couples both at home when they are alone with each other and away from home? How many of the rules are negotiated in direct communication, and how many are left to assumption or inference?

The majority of the negotiations of nontraditional couples concerned home rules. This concern was surprising since while living together they had had to address the problems that usually surface during the first year of marriage — a time typically consumed with working out the pragmatics of household management and struggling to achieve personal and sexual compatibility.

Most couples were overwhelmingly casual about the division of labor necessary to household management. This pattern seems to have been a carryover from their life-styles before marriage. While the quantity of these couples' home-centered interactions equaled that of the traditional couples, the quality of their interactions was different.

Financial responsibilities were consistently divided. All the couples maintained separate checking accounts, and when two salaries were earned, the money was pooled, and the husband paid the monthly bills. Pooling the money monthly was the only apparent modification of the premarital financial arrangement. Couples stated that they had retained the financial division because "it worked before."

Aside from finances, most couples had difficulty identifying specific tasks that were the responsibility of one partner or the other; rather, they said the housework just tended to "somehow get done." None of the individuals remembered ever having formally negotiated these rules; nor could the couples account for how the rules came about. For example, they would say: "When the clothes need washing, I guess we wash them." When pressed for a delineation, several couples stated that "more often than not" the woman did the cooking and the man maintained the car and the checkbook. Tasks most frequently shared were washing and drying dishes, vacuuming, dusting, and grocery shopping. Much of the division of labor was dependent on the particular couple's situation. Men and women alike were willing to take on additional chores to accommodate the changing needs of the other. In this sense, the informal to absent negotiation process served these couples well in fostering a flexible, dynamic adjustment. One of the women, who had returned to school full-time, stated that her husband now did the laundry, all the cleaning, and the cooking to give her more free hours for study. Another woman, who was in the process of changing jobs, said she now assumed almost the entire responsibility for the apartment because she "was home all the time." Clearly, task allocation for these couples was contingent on their skill and personal preference. No division on the basis of sex was evident.

Several of the women did identify, however, very clear differences between themselves and their husbands in their approach to household management. They typically felt that their husbands never saw what needed to be done or anticipated a job. One woman explained this difference in approach:

We have a different style of doing things. W. will watch things deteriorate until they're ruined and in real shambles, and then . . . like he'll let the dishes stack up for three weeks and then do them, and I can't tolerate that. Not that I'm so neat, but it gets to be a hassle keeping things neat when he doesn't even see it as messy.

Usually the men responded to such differences by ignoring them, clinging more rigidly to their own styles or making gestures to compromise. One husband said:

I told her it's not all up to me. She doesn't have to do the damn vacuuming every week. She can do things a little less thoroughly, and I'll try to be tidier.

Throughout the interviews, only the women expressed any dissatisfactions about mutuality of rules. In addition to wanting their husbands to approach housework as they did, all the women identified what behavior they expected from their husbands. These expectations ranged from "keep things from becoming boring" to "be more forceful with me and his family." The universal unfulfilled expectation of women was that their husbands should be "more open with his feelings." For example, one woman remarked:

I wish that G. would be more open or direct about his feelings. I guess it's partly 'cause he is just not used to talking about how he feels, and it's hard for me to tell what is really going on with him. . . . I can't always tell what he's really trying to say or what's really going on.

The request to be more open was often interpreted by the men as an expectation that they be more like their wives are. For example, one woman demanded that her husband be "just as ecstatic" as she was about the china she had found. As might be expected, the women who verbalized one dissatisfaction or expectation tended to be the same ones who verbalized others.

129. Nontraditional Marriage

They were also the women who had high expectations for themselves and their own role performance. One woman said:

I know it's irrational, but every once in awhile I still expect myself to work all day, keep the house clean, and have all these meals arranged all by myself.

The men generally wanted their wives to be "less sensitive" to what they see as trivial issues. The women generally expected more expression of feeling while the men wanted less. One man summed up the husband's attitudes well:

She doesn't allow me to ignore all these things, which I don't think are important. When she starts bringing up stuff about the house, I'll ignore her as much as I can 'cause I don't think the issue is worth discussing. I say, "Lay low and forget about it. You don't have to discuss every little thing that comes along."

Another man said:

I don't expect much, that way I'm never disappointed.

The women were consistently more outspoken in regard to sexual relationships. Although all the individuals agreed that the relative importance of their sexual relationship had not changed after marriage, the women were vocal in registering dissatisfaction and in contrasting the actual with the expected or desired. One woman remarked:

You know, you read all these statements, and I kind of think we're below normal, and this used to bother me. I'd think, my God, how could we be this way already, we've only been married a year. I'd really get upset about this, you know. Everyone else in the country is having sex but us.

This woman and several other women recognized their tendencies to compare their sexual practices to childhood notions of married sex, society's standards, and premarital experiences with other men. One woman felt that her diminished need for outside liaisons was a sign of a "successful" marriage. Like Montgomery's couples who demonstrated flexible attitudes toward extramarital liaisons, the majority of the women admitted to thinking frequently about the conditions that would justify seeking additional sexual partners. Each of them felt that continuing in the rut they were in would be sufficient grounds for having an affair.

In contrast to popular opinion, which characterizes the male as dissatisfied with the frequency and variety of sexual activities, the men in this group were noticeably devoid of complaints and usually made little response when their wives characterized their sex lives. As with other concerns, they were seemingly tolerant and accepting of their wives' role as the initiator and barometer of the level of satisfaction of the marriage. These women were at a different point in their sexual relationships with their husbands than were their traditional counterparts.

All of the women who expressed dissatisfaction with the sexual aspect of their marriage relationship also showed signs of independently trying to come to terms with their feelings. One woman commented:

I'm trying to accept our sexual life as normal for us. . . . I think it bothered me intellectually more than it did emotionally, if that makes sense. I guess I was looking at somebody else's standards, and I think I'm coming around to, if we still feel comfortable with each other and don't have kind of negative feelings or feelings of animosity or whatever, then I'm coming around to thinking it's not a bad thing. It bothered me for awhile, but it's not as if we're abnormal I guess.

In such resignation we may be witnessing both the seed of sexual dissatisfaction and the means for its perpetuation.

The couples unanimously considered procreation to be a function of marriage and had clearly formulated plans for when and how to begin parenthood. All were currently practicing birth control and agreed that two to five years after marriage was the ideal time to have the first child. Parenthood was typically viewed as a "big responsibility" and a "drastic change in life-style," and all the couples felt themselves unwilling to make the "sacrifices" involved at this point in their marriages. This decision was based more on the need for personal freedom than on financial or occupational constraints.

The couples generally experienced slight to no differences after marriage in the way they disagreed and resolved conflict. They usually said that they "fight about the same things." Only one couple could identify an issue about which disagreement was recurrent. They were unique among the others in their chronic inability to budget. The woman described the result of their mismanagement:

. . . me yelling at him because there's no money again, and we have these bills to pay. We make all these resolutions, but somehow every month it still falls through our hands.

The others attested to their ability to talk periodically about money matters and to decide on priorities among purchases and savings. This process was reciprocal, with both partners assuming equal responsibility for being informed because, as one woman stated:

"Half in that pool's mine now and I want to know where it's going."

When conflicts did arise, the majority of couples relied on conflict resolution strategies ranging from "yelling and screaming that this is the way it should be; I'm right, you're wrong," to "rationally discussing my opinions and needs and asking if it can be changed" to "trying to make compromises rather than one person changing completely." No particular pattern of resolution emerged as typical of the women, although the men again reflected a pattern of "avoidance — hoping it will go away." One husband admitted that he always tries to "ride out the storm — sometimes I get lucky and it blows over."

It was evident that the women initiated most of the conflicts. While on several occasions husbands appeared quite willing to discuss a situation, the wife almost always broached the problem and pushed for a resolution. One husband aptly commented:

We have a fight and get things decided whenever she gets upset.

The slight differences noted by some couples in conflict patterns after marriage were on the side of fewer disagreements. One partner attributed this decrease in conflict to an increasing ability to:

. . . become oblivious to the small things and anticipate the larger ones. I still get hyper about the same things, but I have a tendency to let it go by unless it's a major issue, and I know the difference now.

This couple may have had more invested in paying attention to conflict patterns because they also stated that marriage was different from living together in that disagreements in marriage must be better reconciled.

Indeed, paying attention is at the crux of rule establishment in a relationship. Some couples paid more attention to and were more aware of certain aspects of their relationships than others. While this awareness could easily be interpreted as the pattern of rules the couple maintained, it is doubtful that they would be so labeled by the couple. Since so many rules depended on the particular situation and the prior experiences each partner brought to the relationship, perhaps the only rule that could be considered common to all couples is that the situation determines the outcome.

Most nebulous of all rules were those that stemmed from needs of which the individual was least aware. For example, one woman who had been feeling sexually frustrated and had kept it to herself described taping an article to the bathroom mirror listing all the causes of male impotence. She was initially upset when her husband ignored it, realizing only much later that her real anger was directed at herself for not making her needs known in a direct manner. The woman's unawareness of her own behavior almost resulted in the couple's recognizing an implicit rule not to communicate directly about sex.

All the couples tended to change their expectations and establish rules by discussing what other people did. Here again, it is doubtful whether the couples themselves realized how much they were being influenced by others. Many individuals frequently lapsed into an elaboration of how filthy a friend's apartment was, or how one man never tells his wife where he's going, or how one woman "really takes care of her body physically," all of which provided a commentary on the needs and expectations of the speaker and set a standard for performance in his or her relationship. Despite their ambiguity, the nonthreatening nature of such exchanges may be an important means by which couples can transmit expectations and establish norms for their relationships.

NEGOTIATING EXTERNAL RULES

The couples spent considerably less time discussing their role performances outside the home, perhaps because all the partners were emancipated individuals with well-established careers at the time they met. Nevertheless, once married, couples usually project a new image to others. We therefore predicted that new issues would have to be negotiated. In fact, all the couples had to address issues stemming from work or school, religion, and relationships with friends.

Each of the partners, with the exception of one couple, felt that religion played little role in their relationship. All agreed, however, that religion would become important once they had children. They felt that then they would have to find a mutually agreeable church and begin attending. Two couples claimed little need for organized religion but did believe mystical experiences to be an essential part of their personal lives. Several others practiced yoga. The couple who identified religion as important qualified their statement by saying that although they were not avid churchgoers, they discussed religious beliefs frequently. These nontraditional couples' views about religion contrast markedly with those of the traditional couples.

These couples characteristically relied little on their parents and family relationships. Some anticipated that their parents would exert more of an influence on their lives after they had had children, but these couples tended at present to do "what's politely required and that's that." Distance between homes influenced parental contact; those couples with parents nearby called or visited them on a regular basis. Only one couple stated that they saw both sets of parents more after they were married. They explained that the parents "don't mind coming here now." Only one woman reported having family problems, and they were with her husband's sister. Her description of the recurring grievances and her varying approaches to motivate her husband to take action reflect her efforts to establish rules for "getting along with family." She stated:

It was so many things with [her husband's sister], something that would turn me off. Then I'd really feel like a martyr, which is not my basic character. Then I thought, hell, I don't have to take that from her. I don't take that from my own family or friends. I think he recognized that too; he learned to cope with it. I think he's learned to live with it 'cause I keep insisting he be angry with her too, . . . which I thought was very fair. He said no, he wouldn't get into that. Even though it increased my anger, it made me respect him more. He said, "I've lived with her and I can deal with her; I'm sorry you can't." Made me feel abandoned at the time, but I think he did the reasonable thing. I'm glad he didn't let me dominate him in that instance, and that's fine.

133. Nontraditional Marriage

This solution established a rule that governed their dealings with his sister in the future. It reveals the benefits of a long-lasting relationship. For example, the woman concluded:

I could have never gotten that far with her or him when we first started going together.

Since in the majority of these marriages, one or both of the partners had returned to school either full-time or part-time, adjustments in schedules were a frequent point of negotiation. All the couples seemed to rely on each other for feedback about developments that occurred at work or at school. Shifts in household responsibility, getting up earlier or later, being separated more, and going out less were frequently discussed. Such topics could be regarded as part of interpersonal rule establishment, since working out a problem about a homework assignment often became transformed into a gripe session involving study habits and general procrastination. In other instances school- or work-related issues were transformed in the course of conversation into unfinished business involving other aspects of the marital relationship.

All the couples expressed an appreciation for new opportunities (school, job change) to learn how supportive and accommodative to their needs and interests their partners could be. In this way, the partners were given personal validation regarding the other's degree of commitment to the relationship. One woman explained:

He watched me struggling through this and failing so miserably, and several times during those two weeks I asked, "Would you love me even if I didn't get a master's [degree]?" You know, I had to be reassured. He kept saying "Of course I would. I'd love you if you didn't have your bachelor's [degree]."

The apparent autonomy of the partners was striking; each seemed to believe that the other's work or school career was essentially a personal affair. There was no evidence of attempts to maneuver one or the other toward or away from particular occupational achievements. Nor was there evidence of subtle efforts to influence the other in any particular direction. A partner would offer his or her opinion if it was requested or if the issue involved mutual needs or schedules.

Perhaps because all the couples devoted so much time to their educations and occupations, the majority of them spent their free time at home. Joint activities or "just being together" were priority for all. Many couples described their evenings and weekends as "just sitting around, maybe talking, watching TV, and going to bed early." Most were active in sports; the men in particular followed weekly routines involving tennis, swimming, or other sports. The women usually took the initiative in contacting friends and setting up social activities. The most typical form of social life was small dinner parties with friends. Almost all of the couples' friends were couples they had been close to before marriage. None of the couples had many single friends because, as one woman said, "Singles are too much of a hassle; you gotta find somebody for them and all that." The majority of contacts with friends were as a couple, although several of the women reported lunching or shopping with girlfriends. None of the couples seemed particularly concerned about social activities. They lived predictable, routine existences that they construed to be a haven of stability against the many pressures of work and school commitments.

TRADITIONAL VS. NONTRADITIONAL COUPLES

This chapter has examined the early stages of married life for a small group of nontraditional couples. Obviously, it would have been beneficial to have interviewed these couples at the time when they began living together in order to effect a sharper contrast between the adjustments made then and the adjustments made following marriage. Nevertheless, using the data available — the couples' statements that being married in itself constituted no adjustment crisis — we may speculate that the process of actually setting up housekeeping with another person requires a more significant change and adjustment than does marriage. The statements of the traditional couples seem to confirm this same conclusion. Yet setting up housekeeping with another person may be the critical factor only when such a living together arrangement is as complete and mutually exclusive of other relationships as it apparently was for these couples. These couples evidently began with a semblance of reciprocal commitment and moved toward greater permanence. As one woman stated: "Marriage is a nice formality, but no difference."

A more interesting, although much less obvious, question is whether the time the nontraditional couple spent living together somehow gave them an advantage over, or put them ahead of, the traditional couple who had not lived together. Certainly, the nontraditional couples had to negotiate fewer issues, their having been negotiated already, prior to marriage. But whether such matters of negotiation give one group an advantage over the other is too complex an issue to be settled with these data. Although the nontraditional couples did not need to adjust as much to in-laws, for example, distance, not length of cohabitation, was the crucial determinant. Other differences between the two groups of couples, differences such as sexual adjustment, reflected individual personality differences and relationship quality and cannot be viewed simply as a function of cohabitation. Even within the nontraditional group, the couples emerged as unique rather than similar. Their relationships changed and evolved as their particular life circumstances shifted in planned and unpredicted ways. The fact that their early months of marriage did not reflect as many crises as those of the traditional couples, particularly in relation to in-law problems and conflict resolution may be an indication either that these issues were irrelevant for them originally or that they did do some initial rule making while living together. To risk a generalization, we may say that the longer they were married, the more the traditional couples began to look like the nontraditional couples had been all along. In other words, the traditional couples at the end of one year were most like the nontraditional couples when they began marriage. Why this is so is a fruitful path for further research.

The tendency of the women in the nontraditional group to be more aggressive and to take the initiative in defining the boundaries of the relationship is difficult to interpret. It could well be that the women tended to give this impression simply because they habitually answered the interviewer's questions first and the husbands came to rely on their assumption of this role. The wife's initiation during the interviews may, then, in no way reflect the character of their daily interactions. In fact, it is impossible to draw any conclusions about the couples' styles of interaction based solely on their interactions during the interviews. It is tempting to conclude that the women, on the basis of their offering more opinions and verbalizing more expectations for marriage and husband-wife role behavior, determine more of what happens in a marriage relationship. Nevertheless, the application of a concept from systems theory — "equilibrium is entirely relative" — guards against such hasty conjectures. Not only does the woman's apparent dominance characterize the relationship at only one given moment in time, but it depends on the husband's compliance to the wife in that role. It could just as aptly be said that the husbands were really in control of what happened in the relationship by allocating the control to their wives. Any role behavior is the product of both individuals.

The most obvious implication of our data for nurses who must counsel couples who are living together or who are newly married and have lived together is to attend closely to the uniqueness of the particular couple. Since the duration of the relationship and the experience of prior living together result in only slight differences in the adjustment process of nontraditional couples, nurses must assess the particular stresses impinging on the couple as identified by the couple at that time. The demands of real life stimulate discussion and elicit change in the early marriage relationship. Nurses cannot rely solely on globally generated norms to guide their intervention. Instead, they must approach each married couple first in light of the adjustments they themselves are experiencing at the time of intervention and only secondarily in light of particular normative changes believed to characterize marriages of a particular duration and background.

REFERENCES

1. Arafat, I., and Yohurg, B. On living together without marriage. *Journal of Sex Research* 9:97, 1973.
2. Joesting, J., and Joesting, R. Attitudes about sex roles, sex and marital status of anti-war demonstrators. *Psychological Reports* 31:413, 1972.
3. Montgomery, J. Toward an understanding of cohabitation. Unpublished Ph.D. dissertation, University of Massachusetts, 1973.
4. Morrison, J.L., and Anderson, S. College student cohabitation. *College Student Journal* 7:14, 1973.

10. The Black Wife. Bette L. Morrison

In previous chapters we considered family roles in a generalized way, disregarding such issues as race and how general cultural attitudes about race influence family roles. This chapter examines the factors that influence relationships between black men and women while focusing on the black woman's own view of her marital role.

The role of the black woman is frequently stereotyped. Black women are often characterized in terms that denote power. For example, they are said to be "strong," "domineering," "matriarchal," and "emasculating." These qualities, when ascribed to black women, reflect the nature of the roles they are presumed to play when relating to black men. Such characterizations of black women have been popularized in a highly publicized work on the black family by Moynihan [8]. Other authors such as Frazier [3] and Battle and Barnett [1] echo the theme of the "matriarchy" or the domineering black woman. This chapter explores these labels in an effort to determine to what extent they reflect the black woman's reality.

Historically, the black woman in her role as a wife and mother has assumed many nontraditional duties out of economic need. Some authors such as Rainwater [9], LeMasters [7], and Brink and Harris [2] have traced the black woman's family role and her relationship to the black man to the institution of slavery wherein the woman was the acknowledged head of the house and her associations with the man were seldom stable. However, other authors such as Herskovites [5] and Ladner [6] have studied black families in Africa before the introduction of slavery in order to understand what happened to black families after they arrived in America as slaves.

The African woman who was transported to America as a slave came from a culture in which she was respected by male as well as female members of the community. Her role was diversified in that she worked outside as well as inside the home and had economic as well as political significance. Her relationships with the man were egalitarian, but he was revered as the basic provider and protector of the family, with custom dictating that the rearing of children be a shared experience. The institution of slavery disrupted this stable, structured African family pattern as family members were sold separately instead of as family units. The black man's role changed most noticeably. As a slave, he was by law unable to provide for or to protect his family. As such, he was helpless. Black women therefore assumed those duties that black men could not perform. In America, the black woman became the provider, protector, and nurturer of the young. The strengths that the black woman brought with her from Africa were magnified during slavery and are still apparent in the twentieth-century black family.

The modern black woman continues to work outside the home and is still the primary nurturer of the young. Yet her strengths, which contributed to the survival of the black family, have labeled her a matriarch. In some instances her role is being challenged by black men, and she is being asked to relinquish her strengths. Such issues as black liberation, women's rights, and matriarchy, which permeate much of black literature today, could directly affect the future of the black woman's family role.

Most studies of black family life have focused on those families from which the father is absent. However, the majority of black families in the United States are comprised of two parents. This study therefore focuses on black women who are members of intact families. The twenty women studied ranged in age from 24 to 48, with a median age of 36. All but one had completed high school and thirteen had attended college. Fifteen were employed outside the home at the time of the study. Although the findings provide insight into intact black family life and the black woman's role in the family, the small sample size obviates application of our findings to the black population as a whole.

THE DISCREPANCY BETWEEN ACTUAL MARRIED LIFE AND PREMARITAL EXPECTATIONS

When asked to describe their premarital expectations of their own and their husbands' family roles, most of the women interviewed pictured a strong, masculine husband who would provide for the family economically and have a voice in decision making. All the women expected to be homemakers, and some also expected to be employed outside the home. Most expected to share equally in decision making while a few expected their husbands to act as primary decision makers.

For the black woman, the actuality of her married life is often very different from her premarital expectations. One woman who had been married six years, had one child, and had been employed full-time throughout her married life referred to this discrepancy when describing her frustrations with a marriage that offers her little affection or verbal communication. She commented that prior to marriage she had expected to be:

. . . the typical wife you see on TV. I would be in the kitchen making apple

*pie, and my husband would come in from work everyday, and everything
would be rosey-dosey. We would plan everything together, and there would
be a lot of love. That good old storybook thing.*

Another woman, a mother of four children, who had worked all of her
married life and was in the fifth year of her second marriage, traced her discrepant attitudes to her experiences as the child of parents who were live-in
domestics. Referring to her premarital expectations, she stated:

*I have lived a very sheltered life in that I was always around wealthy white
people whose mothers' obligations have always been to do fun kinds of
things with their children. . . . I thought I would grow up and get married
and live in a beautiful home and go out and play tennis and things of this
sort. Being a working wife didn't enter into the picture, not at all.*

This woman had assimilated white upper-class role expectations even though
her mother had been a domestic.

A woman who had been married for twenty-two years and had one child
emphasized her dislike of the domestic role she acquired with marriage:

*I'm just learning now what marriage is all about. I guess I thought more of the
social life. I've always disliked cooking and washing, and I probably thought
about trying to get out of as much housework as I could. For several weeks
after I got married, I didn't realize that I couldn't go to the movies instead
of fixing dinner. He had to stop me. He said, "You have to come home and
cook, and do this and that." I'm really just learning my role now.*

Nineteen of the twenty women spoke of the differences between their
premarital expectations and the reality of being a wife. All of the women had
to adjust to changes in role expectations after marriage. Many of these adjustments were related to employment outside the home.

Tradition dictates that a woman's place is in the home, and many of the
black women interviewed expected to remain at home after marriage. However, black women have usually worked outside the home, and the majority
of the women interviewed have followed this nontraditional pattern, some
by choice and others by necessity. Most of the women modified their expectations to include the role of partial provider for the family or economic contributor to the advancement of the family to middle-income status. In most
instances, the women regarded their work as a means of personal fulfillment
as well as a source of economic security. They did not consider themselves to
be confined to basic household tasks but actively sought employment outside the home.

When the women were asked to specify their premarital expectations about
working outside the home, twelve stated that they had expected to work only
until their first child was born. Only one woman had expected to work all of
her married life. Seven of the women had expected to be housewives after

they married. Yet fifteen of the twenty women are working wives and mothers.

One woman who had a small child and had worked throughout the five years of her marriage described her job as "challenging" and "useful." Even though her husband requested that she stay at home after their child was born, she intended to continue her professional career. This woman had found satisfaction in her work and had decided to continue working outside the home for her own personal satisfaction. However, another working mother of two children stated:

> I thought I should be a housewife, take care of the house and children, and be home when my husband got home from work. I never dreamed that I would go out and have to earn part of our livelihood.

Yet this woman has adjusted to her role as partial provider. Later in the interview she cited the advantages of working outside the home, describing the housewife role as "remote" and "unreal."

Most of the women interviewed modified their expectations to include the role of partial provider for the family. This modification was easier for those women who had what they considered to be good jobs that paid adequate salaries.

The fifteen women who were working wives and mothers had in common their expressed attempt to expand their husband's role in the family by sharing with him not only the socialization of the children but household tasks and family decision making. Even though these black women remained the primary nurturer and authority figure in rearing children, they described their husbands as sharing more of the nurturant role than has been reported in past studies on black families.

DIVISION OF LABOR FOR HOUSEHOLD TASKS

Although fourteen of the women to some degree shared household tasks with their husbands, they made clear distinctions between male and female tasks. The women seemed to agree that black men are more role-conscious than black women, that is, black men tend to avoid female tasks whereas black women will do whatever needs to be done regardless of the role connotations.

Most of the women perceived themselves as doing most of the routine household tasks that must be performed for the family. They often stated: "You name it, I do it." Yet when asked to identify those tasks that are "theirs," seven of the women cited their duties as workers outside the home and the fact that they assume "male" roles. For instance, one employed woman spoke proudly of her performance of other than traditional female tasks:

> Making the beds. That's the only thing I do every day, because my husband shares with the washing of the dishes; he shares with the cleaning of the

house, the washing, and ironing. So, the only thing I do that he does not do is make the beds. After all, a man has to eat, wear clothes, see the dust in the house. So, if we both are working, the one who feels the most rested should get on with the business of taking care of the house. Well, I can get under the hood of the car too. I cut grass and trim hedges, and change tires, and I like doing it because I think these things belong to us, and it should be "we" doing these jobs. Somehow, when you start saying this is your job, and this is my job, you are going to come out unequal. Now he does do those things that I don't have the muscle to do.

While this woman expected her husband to help her with household tasks, she reciprocated by performing tasks normally performed by men.
Another employed wife and mother of two children stated:

I'm a working mother, and we share this whole thing. Tonight he cooked dinner because he was off, but I washed the dishes. I don't really have any regular tasks. The only thing that he depends on me for is to supervise the children's homework, and I do this every night. Now everything else, it might not be expected of me. Now that does not sound like a housewife, but I'm a working housewife.

Another woman who is also employed outside the house noted:

I do most of the housework and cooking; my husband does the grocery shopping. I guess most of these things are shared at times because sometimes he will cook dinner, too, and clean up a little bit. I don't think that any job here is exclusively mine or his. But I feel that there are some things that we can each do better.

In these families the roles assumed by the husband and wife are flexible; the couple's predominant concern is the work to be done; so each person feels responsible for assuming a wide range of tasks.
Other women described distinct male and female roles. One employed woman, when asked how she happened to take on certain household tasks as part of her role, stated in a laughing but somewhat angry manner:

Are you kidding? Some things are self-explanatory. Women cook, clean, and wash diapers, and men sit around and look. We [women] are all conditioned that this is what we are going to do.

Another woman who had three children and was employed irregularly stated:

I'm sure that if I left certain things undone long enough he [husband] would probably do it, but it would have to be a monumental thing. I think that no matter how we try to get away from tasks labeled male and female, I just don't think that we can get away from it that easy. After all, he goes out

141. The Black Wife

and he works. I don't work that hard that often; so I have more time to do these things.

All the women in the sample expected some sort of male participation in household chores. Those women who were employed full-time expected more participation than those who were unemployed or working part-time. The working women all sought equality in work within the house, mutual sharing of responsibility, and a disregard for "male" and "female" labels on tasks.

FAMILY DECISION MAKING

The black woman's role is in part determined by the degree to which she participates in family decision making. Major decisions often entail conflict and negotiation. The women interviewed generally believed that major decisions should be discussed and agreed upon by both parties and that neither party should act independently of the other. The women identified major decisions as those actions taken to enhance the upward mobility or internal harmony of the family. For instance, the women regarded the decision to make major purchases or to change residence as tangible evidence that the family is upwardly mobile.

Some of the women described their husbands as being "too passive" in moving the family forward. These women chose not to override the man's position in the family but instead sought other means to gain his approval before taking any action. Twelve of the women stated that the decision to move or purchase a home was discussed and eventually shared by both parties. In seven families moves or home purchases were initiated by the wives. The tactics used by these women often required years of patience coupled with subtle manipulation designed to persuade the husband to act. However, one woman's frustration with her husband's passivity and failure to move the family to a safer environment caused her to take much more direct action. When asked how the family decided to move to their current residence, she stated:

Well, for five years we were living next door to my in-laws in an apartment over a tavern, and I just got tired of it; so I made up my mind that I was going to move. I had got tired of living next door to his relatives, and over a tavern. I have two little girls, and men would be around at the back and front. You couldn't step out of the door without meeting them. So I just told him that I was going to move, and it wasn't decided between both of us because it was my decision. I told him that he could come if he wanted to, and if he didn't, he could stay where he was. So I found this apartment, and he came along with us.

Another woman, with a professional career and four children, described her attempts to change the family's place of residence:

My husband's family owns this building. I came here with the idea that we
would only be here for a year or so. . . . At one time I was all gung-ho to
move; so I took my husband to look at a nice apartment in a big building.
He just could not see himself living in a big building; so we retreated and said
we would go on and buy a house. At that time they had this money available
for black families to move into white neighborhoods. I went and processed
that loan and got that together, but he would never want to go and look for
a house. I really got depressed, and we lost the loan because we didn't use
it. So, I just said, if he wants to move, then he's going to have to go through
all of the changes and all of the work. So, whatever he wants to do, I'll do
it, and wherever he says he'll go, I'll go, but he's going to have to go looking
for it and arrange it. I have reset my goals.

In contrast to the woman who took direct action, this woman adjusted her
goals. She responded to her husband's passivity by becoming passive herself.
She has no interest in furnishing or cleaning the current residence. She spends
little time, energy, or money in keeping the apartment the way her husband
likes. Frequently she takes her husband to visit friends who have new or
beautiful homes in an effort to reinforce her belief that they too can live
better. Women who viewed their husbands as overly passive criticized black
men who are not aggressive in making decisions for the family and expressed
their resentment at being forced to make decisions for the family.

In most cases, however, major decisions such as a change in place of residence were discussed and negotiated. Even though the element of conflict
was present in the beginning phase of discussion, the final decision to move
was by mutual agreement. For instance, one woman who was a housewife
with two small children at the time of the change to the current residence
stated:

I agreed to move here to save money. We lived someplace else, and he said that
this flat was vacant, and we discussed all the money we could save. I wasn't
gung-ho, but I said okay. I just thought it was too small. I agreed to move
here to save money.

Another woman stated:

We were interested in buying a home, and I had a friend who lived in this com-
munity. We had driven around different communities looking, but we never
really liked the location or the house from the outside. This one was really
the only house that we came inside of. We both liked it, and it was within
our means; so we decided on it.

For families such as these a change in place of residence was achieved by
mutual agreement and a joint decision making process.

Decisions to purchase major household items are usually shared. Major purchases include such items as a piano, an automobile, a stereo, and large pieces of furniture. Small items are purchased by the women without consulting their husbands. However, when the woman is not working outside the home, she is dependent upon her husband, and quite often the man exerts his authority to keep the family living within his economic means. One unemployed wife described her experience in attempting to live within her husband's salary:

> I dragged him to all of the stores with me, and we decided what we wanted, except for the record player. I wasn't supposed to get the record player, but I got it anyway. When I buy something big, I drag him along because he has to pay for it. He thought the record player was too expensive, but I got it anyway. They were bringing it in and he was saying, "Where did this come from?", and I said, "Well . . . [laughter], and he said, "If you don't stop I'm going to take your charge plates from you."

Even though this woman took her husband along, she made the decision to buy one major item against her husband's wishes.

Another housewife who occasionally works part-time stated:

> I do a lot of suggesting but the final decision is a joint venture. Usually he is going to be saddled with the bulk of the payments.

In general, working wives are granted a larger role in the decision making process. Probably because most of the women interviewed work, they see themselves as equal partners in the decision making process and seek to maintain an egalitarian relationship in which neither partner has more control than the other.

SHARED ACTIVITIES AND INTERPERSONAL RELATIONSHIPS

Shared activities are defined here as those periods during which the husband and wife enjoy each other's company either alone together or with other people. Fifteen of the women interviewed stated that they engaged in some form of activity with their husbands outside the home, but only six of the women described the time spent with their husbands as mutually enjoyable. One of these six women, a woman who had been married for twenty-six years, stated:

> I guess we have gotten in a rut in the last few years, as far as going out is concerned because we haven't done too much. But, say for fun, as such, we can buy a box of crackers and a can of sardines and curl up in the middle of the bed and have a good conversation. Just talk to each other, and that can be fun. Just the peace and quiet with nobody to disturb us. To talk to each other about whatever is on our minds. We have gotten to the age now where we have given so much of our time and of ourselves that we need some time alone.

144. Family Beginnings: Marital Interaction

Another woman, who had been married for twelve years, stated:

We enjoy watching TV together on weekends. I think the nicest times that he and I have together are when he sits in the kitchen with me while I am cooking and in the summer when we sit on the porch together. We always seem to have good things to talk about at those times.

Another woman, in the third year of her second marriage, stated:

There's nothing that we don't do together. We belong to two bowling leagues, and he's involved in an organization for boys, and I go to the meetings with him because I am on one of the committees. And we've joined church together since we've been here. I very seldom go anywhere without him, and vice versa, except, of course, to work.

These three women described strong emotional ties to their husbands and enjoyed the companionship of marriage. Each of the women who spoke of their relationships with their husbands as being mutually satisfying cited the ability to communicate and to share in activities outside the home that were mutually enjoyable. They most frequently said: "We talk to each other." In contrast, those women who spoke of their relationships with their husbands in negative terms described a lack of mutual friends and interests and an inability to communicate individual needs.

Marriages remain intact for a variety of reasons, one being the positive nature of the interpersonal relationships. When asked why they remained married to their husbands, eight of the women interviewed responded in affectional terms, stating that they loved their husbands and felt loved in return. Seven expressed a dependence on their husbands to provide for the family. Five had remained with their husbands because it gave them a sense of freedom — freedom in the sense that they could spend time away from the house without their husbands objecting. This latter group of women did not feel that marriage had imposed social restrictions upon them.

One woman who had three children and had been married for fourteen years stated that "understanding of one another is the main reason we are still together" and that she and her husband accepted each other as less than perfect. She cited the importance of tolerance, adding:

And you also have to like the person. I think my husband likes me and I like him, and I certainly hope that we love one another.

Another woman, who has been married for ten years, stated:

I guess after all the hollering and shouting is over, we can sit down and talk. And then, I still love my husband.

Another woman, married for eighteen years, when asked why she and her husband remained married, stated:

145. The Black Wife

I asked my husband that, and he said it's because I need him. He's probably right. I think I do need the kindness and consideration and the willingness to share that he has to offer. I, in turn though, think he needs me too. He probably needs me for a different reason, but I think he needs me too for some support.

Couples who remain together have developed mutual respect and value each other's company. Their interpersonal relationships are enhanced by open communication and the ability to form strong attachments to each other.

The black women interviewed perceived their relationships with husbands as egalitarian. They actively attempted to involve their husbands in household work and in major decision making. Moreover, they valued interpersonal sharing and communication between marital partners.

OPINIONS ABOUT BLACK FAMILY LIFE

Most of the women interviewed expressed definite opinions about black family life today, especially the economic suppression of black men and their roles as providers in the family. Much of their thinking had been influenced by their own life experiences as well as by the mass media.

The modern black woman does not see herself as "the boss" or "main authority figure" in the family, but she also rejects the idea of being subservient to her husband. As one woman said, "We are both equal in our thoughts," meaning that each partner is capable of making decisions that are beneficial to the family.

Since the abolition of slavery, black family patterns have continued to emphasize the woman's role. But the black woman does not dominate the black man. The black family pattern is egalitarian; power is shared by both partners, and black women regard such a relationship in marriage as an ideal.

Black women are strong because the history of black people in America has dictated that they had to be so. Their internal strengths have enabled black families to survive in a society that has economically discriminated against the black man, preventing him from assuming the role of total provider for the family. Although cognizant of the discrimination black men have suffered, the black women interviewed felt that they were not always receiving what they should from their marriages. For instance, when the women were asked to describe black men as providers, the majority of them chose to redefine the word "provider" in order to express their thoughts about black men and what they should provide for black women. One woman stated:

Because of my education I don't need anyone to provide a salary or money for me; I am capable of doing that myself. I think black men are able to provide for their families, but I think it's how we, as black women, see the word "provide." What do we expect out of them? What I want is understanding and to feel that I can lean on him, to reach him when I need him. He doesn't see this. He feels that if he doesn't give me material things, then he isn't providing for me.

In this instance, the man's definition of what he should provide was divergent from his wife's need.

Another woman spoke about the influence of television on the aspirations of the black family. She said:

Fifteen or twenty years ago, taking care of a family didn't include all of the luxuries that you see on television now. It included the essentials of life, like rent, food, clothing, and utilities. These things were provided for the black woman, even with the black man's menial job. Now it seems that black women want all of these things they see on television. If the black woman would accept what he [the black man] can provide, at his own level, he could provide for his family. But the black woman is not satisfied because it is portrayed on television that they shouldn't live this way. The black man watches television too, and he would like to provide all of these things, and it causes frustration on his part because he can't.

Another woman stated:

I think the black man is responsible and capable of providing for his family if he would work with what he's got and hang in there and look toward a future in which things would not always be this way. In generalities, you find them [black men] saying, "I would if I had a job." "If"; there's always an "if." Now the black woman, she doesn't do this. She says, "I'm going to provide," and she provides. She's keeping the family together whereas the black man has not matured enough. I think this comes from his not liking himself. He starts to say "If I had a better job, . . . if I didn't have all these children. . . . I'll split because she can make it better on ADC. If the establishment would let me . . . if the man would get his foot off my neck . . . if I had the education . . . ." All of the ifs. I believe that they are capable of providing for their families, but until black men learn to like themselves they will continue to use these cop-outs.

These three attitudes, which are representative of the thinking of the black women interviewed, reflect the gamut of attitudes found in the literature on black families. In essence, black women speak of and relate to black men from their own personal perspectives or observations. No one attitude reflects a general consensus. However, the majority of the women interviewed believe that black men are capable of providing their families with those things that the women consider to be essential to a stable and harmonious family life.

THE ATTITUDES OF BLACK WOMEN TOWARD BLACK MEN

Black women have never been able to assume the traditional role of wife and mother because they have always had to work outside the home to help provide for the family. Fifteen (75 percent) of the women in our study are employed outside the home. Their earnings contribute to the economic stability of the family by providing luxuries as well as necessities. When both partners work, the family enjoys a standard of living that would not be possible on the man's salary alone. Very few black men earn enough money to support their families in a manner that is considered adequate by middle-class American standards.

The black man's inability to assume the total provider role is mainly a result of society's continued economic suppression. Census bureau reports have consistently indicated that the median earnings of black men are substantially lower than those of nonblack men. The black man is the most likely worker to be unemployed, and when he does have a job, the pay he receives is likely to be low. Most black women therefore must work in order to keep the family life-style above what they consider to be a poverty level.

Black women who work outside the home must make concessions in their role as wives. Some of the husbands of the women interviewed shared some household chores, but in general such tasks fell to the women. The black working wives interviewed rejected the notion that a specific division of labor should be established when both partners are working outside the home. One woman's comment is representative: "There should be no handmaidens around the house." In effect, the black women sought equality in the home by encouraging their husbands to assume more responsibility in the total functioning of the household, including the socialization of children. A recurrent attitude among these women is congruent with that of Glaser-Malbin [4], who speaks of the wife's role as a caste system in which women are expected to assume the role of housewife by virtue of the fact that they were born females, regardless of whatever other roles they assume. Even though the black women in our study have not assumed traditional female roles, they have been victims of a caste system that dictates male and female tasks within the family. Black women seek to disengage black men from this system by encouraging them to participate fully in the management of the home and by convincing them that such participation is part of their role in the family. In spite of the black man's expectations about not sharing the domestic role with his working wife, the women interviewed respected the man more when he was actively engaged in all aspects of family life.

The issue of women's rights was raised by half the women interviewed. One woman stated quite strongly:

If I had to make a choice between women's rights and the black man, I would choose the black man.

The women seem to perceive a conflict between the feminist movement and the effort of black men and women to meet the needs of their families. The black women in this study considered their quarrel with black men to be in the area of family life. They seek to strengthen the family unit by expanding the man's role, encouraging him to share in those duties that have been traditionally held by women. They want black men to become true family men who not only share domestic duties but spend more time at home, giving more affection and attention to their wives and children.

In spite of their lack of active support of the issue of women's rights, the women interviewed tended to incorporate certain elements of feminist views in their manner of relating to black men. For example, they often expressed their belief that women are mentally equal to men and are capable of sharing authority in the family. The right that the black women in the study sought was equality in the home by liberating black men from the local bars, street corners, pool rooms, and other activities in which they spend time away from their families. Black wives seek equality in sharing the responsibility for maintaining a home in which each partner participates in meeting the individual needs of every family member.

The duties and obligations that have been thrust upon black women have made them strong persons, but they are also aware of the plight of black men. Black women are therefore quick to defend black men when the issues involve the larger society. Thus the women interviewed assumed the dual role of severe critic and staunch supporter of black men. While they supported black men in their fight for economic equality, they criticized them for their failure to perform their familial roles. They also criticized black women, such as their own mothers, who assume too dominant a role in the family, as well as black women who assume passive roles in relating to black men. In general, the women in the study adhered to the concept of egalitarian relationships between black men and women in which power or authority is shared equally.

Most of the research on black families has focused on families in which the father is absent from the home or families in which delinquency or illegitimacy rates are high. These facts are well-known to those who read about black family life in the United States. Yet very little is known about the stable, intact black family, which comprises the majority of the black population. In these cases, self-perceived as opposed to stereotyped roles must be foremost in the minds of those who attempt to assess family problems.

These findings indicate that black women who are members of intact families experience problems similar to those experienced by other women in society. Yet very little, if anything, is known of the affectional ties between black men and women that are the basis upon which most two-parent families have been sustained. Strong bonds are often developed and strengthened by the hardships that the partners endure in a society that still makes the survival of black family life difficult. Black families are measured by Western standards that fail to take into account the strengths inherent in those black men and women who, in spite of social constraints and pressures, produce children who do not become social deviants. We must learn more about the strength as well as the quality of black family life that allows black individuals to survive and advance in a society that still does not accord them first-class citizenship.

REFERENCES

1. Battle, M., and Barnet, J.   The Negro Matriarchy. In J. Hadden and M. Gorgatta (Eds.), *Marriage and the Family*. Itasca, Ill.: Peacock, 1970.

2. Brink, W., and Harris, L.   The Negro Family: Chapter 7 in *Black and White*. New York: Simon & Schuster, 1966.

3. Frazier, E.   New role of the negro woman. *Ebony*, 1966, p. 88.

4. Glaser-Malbin, N.   Housewifery as a caste status: The public and private worlds of women. Unpublished paper presented at Northwestern University, 1976.

5. Herskovites, M.   *Dahomey: An Ancient African Kingdom*. Evanston, Ill.: Northwestern University Press, 1967.

6. Ladner, J.   *Tomorrow's Tomorrow: The Black Woman*. New York: Anchor Books, 1971.

7. LeMasters, E.E.   *Parents in Modern America*. Homewood, Ill.: Dorsey Press, 1974.

8. Moynihan, D.   The Negro Family: The Case for National Action. Washington, D.C.: Government Printing Office, 1965. (Reprinted in J.H. Bracey, Jr., A. Meier, and E. Rudwick (Eds.), *Black Matriarchy: Myth or Reality?* Belmont, Calif.: Wadsworth, 1971.)

9. Rainwater, L.   Crucible of Identity: The Negro Lower Class Family. In J.H. Bracey, Jr., A. Meier, and E. Rudwick (Eds.), *Black Matriarchy: Myth or Reality?* Belmont, Calif.: Wadsworth, 1971.

11. Negotiating a Divorce. Joan M. King

Marital dissatisfaction is not new, but the way in which unhappily
married couples are resolving their differences is changing. Americans are
increasingly choosing to divorce when they judge their marriages to be
painful, problematic, or unrewarding. Glick and Norton [3] predict that
25 to 29 percent of all women near 30 years of age have terminated or will
terminate their first marriage in divorce.

This chapter examines the interactions of individuals in their first marriages
during the period when they were headed toward divorce. Data were obtained
from eight men and nine women, all of whom had remarried. The majority
were college graduates and were working at the time of their divorces.
Although many experienced financial constraints during their first marriage,
none were faced with a struggle for daily existence or other overwhelming
problems. Their educational, professional, and family accomplishments
indicate that these individuals are able to cope effectively.

All the individuals interviewed had experienced continuously unresolved
problems in their marriages. In some instances, problems were present at the
beginning of marriage; in other cases, difficulties arose after a short period
of relative satisfaction with the marriage and spouse. Both the men and
women interviewed attempted to cope with stresses, but their actions did
not resolve the problems.

When individuals live together for long periods (two to fourteen years
for the individuals interviewed) during which at least one spouse experiences
stress and is dissatisfied, what finally impels one partner to seek a divorce?
Those occurrences that the individuals interviewed identified as the "final
straw" were essentially ongoing marital problems. The difference between
the problem requiring action and preceding problems was the presence of a
new element that altered the meaning of old problems. This redefinition and
its import were the critical factors impelling individuals toward action re-

sulting in divorce. Such a process is illustrated by one young woman who realized that the new element was tangible evidence that her perception of an improved marital relationship was inaccurate. She explained:

I thought that he had quit seeing other women, and we seemed to be getting along better, much better. And then we started getting these phone calls, and it was just like in a movie, whenever I'd answer, the person would hang up. And so finally one night I, you know, the phone was ringing and I said, "Answer the phone." And I guess in a way he wanted me to find out. He answered the phone, and I picked up the other phone, and I listened. I listened to a 16-year-old girl! And she was saying, "Don't come into the bar again" — her father owned some bar — "because Dad knows," and all this stuff. And I just hung up. I said, "I'm leaving." And it was funny, by the time that happened, I didn't cry. It was not a traumatic night or anything. I just felt like I knew what I had to do, and I did it. The next day I rented an apartment, and I left.

Thus it was not a specific occurrence that constituted the turning point but the meaning attached to the occurrence. The individuals could no longer cope with long-standing stresses once this redefinition had taken place. New meaning required a new approach, and divorce was the solution chosen.

Individuals explained their marital failures in several ways. Most focused on their own youth and limited experience with life. They indicated that greater maturity or experience would have helped them recognize during courtship those characteristics of their spouse that caused problems in marriage. These characteristics included alcoholism, irresponsibility, and immaturity. Others admitted that their own immaturity contributed to their inability to deal effectively with marital issues; they were unable to see or were too insecure to try other solutions to problems. Many of those interviewed focused on the youth and inexperience of both spouses. One person said: "We were like children growing up together." These individuals now consider divorce to have been inevitable. Illustrative of these problems is one woman's description of her ex-husband as totally unconcerned about others and of herself as passive and accepting. Some cited changes that occurred in themselves or their spouses after marriage. These changes led to incompatibility or a drifting apart because of different interests. The changes were directly related to such experiences as education, career, and social opportunities.

These explanations of marital failure are similar in that they do not place blame. The individuals either accept their own responsibility, share it with their spouses, or externalize it to situations over which they and their spouses had no control. But these explanations are so general that they provide only a vague understanding of what occurred in the marriages of the individuals interviewed. Obviously, many immature and inexperienced individuals marry. Many remain married, some unhappily so and others happily enough after negotiating a mutually satisfactory relationship. Why then did these particular individuals divorce?

The individuals interviewed saw no possibility for change or improvement in their marital situations. They were caught; both spouses were locked into roles they could not alter by their own effort or with their partner's help. Separation or divorce was the only alternative. Many individuals tried separation with the hope of solving marital discord and obtained a divorce only when no change resulted. But what process froze these individuals into unrewarding roles?

IDENTIFYING FIVE PATTERNS OF NEGOTIATION IN THE TROUBLED MARRIAGE

Marriage requires a number of adjustments for both partners. Each must adapt his or her predominantly self orientation to one of mutuality without compromising his or her individuality. Dissatisfaction or conflict is inevitable, and the decision making process can be a major source of such dissatisfaction and conflict.

Individuals who differ on an issue must come to a mutual understanding if required to pursue a joint course of action or if the behavior of one impinges on the other. Both situations occur frequently in marriage as the individuals reach mutual understandings through negotiation. Negotiations may be directed toward changing the beliefs of one individual so that differences no longer exist, or they may focus on establishing some workable compromise that requires neither party to alter his or her beliefs. The ways in which couples interact to negotiate change and resolve conflict influence their ability to find mutually satisfying or tenable solutions to everyday problems and issues. Moreover, a couple's flexibility and experience with negotiation processes influence the effectiveness of their negotiations. Learning to negotiate with one's partner requires practice and considerable thought. Ideally, individuals modify their own behavior and persuade others to change their opinions on the basis of personal goals and an accurate understanding of the situation and the other person's point of view. However, this process may go astray at any point. It is influenced by the individual's and the couple's current and past life situation. The inflexibility of roles experienced by the divorced individuals interviewed arose from patterns of negotiation that reinforced and maintained existing patterns of behavior; these existing patterns in turn interfered with the individuals' ability to develop alternative courses of action. Thus, for them, negotiations tended to be repetitive in nature.

During the interviews, four major patterns of negotiation were identified: (1) I'm not responsible; (2) there's something wrong with you; (3) blackmail; and (4) let's not talk about us. Spouses demonstrated numerous variations of these patterns, but the basic patterns could always be identified. A fifth pattern, unilateral decision making, was also identified. However, this method forestalls negotiation and is qualitatively different from the other four patterns. It is therefore discussed first below.

These negotiation patterns exhibit many of the characteristics of games [1, 2]. Partners involved in negotiations follow predetermined steps or "moves" that serve to establish predictability and repetition. Spouses are often unaware of the patterns of their negotiations and are thus unable to recognize their effect on roles and relationships and to employ other, more effective interaction patterns. Negotiations reflect the serious attempts of spouses to alter situations that have caused problems. But the element of control inherent in many negotiations often rules out novel approaches and makes roles static.

The individuals interviewed tended to use more than one negotiation pattern and to be unaware of the relation between their own and their spouses' patterns. The behavioral response of one spouse to the other's negotiation tends to reinforce use of a particularly effective pattern. Divorced individuals frequently are able to identify an ex-spouse's particularly frustrating patterns of negotiation while remaining unaware of their own use of these same patterns.

Unilateral Decision Making

Unilateral decision making precludes negotiation between partners because decisions are made by one party alone. When these decisions involve spheres that affect both partners, conflict often results.

The individuals interviewed often referred to unilateral decisions involving violation of a prior agreement. The agreements were not renegotiated; instead, one partner decided not to abide by the previous understanding and chose not to consult the other partner about the decision. One woman explained:

He wouldn't pay the bills and debts that he owed. He just wouldn't pay them. There were bill collectors coming by, the electricity turned off, and letters about the debts. We talked about it and agreed that I should take care of the bills since it wasn't working out with him doing it. So I'd write letters to the companies saying we would pay, and started paying bills as we could, a bit at a time — we were so far in debt. After awhile he'd start questioning what I was doing and start a fight. He'd agreed I should pay the bills, but he couldn't stick to it, and he'd take over again. We'd be back where we started. The same thing all over again.

This woman reacted to this unilateral pattern with resignation, a frequent response. Spouses generally were unable to cope effectively with this pattern, a result in part perhaps of their insufficient attention to the structural assumptions of negotiation: one spouse may choose to ignore the ground rules of negotiation when it suits his or her purposes; decisions that are binding for one partner may or may not bind the other. One partner's behavior may reflect a clear effort to gain control of the relationship, and the other partner's efforts to equalize control are in these cases resisted.

A less direct approach at gaining control involves making unilateral decisions and then concealing them by acts of deceit or intentional omission. The husband of the woman quoted above used this tactic. Her own use of the same tactic may partially explain her compliance with her husband's behavior. She further stated:

I just hated to come home to an empty house all the time. So I started to go out for a drink or dinner with people at work. He didn't like that at all and told me not to. I didn't for awhile, but then started to again. It was lonely and depressing being alone all evening when he was working. One night I came home about ten, and he'd come home early. I hadn't expected him. He was angry, started a fight.

This couple experienced so much conflict that they were at times unable to make relatively simple decisions. The woman described their solution to these impasses:

We fought — that's what happened! Sometimes we wouldn't do anything [for recreation] because of the fighting. It was impossible. I'd say, "Take me home," or he'd say, "I'm leaving." Sometimes we could decide, though. What would happen then was we'd get into some abstract argument that we could never resolve. Then we could decide what we wanted to do because it was so much simpler than the abstract argument. It was easy to decide then, but we still argued.

The use of unilateral decision making patterns contributed to this couple's inability to resolve differences. Yet this pattern may be the only method by which couples who cannot negotiate with one another can make decisions. Thus unilateral decision making may both contribute to and circumvent a couple's negotiation difficulties.

In some instances, couples use what appear to be unilateral decisions to prevent conflict or conserve energy. These decisions generally create no difficulties and are clearly distinguishable from the above pattern by the negotiation or tacit permission that precedes them. Women make unilateral decisions about routine household matters such as grocery shopping and meal planning without consulting their husbands. Sometimes spouses even request that their partners make such decisions when they have no preference concerning an action.

"I'm Not Responsible" Negotiations

With this pattern, one partner, at the explicit or implicit request of the other, assumes responsibility for decisions and actions or the consequences of these decisions and actions. One man's comment is illustrative:

. . . when she said it, you know, she decided we should have a divorce, I said, "That's fine." I didn't put up a fight or anything. You know, I was rather relieved if anything. You know, it was as if somebody else had taken that decision out of my hand.

This negotiation pattern is effective when the partner who is stronger at a certain moment assumes the abdicated responsibilities of the weaker partner, but if this pattern continues, the spouses become locked into roles from which there is no escape. The partner who has continually been defined as unable, irresponsible, or inadequate both acts and is treated accordingly.

One couple had agreed that both partners would work while attending school, but the husband was not doing well academically. The woman explained the failure of her attempts to change the situation:

Well, I think the things I did just made the situation worse, because I tried all different kinds of things to motivate him to try to find out what was wrong, why he wasn't motivated, why he wouldn't do things. We talked about it, and we decided what we would do to help him. This was kind of a mutual kind of thing. We decided that he would just go to school and he wouldn't try to do as much, you know, working and going to school. Maybe the extra pressure was making it too hard for him to concentrate on studying. So that's when I picked up the two extra part-time jobs so that he wouldn't have to work at all.

If one partner is thus judged unable, the partnership is no longer equal; yet the less able individual may control the relationship by delimiting its nature. The man referred to above demonstrated more irresponsibility as a means of gaining control. The woman continued:

Well, after about two and a half months, I found out that he wasn't going to classes and like he was home all day long and told me that he had evening classes, that he had independent study type classes where he didn't have to go to class. Well, when the grade reports would come, he'd be home to get the mail, and I wouldn't even know that he was getting incompletes and warnings and all this other kind of stuff. So then when that happened, I got extremely upset. I suggested maybe he would like to work. [Laugh] Well, he didn't like that idea too much, but then he got a part-time job. Then he started calling in sick and wouldn't go into work. I still, of course, did not drop my jobs. I told him that I had dropped one of them, but I wasn't feeling secure enough really to do it.

Both the husband and wife in this situation maintained some control by employing unilateral decision making and deception. As long as the wife continued to work, she indirectly supported the husband's lack of responsibility and the pattern attendant on it. This couple and others often employed several negotiation patterns and changed from one to another with ease.

If repeated frequently, these negotiation processes will have an impact on the individuals as well as on their relationship. These negotiations convey messages about how each person views the other. Each partner's view of self, spouse, and their relationship will be influenced by such messages. The two individuals may eventually become locked into roles they cannot escape. As the established patterns are repeated, the partners are less able to recognize options that might change existing patterns. Furthermore, their relationship becomes tinged with resentment and anger that escalates conflict and dissatisfaction. One man admitted:

I resented those things [assuming full responsibility]; I resented money, handling the money. Basically I think I was put into a role, which I accepted readily, of taking care of her very father-daughter type thing.

Partners assuming an "I'm not responsible" stance minimized their own sense of blame or responsibility for the divorce.

"There's Something Wrong With You" Negotiations
These negotiations convey the very clear message that one spouse believes something is wrong with the other. One partner defines the other as "inadequate," "sick," or "immoral" on the basis of his or her beliefs and actions. Although some spouses were receiving medical care for long-term illnesses, their behavior rather than the illness itself was cited in the definition. Some definitions incorporated value judgments apparent in the demeaning tone or terms in which the partner was described. In these cases, the interactions reported were consistent with this definition. Other individuals did not appear to attach value judgments to their definitions.

Sometimes both partners clearly believe something is wrong with the other and that his or her position is correct. Neither can place himself or herself in the other's position in an effort to gain a greater understanding of the opposite point of view, an action that might permit resolution and greater role flexibility. One woman remarked:

We fought all the time because he thought that we should both work but I should do all the housework and take care of all the bills and all of the home responsibilities should be mine. And we fought bitterly over that, because I thought that was really ridiculous. I think he thought I should be an asset to him . . . go to parties and be what he wanted me to be. It didn't matter what I thought, you know, and I resented that, terribly, because I didn't feel as though he thought he should give me any consideration. He started drinking a lot. At the time, I did not drink at all.

This woman believed that her husband made unreasonable demands of her. Moreover, she felt his excessive drinking seriously impaired any attempts to negotiate a mutually satisfying relationship. Mutual change or adaptation is ruled out when one spouse defines the other as flawed. The partner so defined also has his or her options limited. He or she may resist any attempt to change this definition, and such resistance may take the form of avoidance. Of course, the partner may also accept the definition.

A variation on the "there's something wrong with you" pattern occurs when one spouse is defined as flawed while the other is defined as a helper.

Problems arise when the partner defined as flawed and needing help fails to accept the other's help and definition of the situation. One young woman experienced a change in values and preferred life-style as a result of new experiences. Her clearly and repeatedly stated beliefs conflicted with those of her husband, and he was unable to accept this change. He defined her as sick and himself as a helper. He commented:

I would try to sit down and talk to her about, "What do you want out of life; what do you want to do; what do you want to be?" And all I would hear is "I don't know." Just a big ball of confusion. She said it with such vehemence, like I had transgressed some law, that I decided I'd better cool it. I tried it about three times, I think, three or four times to have a real basic type of conversation, and I was always turned off.

The husband's decision to ignore his wife's position and to define himself as a helper met with resistance and his wife's refusal to communicate. Her response avoided confrontation but offered no hope of clarifying the situation or developing other options.

Blackmail Negotiations

Spouses may control the marital relationship by threatening their partners. These negotiations derive their effectiveness from pain. Fear and guilt are two painful responses common to blackmail. One woman feared physical violence. Another sought to avoid guilt. She explained:

I would have left him a lot sooner, but he kept threatening that he would kill himself.

Threats of this nature separate responsibility and action. One individual acts while the other is assigned responsibility for this behavior.

A variation of blackmail negotiations might be called the "prove you love me" pattern. One man described such negotiations:

When we first got married, she did an awful lot of crying because [she thought] I didn't really love her and so on and so forth. I would always comfort her, and eventually she came around to where she wasn't crying all the time. So I went in the Army; she left me two or three times. I got letters, and she really started to do some running around, although she denied it at the time. And then I would come back, and I would get her back.

The wife in this instance used her husband's love to force the kinds of demonstrations of affection she preferred. She controlled the relationship by tears and threats, and her husband complied to prevent the loss of his wife.

Blackmail involves acting out or threats of acting out anger over interpersonal issues. Acting out relationship issues rather than discussing them holds little promise for resolution. Blackmail is effective, but its effectiveness is limited. Blackmail loses its power if it fails to stimulate pain. It becomes ineffective when the partner being blackmailed no longer cares about the issue involved. His or her initial helpless response to the blackmail negotiations may soon be overcome by the resentment and anger they also provoke. Then the blackmailed partner is no longer willing to be victimized and may openly declare his or her freedom. One man did so in this manner:

The last time she called up she said, "I'm married, but I can't stand the guy, and I want to come out to you." [I said] "There's no reason to, just forget about it." And that's the last time I heard from her.

The strong effect of blackmail makes couples unable to openly discuss their relationship and thus limits their ability to find new ways of relating. Divorce, separation, or emotional isolation may provide the only release from these rigid roles.

"Let's Not Talk About Us" Negotiations

When they were married, the individuals interviewed seldom communicated directly with their spouses about himself or herself or their marital relationship. In some instances, the avoidance of open communication had the implicit support of both partners. In others, avoidance was negotiated by one partner. The purpose of avoiding communication was not always clear. Sometimes it prevented conflict and confrontation. Occasionally it shielded the partners from intimacy. One partner admitted:

Right at the end, when we had finally confessed to each other how rotten the whole thing had been, was about the closest we ever came [to intimacy]. That was the first time we ever admitted to each other that sexually we did not enjoy each other the way we thought we could. That was the first time we even began to admit that maybe we had been at fault. . . . It was the first time . . . that we had been honest with each other, direct.

Lack of communication prevented many partners from identifying relationship problems and sharing responsibility for clarifying matters and finding alternative courses of action.

The individuals interviewed functioned in such closed systems that they supplied neither themselves nor their spouses with new information necessary for change and adjustment. The partners did not give one another direct, clear messages about their feelings, thoughts, and personal preferences. Consequently, each partner was unable to view the marital situation from his or her spouse's perspective in an effort to discover more satisfying negotiations and solutions. One partner remarked:

You know, we never did tell each other where each other was at. We never really had any big fights or anything; it was just kind of an impasse. I think it would have been nicer to fight.

159. Negotiating a Divorce

Some couples considered absence of conflict to be more a source of problems than constant fighting.

In an effort to resolve disagreement while avoiding discussion of their relationship, couples found ways to spend less time together. One woman described such an effort:

I was working then, but I'd also come home and make nice meals and try to keep the house clean and do all these tasks myself. I never asked him to help me, and he never offered, and I never thought that was wrong. I would then go out many evenings to play bridge and generally be furious that he would not understand I needed to be in bed asleep at 11 o'clock. It evolved into my encouraging him to go ahead and play sports on his own. So we'd end up with him not being home a lot and me being home and liking being home alone [Chuckle] and still keeping up this facade of having a good marriage.

Some couples carried this avoidance to the point of playing "keep-away." The reasons the individuals gave for avoiding one another were socially acceptable ones: work, school, and other responsibilities. One man described such a relationship:

So we just never saw each other. One time I was wrapped up in school and then she was. And the last few years, especially, she would be out all night at the library. I would get home at 5 o'clock and throw a TV dinner or something in the oven for myself. She would come in later when I was in bed, and I would get up and go to work while she was still sleeping.

By avoiding one another, the couples could postpone having to confront the realities of their marital situation.

The couples were quite inventive in discovering reasons for not discussing relationship issues. The readiness of the spouses to comply with negotiations closing communication suggests the existence of a family rule forbidding open, direct communication between partners. One man defined his wife's desire to discuss his extramarital involvements as an intrusion of privacy. His wife's acceptance of this explanation obviated communication. If the wife pursued the discussion, she would be accused of prying.

Other couples developed complex patterns to prevent dealing directly with relationship issues. One woman was somewhat aware of the purpose of the patterns established in her marriage. She remarked:

He taught me to be articulate, and then that was a problem. As I became more self-assured and more articulate, I could hold my own and then beat him in a discussion. He didn't like that; he had to be dominant. All the discussions were abstract arguments, but it was really more than that. It was talking about ourselves that was going on. Someone always won and someone lost.

Some partners desired communication but were discouraged from it by their spouse's response. One man said:

She always asked for open lines of communication but was very unwilling to give them. You know, open your mouth and talk. Any of my problems were paranoias and neuroses. I would not, after awhile, say things that I was feeling inside. I didn't trust her [enough] to say the things that were really inside me.

"Let's not talk about us" negotiations were present in the marriage of every divorced individual interviewed. This negotiation pattern appears to be an essential component of the process by which spouses become locked into roles. Open, direct communication provides an opportunity to discover other, more effective negotiation patterns.

The four major negotiation patterns identified during the interviews focused on verbal interaction. With rare exception, those individuals interviewed mentioned only verbal negotiations, probably because they were more aware of verbal than of nonverbal messages. Videotaped marital negotiations might well demonstrate many patterns that are nonverbal in nature.

Positive or mutually rewarding negotiations were omitted from this chapter because they facilitate flexible role definitions. Surprisingly few of these patterns were mentioned by the individuals interviewed. Such negotiations probably were never a focus of attention in the relationship because they were not a source of problems.

No differences were identified in the negotiation patterns of men and women. Numerous examples of each type of negotiation were demonstrated by both sexes. Both sexes also showed considerable variability in patterns used.

NEGOTIATING A DIVORCE

Occasionally spouses had difficulty negotiating a divorce. In these instances, rather dramatic turning points were identified. These turning points, always initiated by one partner, take on greater significance when viewed from the other partner's perspective and the particular marital situation. Were these turning points designed to impel the partners to action? Did one partner use his or her understanding of his or her spouse to devise events that could not be overlooked and would call forth a predictable response? It is not possible to answer these questions about motivation from available data. However, the individuals interviewed cited numerous examples of dramatic and individually meaningful turning points.

A student of ministry had been separated from his wife for a year with no decision to divorce. He described himself during this period:

I think in political and moral [areas] . . . I saw things in terms of black and white.

The turning point he identified is related to this self-definition. He described what had motivated him to seek a divorce:

She called me up one night and said she was pregnant and wanted me to pay for an abortion. Immediately my initial conviction was okay, but then I started thinking what this meant for me. Now the fact was we had been separated for such a time I knew there was no way that it was my own.

He decided to divorce soon after.

One young woman repeatedly emphasized the pleasure she derived during marriage from knowing that she was the most important thing in her ex-husband's life. She saw herself as well understood and loved. She and her spouse had separated, returned to each other, and still had experienced severe conflict. Her turning point had been her husband's attempt to negotiate sanctioned infidelity. She said:

It occurred after we'd been trying to work it [marital discord] out. But it was still all wrong. My husband wanted to go to Denver. He had just finished reading Open Marriage *[4]. He was all excited about it. He suggested one night he wanted to go and live apart and have affairs and try to work it out that way. I was shocked! What an idea! I told him that if he went I was going to get a divorce. I don't think he believed I'd do it. He went to Denver.*

Of course, such negotiations would be unnecessary if partners could openly request a divorce from one another, but then the request itself might be unnecessary.

Couples who repeatedly employ the restrictive negotiation patterns examined in this chapter probably cannot discuss their differences openly and directly. They may in fact have established a family rule that prohibits communication, particularly if it concerns their relationship.

The negotiation patterns identified in this chapter have serious consequences for couples. There is no doubt that the repeated use of the four major negotiation patterns identified in this chapter will lock marital partners into rigid, restrictive roles. Divorce or separation may then offer the only opportunity to escape these roles. Yet the individuals interviewed considered divorce only after extensive efforts to resolve long-standing conflict had failed and the partners were unable to think of new approaches to their marital problems.

These serious consequences might be prevented if individuals become aware of their communication patterns prior to marriage. Preventive measures could include discussion groups focusing on marriage and marital adjustment. A free, open, group-centered atmosphere would facilitate questioning, exploration of negotiation patterns, and "trying on" new responses in role playing situations. This experience would provide a more accurate understanding of personal negotiation patterns and offer an opportunity to refine these skills. Group members would benefit from being exposed to other members' suggestions. The negotiation repertoire of all members might be increased through this exposure. What is learned at the discussion group might be transferred to other relationships encountered in daily life.

REFERENCES

1. Berne, E. *Games People Play: The Psychology of Human Relations.* New York: Grove Press, 1964.
2. Chapman, A.H. *Marital Brinksmanship.* New York: Berkley Publishing, 1974.
3. Glick, P.C., and Norton, A.J. Perspectives on recent upturns in divorce and re-marriage. *Demography* 10:301, 1973.
4. O'Neill, N., and O'Neill, G. *Open Marriage: A New Life Style for Couples.* New York: M. Evans, 1972.

IV. The Expanding Family. Parenthood

marks an important turning point in the marital relationship. Part 4 examines the repercussions of a couple's becoming parents. Chapter 12 reports the fears of women whose childbirth is managed and coordinated by the obstetrician within the hospital setting. Pregnancy obviously constitutes a transitional state in which relationships and self-perceptions are altered markedly. Mothers describe in detail in Chapter 12 their fears for themselves, their babies, and their relationships with significant others. Concerns for their inability to predict or control their emotions or physical responses and for their helplessness in the medical care system generate multiple anxieties and fears. Feelings of helplessness and vulnerability prevail. Women who recall their hospital deliveries remember most vividly their being treated as an object rather than as a participant in the birth.

Chapter 13 presents a very different picture of the same period of time in the lives of expectant parents who chose home delivery. In these cases, the parents controlled the childbirth while the physician merely assisted in the process. Parents who chose home delivery sought to avoid the hospital setting. Peer group support strongly influenced these parents' decision. The decision elicited problems with future grandparents that required negotiations similar to those described by couples planning a wedding. The grandparents generally opposed the decision to have a home delivery. The couples' descriptions of childbirth at home are characterized by their being in control and being relaxed. According to the couples, the shared experience brought them closer together.

Chapters 14 and 15 focus in a more general way on the development of parental roles, contrasting parents who make parenting a profession (Chap. 14) with professionals who become parents (mothers) (Chap. 15). The home delivery parents were the subjects for Chapter 14. Transition to parenthood for these parents signals a dramatic change; the mothers leave the world of work in exchange for motherhood as a full-time occupation while the fathers take on additional work to support the family. Fathers even assume additional roles within the family in order to better support the mothering process. A clear division of roles occurs, and the parents become almost totally invested in child rearing.

For professionals who become mothers, the process is somewhat different. Instead of surrendering one role and replacing it with another, they add an additional role and establish the entirely different pattern reported in Chapter 15. These mothers, like those described in Chapter 14, set high standards for themselves in terms of both childbirth itself and subsequent child care, but they are highly dependent upon the support of others to achieve their goals. The lives of mothers who are professionals reflect the heavy managerial demands of their multiple roles and the high expectations they set for themselves and for others.

165

Entrance into parenthood may be equated with promotion into a supervisory position in the occupational realm. Parents are the overseers of the development of their children. Movement into such a role constitutes a major transition in which the predominant themes become management and control.

12. Fears During Pregnancy. Dale S. Cohen

Unexpectedly I became pregnant for the first time after having
had an intrauterine device properly in place for almost a year. I noticed I was
becoming emotionally labile, and gradually the reality of my pregnancy registered. I also noticed I was becoming very sensitive not only to others and to
the external environment in general but also to my inner thoughts, feelings,
and physical changes. I became mother- and baby-oriented in my thinking,
probably out of initial curiosity blended with a spirit of adventure rather
than out of pride and love. Being a rather introspective person, I questioned
my attitudes, fears, thoughts, and general emotions constantly. From this
state of affairs evolved the study problem for my thesis research, that is,
what constitutes the emotional experience of becoming a mother for the
first time. This chapter focuses on fears of pregnancy which were one aspect
of my more general thesis research on becoming a mother.

With the exception of one woman who had experienced a spontaneous
abortion, the data reported in this chapter were obtained from nine women
who were pregnant for the first time. Each of the women was interviewed
intensively four separate times, once during each trimester of pregnancy and
once three to four weeks after giving birth. The interviews were conducted
in the women's homes, where they would be most comfortable and least
threatened. When the content of the interviews was analyzed, fear surfaced
as a major issue.

Fear is an emotional expression of a perceived threat posed by a specific
object or definable source [1]. When such fear becomes anxiety the perceived
threat "engulfs the whole personality so that the person feels his very existence is endangered" [1, p. 324]. The anxieties of pregnant women, which
increase progressively throughout pregnancy, are most often expressed as fear
[10]. Three categories of fears during pregnancy have been identified: (1)

fears concerning self, (2) fears concerning the baby, and (3) fears concerning significant others such as mother, father, and husband.

During pregnancy, women experience the gamut of emotional changes, crying and feeling depressed and irritable one minute, then laughing and feeling perfectly fine and happy a few minutes later. This rapid fluctuation of emotions itself can be frightening and confusing. It is not uncommon to hear women express the fear that they are losing their minds. No one knows for sure why pregnant women experience such emotional changes, but hormonal, metabolic, situational, and psychogenic reasons have been cited.

The emotional changes of pregnancy are also characterized by introversion, passivity, and primary narcissism [2]. Shields [10] has argued that this turning inward or preoccupation with self is necessary to accomplish four psychological tasks of pregnancy: (1) accepting the actual fact of pregnancy, (2) believing in the existence of the child, (3) visualizing the child, and (4) preparing to mother the child. Shields believes that if a woman can accomplish these tasks during pregnancy, she will be able to love, nurture, and care for her baby successfully. Some women fear that they will be unable to love their babies; these fears may or may not be conscious. Other women fear the responsibility of taking care of a child because they feel inadequate and insecure [8]. Some women fear the role changes that their pregnant state supposedly prepares them to assume. They fear changes in their relationships with their husband, family, and friends. Concerns about such changes in lifestyle may be very real, particularly if they involve finances, living conditions, employment, or freedom to come and go at will. For example, if the husband is out of work, or the woman's highly valued career must be ended or temporarily shelved, or the woman feels that she will be burdened with the baby and with subsequent additional work and responsibilities, the woman may develop phobias and fears to rationalize her negative feelings about the pregnancy. As Rubin [9] points out, resistance to the idea of pregnancy "right now," to the idea that "someday" is suddenly the present, may be expressed somatically in fatigue, nausea, foul tastes in the mouth, or general discomfort in the first months of pregnancy. Moreover, if the pregnant woman came from an unhappy, unloving, disturbed family life, she may fear repeating her own mother's poor example of motherhood. She may fear the kind of relationship she will develop with her child. Furthermore, she may fear that the child will be an intruder or rival, as her own siblings were [7]. Obviously, for any woman, the fears related to the emotional experience of pregnancy are many and varied.

The biological changes that take place during pregnancy are not only physically uncomfortable and even painful at times, but may also threaten a woman's self-image, particularly if she values physical attractiveness highly [3]. She may accept that the backaches, swollen feet, and leg cramping will end but still fear her figure will be lost forever. She may fear losing her physical attractiveness to her husband, particularly if the couple experiences the changes in sexual frequency or performance that are very common during pregnancy [2]. These changes, added to the woman's confusing mood swings and increased need for love and affection, may strain the marital relationship. The woman may fear the consequences of such stress and wonder whether it will persist after the child is born.

Personality changes are a particularly interesting characteristic of pregnancy. Caplan [2] discusses such changes in Freudian terminology. He states that changes in equilibrium between ego and id and a general weakening of defenses cause unresolved or poorly resolved conflicts and all kinds of fantasies, needs, and wishes to surface to the conscious level during pregnancy. The term *id* refers to the unconscious part of a person's personality that is concerned with basic, instinctual drives such as warmth, hunger, love, and sex. The id is pleasure-oriented. The term *ego* refers to the "I" part of a person's personality. It is concerned with the activities of the conscious mind such as integration, coherent thinking, reasoning, and reality testing. Under usual circumstances, the ego represses the primitive, instinctual needs and aggressive desires of the id. However, during pregnancy, the ego allows the id to surface more often. Because their defense mechanisms are thus relaxed, pregnant women talk more freely than they usually would about problems that were poorly resolved in the past, such as conflicts concerning their mother and siblings and their sexual development. Most often such anxiety-laden, unresolved conflicts are expressed in terms of fears. Furthermore, the increase in dream activity characteristic of pregnancy provides a ready medium for expression of these unresolved conflicts.

A pregnant woman also has fears for the child. Kanner [6] identifies three such fears. The first fear concerns losing the baby. Such a fear may result from previous spontaneous abortions, miscarriages, or stillbirths or from complications attendant on the current pregnancy. The second fear involves heredity, and the third cross-cultural phenomena or superstitions that supposedly mark the baby's fate or physical being in some way. Caplin identifies another fear, that of giving birth to a monster or deformed baby, which he believes is "linked with old guilts about masturbation, or with death wishes or other primitive emotions toward the mother or siblings" [2, p. 46]. Caplan explains that the woman rationalizes deformity, suffering, or death as punishment for past wrongdoings or at least for what she considered to have been bad thoughts or behavior. Still another fear concerns damaging a child by being unable to care for it physically and emotionally. Finally, an expectant mother may fear for her child if she has had difficulties throughout her life accepting her sexuality and feminine role and has demonstrated somewhat distorted or immature psychosexual development [8]. A woman who has had difficulties accepting her female sexuality, and thus has chosen to assume a somewhat masculine role reflected in her choice of career, for instance, may feel threatened or frightened by pregnancy, childbirth, and child rearing.

A pregnant woman's fears extend even to the significant others in her life. Deutsch [5] details how a woman's pregnancy reactivates many childhood memories and guilt feelings concerning her mother and father, particularly her desire for increased closeness to her mother. Deutsch says of a woman's relationship with her mother: "It can even be said that this relation is at the center of the psychologic problems of pregnancy and of the whole reproductive function. In many women the degree of their freedom from psychologic dependence upon their own mothers decides the fate of their motherhood" [p. 149]. She further states that the course of a woman's pregnancy is related in every instance to the fate of her identification with her mother: "The ego of the pregnant woman must find a harmonious compromise between her deeply unconscious identification with the child, which is directed toward the future, and her identification with her own mother, which is directed toward the past. Wherever one of these identifications is rejected, difficulties arise" [p. 154]. Often a pregnant woman's fears regarding her husband relate to conflicts that once involved her mother or father. The woman's husband-related fears may reflect her uncertainty about her husband's truly wanting a child and being able to adjust to the changes parenthood will bring [9]. The woman may even fear harm coming to her husband as she fears harm coming to herself and/or the child [4].

The data presented in this chapter illustrate the fears women who were expecting their first child felt during each trimester of pregnancy, during hospitalization for childbirth, and during the postpartum period. At each point in time these women's fears concerned self, the child, and significant others.

THE FIRST TRIMESTER

At the beginning of the first trimester the women sought to clarify the origin of strange symptoms, to be definitely diagnosed pregnant rather than ill from other causes. One woman commented:

What I thought was an ulcer had been heartburn, but I had that since last Christmas and just put off going to a doctor, and it got gradually worse. Well, I missed my period, but I was so worried that something was wrong I was most worried about my heart. That's why I originally went to the doctor. It runs in my family, a heart condition does, and I had the pains in my chest.

Another woman stated:

Until I actually found out I was pregnant, I was a nervous wreck! Because if I was, I'd have to stop a lot of things I was doing, but not knowing whether you are or not ... I didn't know ... I waited a week and a half; I was late. I had hot flashes; I was nauseated in the morning; I just didn't feel right. I felt different. I thought I had the flu.

On the other hand, women who did not experience some of the common early symptoms of pregnancy doubted the diagnosis. For example, one woman said:

I am more anxious this week. I was thinking that I would like to have symptoms to make me realize that I am pregnant, 'cause I have none.

170. The Expanding Family

All the women interviewed agreed that knowing they were definitely pregnant helped to abate their fears and that having some symptoms of pregnancy helped them verify their condition in their own minds.

Fears concerning self during this trimester ranged from the concrete to the abstract. One woman was afraid to ride with a friend who drove recklessly. One questioned the adequacy of her rubella titer and expressed her fear of being strapped on a delivery table. One felt she was embarking on a strange, mysterious, lonely voyage, described in terms of a dream:

I usually don't dream but the other night I did. . . . I was going to Europe. . . . I was alone.

One woman feared having an abnormal pregnancy, having once been told by a doctor that she had small pelvic measurements. She dreamed one night that the doctor performed a cesarean section on her in a gravel driveway. (This woman did have a cesarean section after a very long, difficult labor.) Only two women verbalized a concern for gaining too much weight during this trimester. One was worried because she had grown so large so soon that she had had to wear maternity clothes in her second month. Another's husband told her that she had "lost [her] radiance;" this woman became acutely aware of her fear of becoming physically unattractive. Another woman remarked that now that she was pregnant it was very important to her "to always look nice." Only one described present and anticipated financial problems, and only one discussed in detail the changes in life-style and goals created by her unplanned pregnancy.

Three women expressed concerns about fluctuating emotions. These women were aware of an "inconsistent feeling." One woman mentioned being irritable and mean for no reason. Another commented on her recent increase in crying:

I would sit down when [my husband] would leave for school and start crying . . . and I'd sit there and say to myself, "What's the matter with you? There's absolutely nothing wrong." . . . and I'd just sit there and cry.

Other women learned about changes in their emotional behavior from their husbands.

At this time only two women expressed fears associated with natural childbirth, but three expressed fears about not being a good mother. One woman in particular was very concerned about her mothering ability because her parents had divorced when she was a young child. She had lived with her father, who had custody of her sibling and her and was employed by the Army. This woman had seen her mother only four times after the divorce. She stated:

I do worry about it, especially being pregnant. . . . I was thinking about the mother instinct. Would I be handicapped because I wasn't close to my mother, whereas I might have known better if I'd had a mother.

Fears for the child during this trimester focused on either losing it or giving birth to an abnormal or unhealthy infant. In different ways, the majority of the women expressed clear concern about losing the child. One woman was hesitant to talk or think about or in any way get ve.y involved with her pregnancy because she feared that she might miscarry before the fourth month. Two women expressed their fear in dreams. One related:

I dreamed one night about the baby, that it was here sleeping in the crib next to me, and then I looked and was shocked that I didn't find the baby there.

The other woman, an obstetrical nurse, had recently had a spontaneous abortion. When she began having problems during this pregnancy, she dreamed about what had happened the first time, reliving a very unhappy, painful experience. So great were her fears of losing this baby or producing an abnormal one that she dreamed about how dead fetuses were disposed of in the hospital and of very sick, deformed babies. Most of the women interviewed were quite verbal about their conscious, admitted fear of losing the child. A few stated that they had abstained from sexual relations because both they and their husbands were "afraid something would happen."

Three women spoke about fears of bearing an unhealthy, abnormal child. One woman asked:

Is every woman worried that her baby will be all right?

Another stated that she needed to hear her doctor tell her everything was normal and growing properly. One woman bluntly asked the interviewer, who was pregnant at the time:

Do you ever think your baby is dead when you can't feel it moving?

Fears concerning significant others were also present in the first trimester. One woman was concerned about her father's heart condition and deteriorating health. She discussed her parents' high expectations and their requirement that she be the best in everything while she was growing up. In light of the preceding discussion about fears as expressions of unresolved or poorly resolved conflicts, it is interesting that such matters should be on her mind. Another woman was worried about her mother, who had had a lump in her breast for some time and was getting increasingly tired (her mother died shortly before she delivered). The women's fears concerning their husbands centered on being physically unattractive or having diminished sexual activity.

THE SECOND TRIMESTER

My data demonstrated a progressive increase in anxieties and fears during this trimester. Fears concerning self were again varied. Four women felt physically threatened by recent illnesses such as sore throats, coughs, and swollen glands; by discomforts common in pregnancy such as backaches or shortness of breath; or by fears from accidents such as tripping down stairs or falling from a chair. Five women were concerned about what would happen and how they would react during labor and delivery. These fears focused on the duration, painfulness, and complications of childbirth. Others questioned where they would be when they went into labor, how they would get to the hospital, and whether they would be able to reach their husbands and their physician. One woman was extraordinarily frightened of having a caudal block and probably just as frightened to discuss this fear with her doctor. A caudal block represented to her the possibility of paralysis or death. She explained her fear:

I was afraid to go in and tell him I didn't want to have a caudal. . . . I was just panic-stricken . . . it seems when I first learned I was pregnant . . . I went to a funeral of a lady who just had a baby . . . she had a blood clot; she died . . . everybody was blaming it on [the fact that] she had that caudal.

These fears were part of a general fear of the unknown, to which all the women attested. To lessen these fears, the women either began reading books as soon as they knew they were pregnant, read pamphlets their doctors provided, signed up for infant care or Lamaze classes, or presented lists of questions to their doctors, the doctors' staffs, or knowledgeable contemporaries. They generally followed their doctor's advice not to listen to other people. Well-meaning relatives did more to frighten than console. Learning the results of routine tests and examinations was very important to one rather anxious young woman. Another woman's anxieties and fears increased after she heard the moans and viewed the discomfort of a woman going into labor in her doctor's office.

Three women experienced some bizarre and frightening emotional behavior that could be characterized by supersensitivity, overreaction, irritability, and hysterical crying. Perhaps the most frightening aspect of the various incidents was the extent to which the behavior was atypical of each woman's disposition prior to pregnancy. One woman who described herself as a very cool, calm person acted out of character when she was caught in a traffic jam, late for a hairdresser's appointment, and almost late for a dinner engagement. She described her reaction:

All of a sudden I could feel myself, you know, explode. . . . I started bawling, absolutely hysterical . . . I have never in my life fallen so completely apart. . . .

Another common fear expressed at this time concerned being a good mother. Respondents questioned whether they would be good mothers, whether they would know what to do in an emergency, or whether they would make the right decisions. One woman stated:

I'm hoping that I can live up to the way I want to be as a mother.

Another woman, more pragmatic and less idealistic in her thinking, stated:

Now I'm starting to get used to the idea that there's going to be a baby when this pregnancy ends . . . a baby, you have to take it with you all the time and take care of it. . . . a baby is a big responsibility . . . you really have to watch it or it'll choke on its blanket or choke on a toy. . . . hope I do the right thing.

Every woman searched her mind and heart and scrutinized the behavior of those around her, past and present, for the right blend of "ideal mother" ingredients to take with her as she embarked on her journey into motherhood.

Becoming physically unattractive or "not looking sexy" bothered a few women. One said she felt like she was "carrying a baby elephant." Another said:

I'm getting sensitive about my body. . . . one day he [husband] called me a beached whale. . . . I felt really bad . . . my breasts are getting all streaked and purple.

Another woman was very concerned about getting stretch marks.

Other fears included the possible dire consequences of not showing by the fifth month; time passing too quickly; being alone, particularly at the time of delivery; and changes in daily life patterns such as not being able to sleep late or stay up late after the birth.

Fears for the baby during the second trimester focused on six concerns: (1) hearing the heartbeat (audibility verified the existence of a live, growing baby); (2) having an abnormal or deformed child even if it was carried to term; (3) delivering prematurely; (4) hurting the baby in some way, e.g., by not eating right, by falling out of bed, or by sexual intercourse; (5) having an "unhealthy" child; and (6) choosing a name that would not be "a subject of harrassment" in the future.

The women's fears concerning significant others involved relationships with childless friends who freely expressed their dislike for children; the health of elderly, chronically ill grandparents; the desire to talk more with their mothers; and the health of ill parents. But the most common fear concerned the husband — his safety, his whereabouts when labor began, his feelings about the baby, his feelings toward the woman, and the marital relationship in general. One woman described her feelings when her husband didn't get as excited as she thought he should upon feeling the baby move for the first time:

I think it was Father's Day . . . the baby had been moving around a lot . . . I told my husband, "Touch it; it's really moving around." . . . he could feel it and that was it; he wasn't as enthused like you see on Dick Van Dyke. . . . he just didn't do the right thing. . . . I was all upset . . . it just ruined the whole day. . . . I told him he didn't love me. . . .

Another woman felt very protective of her husband at this time in her pregnancy. She described her concern for his safety:

I worry more about him lately . . . like if he's not home on time I'll worry, "Gee, what's happened." . . . I want to be with him all the time . . . watch over him.

Still another woman had couple-oriented worries and concerns. She stated:

We went through that "OK let's be honest with each other" thing . . . we suddenly admitted to each other that it wasn't going to be all sunshine and roses . . . the responsibility, the time it would take, maybe the change in our relationship . . . change in life-style. . . . we're going to love the baby, take good care of it, but we don't want our own social life or personal lives to deteriorate.

One woman with a history of marital problems, who had obtained professional counseling in the past, was concerned as much about the course of her marital relationship as about health of the child. Although each woman expressed herself differently, each seemed to say that she needed the love, emotional support, and togetherness her spouse might provide in order to deal with the transition into parenthood.

THE THIRD TRIMESTER

Anxieties about labor and delivery mounted during the third trimester and dominated the women's concerns about self.

One woman described a need to protect herself for fear of being physically hurt. She disliked and avoided crowds or anyplace where she might feel "cornered." She preferred the safety of her home. Another felt threatened by physical difficulties such as swelling, stretch marks, and umbilical bruising. Only one feared gaining too much weight and "being fat." But the greatest focus of fear was labor and delivery. The women wondered what they would experience, fearing loss of control, pain, complications, and even death. Three women feared dying during childbirth. Seven of the nine women were Lamaze-trained. They feared not practicing their breathing techniques enough or losing control. The woman who was an obstetrical nurse was quite concerned about her ability to "perform" well since she now would be a patient in labor among those with whom she had worked and where her reputation as a Lamaze advocate was known. Another woman was concerned about her husband's response to her coping or attempting to cope with pain. A few women were concerned about their ability to work with their husbands as a Lamaze team. Three were concerned about their doctors not being available.

The woman who earlier had expressed fears about receiving a caudal block now expressed fears about an episiotomy, infection, hemorrhage, or tearing; she feared medicines, intramuscular injections, incisions, surgery, and being a patient in a hospital in general. Interestingly enough, this woman was one semester short of completing a diploma program in nursing before she dropped the program. She also had worked in a hospital as a student assistant and as a nurse's aide. She stated:

Now I'm not as worried about labor as I am about delivery and the episiotomy because I just don't care for doctors, medicine, incisions, and surgery and the whole thing. Even though I've been associated with it, I just don't believe in it. I think that they're just human people . . . they're just not infallible. . . . I just don't foresee labor as being that bothersome except when transition comes. . . . I don't know if it'll be the fact that the contractions are harder or that I'll know delivery is coming very soon and that will scare me. . . . I'm afraid of the episiotomy . . . maybe I'll get an infection . . . or maybe something else will happen or maybe it will hemorrhage or maybe it will tear. . . . I think when the time comes for me to be in a hospital that's what is really scaring me 'cause I don't have faith in the hospitals, doctors, or nurses.

This woman's fears, general anxieties, and attitudes may have affected her long, difficult labor, which ended in a cesarean section. She also had some difficulties with the staff during her hospitalization.

Most of the women were anxious to "get everything finished." One woman stated:

I live for this baby to come.

Yet another woman was concerned about the child coming early, before she was "ready." As childbirth neared, the women's fears were very practical in nature. For example, the women wondered: Where will I be when my bag of waters breaks? Where will my husband be? Will my doctor be there? Will I know when it is true labor? Will I get to the hospital in time? Will being nervous make matters worse in labor and delivery?

Emotional changes continued to be a problem for a few women during these last months. These women wondered how upset they could become before it affected the child. One described "blowing her stack" when she usually would not do that, crying for no reason, going to emotional extremes, or being unable to tolerate her husband's joking as she had in the past. Another woman, who felt very vulnerable and sensitive at this time, had a particularly upsetting disagreement with her landlord that left her crying hysterically, emotionally drained, and frightened for her child's welfare. To make matters worse, this same woman's mother died of breast cancer at the very end of her pregnancy. Many old and new anxieties, problems, and fears overwhelmed her. She had gotten to the point of abusing alcohol and stating that she no longer wanted the baby. Fortunately, as a result of professional intervention, she was able to proceed successfully with her pregnancy, labor, delivery, and early months of mothering at home.

The women who had experienced financial problems earlier became even more fearful of them later in the pregnancy, especially when the unexpected happened. One woman's car broke down at approximately the same time the

hospital demanded a substantial deposit. Another who had recently moved into a large new home wondered if she and her husband could afford it.

The fears the women expressed for the child were similar to those described
in the second trimester except for a few variations. Some women were concerned about harming the baby in some way either by becoming emotionally
upset or overly sensitive too frequently in the last months of pregnancy or by
being poked or punched in the abdomen by a playful husband or child. Four
of the nine women were nurses and were concerned that something was wrong
with the child when they felt no movement or kicking. One woman, a nurse
who worked with crippled children, had heightened fears of having an abnormal, deformed child. Another woman had a nephew with Down's syndrome
and stage 1 heart failure. Still another was a special education teacher who
worked with children who had emotional and social problems. In general,
fears for an unhealthy, abnormal baby were most prevalent at this time. One
woman went so far as to question whether the baby would cry spontaneously
and whether forceps would have to be used.

Fears concerning significant others during this last trimester focused largely
on the husband. They ranged from whether the husband could be reached
when labor began, to whether the husband and wife would work together well
as a Lamaze team, to the husband's feelings about the woman's "performance,"
to concern about the husband's maintaining and doing well at his job. One
woman was beginning to feel useless, as if she was a burden on her husband
since she had stopped working. She felt badly about his doing more work at
home and her costing him more money. She feared how the role changes were
going to affect their marital relationship and life-style. Only one woman expressed fears for someone other than her husband. This woman was concerned
about her grandmother's health. The latter, who was chronically ill with a
heart condition and diabetes, became acutely ill and died during her third trimester. Yet this woman was actually more concerned about her mother's being upset about her grandmother's death than about the grandmother's death
itself or her own labor.

HOSPITALIZATION FOR CHILDBIRTH

The women were interviewed for the final time after they had been home
with their babies for three to four weeks. They expressed few fears associated
with the hospitalization experience as compared to those they had expressed
during pregnancy. Their fears centered on either themselves or the child.

Fears for self focused on three concerns: pain, performance, personal harm
or death. Fear of pain focused on pain associated with contractions, medication, anesthesia, and delivery. The pain surprised and frightened some more
than others. One woman described receiving a caudal block:

*I wish she [the anesthesiologist] would have told me it was going to hurt because
when the hurt came it was completely not what I expected. . . . it was the
worst charley horse kind of pain. . . . I just about jumped off the table. . . . it
was just terrible.*

Many women expressed surprise at the painfulness of labor contractions and how "it just wouldn't let up." One woman while experiencing a significant amount of back pain with labor got increasingly more frightened and anxious as she overheard people talking about cesarean section. She remarked:

I got very frightened. I was really scared. . . . I didn't know what was going on; nobody was telling me anything. . . . I could hear mumbling back and forth. . . . they started talking about sections. . . . I was getting scared 'cause nobody was really saying to me "You're gonna have to have a cesarean section." . . . my back was absolutely killing me. . . . I was frightened . . . really scared.

Two women expressed fear concerning their performance in labor and their loss of control. Performance and control were so important to the obstetrical nurse that she was hesitant to consent to a necessary cesarean section because consent meant that she had given up. Three women expressed a fear that harm would come to them in some way, and four expressed fear about dying. One woman said:

I was just so scared; I can't remember everything; all I mostly remember was screaming and about how scared I was. . . . I was just scared of being put to sleep. . . . I didn't think I was going to wake up; I was sure I wasn't going to wake up.

One woman described to her husband her feelings about the labor and delivery experience:

One night I just sat down and cried on [my husband's shoulder]. . . . I had been thinking about the labor and delivery experience. . . . it really made me feel so exposed . . . not physically; I said I feel like I've been hurt. . . . I think it was the pain . . . kind of a reaction to the pain. . . . I really feel like I've been hurt . . . I just felt kind of vulnerable. . . . I wanted somebody to soothe me, so to speak.

Fears for the child that were experienced during hospitalization included: (1) a concern for the baby's welfare after a long labor; (2) a concern about not knowing how to care for the baby during the early rooming-in experience; (3) a fear of harm coming to the baby through carelessness by the staff; and (4) fearing that something was physically wrong with the baby after being told the baby could not be breast-fed for a while due to excess mucus.

THE POSTPARTUM PERIOD

When interviewed post partum, the women again expressed fears concerning self. One woman feared that her episiotomy was not healing properly because it was so painful. Other women expressed fears concerning lack of self-confidence about caring for a newborn baby. One woman described her feelings of satisfaction when her pediatrician told her what she had already discovered herself. Those women who were breast-feeding were concerned with the adequacy of their milk supply. Eight of the women were concerned about what kind of mothers they would be. They questioned whether they would be able to understand and meet their babies' needs. Only one described a fear of not being able to handle the child. She questioned the normality of not feeling love for the baby initially. She feared something was wrong with her because she felt so depressed and frustrated. She admitted that one of her greatest fears was having to experience the same upset again when delivering another child.

All the women were generally concerned about their child's welfare, e.g., germs hurting the baby, getting into an accident with the baby in the car, taking the baby outside where it might get sick, and the baby's becoming spoiled. The mother of one baby who required an operation for a cleft lip correction was particularly concerned with the child's health and welfare. A few mothers still questioned the normalcy of their children. They feared "something might go wrong." Five women feared crib death. One woman remarked:

One thing that keeps going through my mind is I guess I have two friends that each had a child that died of crib death, and I know that goes up to two months [sic] and that keeps going through my mind. I don't know if that is natural or because I have had the experiences with it and have heard so much about it. That goes through my head. I haven't been able to deal with that. This is the first time I verbalized it too.

This remark points up the need a new mother may have to express her fears of crib death.

Fears concerning significant others centered on husbands and parents. The sudden death of one woman's mother caused her to fear that something might harm her husband. She dreamed her baby was stolen from her. She feared that something might happen to "take this happiness away from me." Another woman feared her crying baby was disturbing the neighbors and ruining the health of her out-of-town parents who had come to live in her one-bedroom apartment. But the more common fear concerned the women's changing role relationship with their husbands. One woman said:

The first two years of our marriage we never had anyone around us, and it was a little hard to get used to having a crying baby in the next room while you're in another room. We were used to being alone together. So I worried about this . . . I thought what was my husband going to think; here he wants to have his wife with him as a wife, and she has a crying baby, so she goes to the baby. . . . it was a little hard especially the first week and a half. I don't know if he felt any rejection or resentment, but he kind of felt like an outsider because the baby took a lot of attention.

Practically all the women spoke of the changes and stresses created within the home by the child.

179. Fears During Pregnancy

In conclusion, pregnancy is a difficult time both physically and emotionally. It is more than a simple maturational crisis; it is a biologically determined psychological crisis accompanied by heightened anxieties, fears, and emotional loss of equilibrium. Nurses must help pregnant women be as physically and emotionally comfortable as possible. The well-being of the family, and particularly the early mother-child relationship, is at stake. Pregnant women need a non-threatening, comfortable, unhurried environment and the opportunity to discuss fears and concerns. If a nurse is familiar with not only the common fears but also the subtle anxieties, he or she will be in a better position to acknowledge and alleviate a woman's concerns. Women might cope better during pregnancy if they are encouraged to define, express, and better understand their free-floating anxieties. Women need to know that many of their fears are normal and are shared by other pregnant women. They need to know what to expect so that they and their husbands can prepare psychologically. Nurses can be instrumental in helping a troubled woman obtain the professional counseling she may need. Nurses can help pregnant women grow emotionally at this time in their lives. Fears often stem from unresolved or poorly resolved conflicts. Since pregnant women tend to talk freely about such conflicts, nurses may be able to help pregnant women find better solutions than they were able to devise in the past. Nurses must accept the responsibility of helping pregnant women lower their anxiety levels so they can cope with their fears successfully and give birth with as much security, confidence, and maturity as possible.

REFERENCES

1. Peplau, H.E. A working definition of anxiety. In S.F. Burd and M.A. Marshall (Eds.), *Some Clinical Approaches to Psychiatric Nursing*. New York: Macmillan, 1963. Chap. 40.
2. Caplan, G. *Concepts of Mental Health and Consultation, Their Application in Public Health Social Work*. Washington, D.C.: U.S. Government Printing Office, 1959. Chaps. 4, 5.
3. Carty, E. My, you're getting big! *The Canadian Nurse* 66:40, 1970.
4. Colman, A.D. Psychological state during first pregnancy. *American Journal of Orthopsychiatry* 39:788, 1969.
5. Deutsch, H. *The Psychology of Women*. Vol. II. *Motherhood*. New York: Bantam Books, 1973. Chaps. 6, 7.
6. Kanner, L. The mental hygiene of pregnancy and childbirth. In E. Fitzpatrick, N. Eastman, and S. Reeder (Eds.), *Maternity Nursing*. Philadelphia: Lippincott, 1966. Chap. 9.
7. Flapan, M. A paradigm for the analysis of childbearing motivations of married women prior to birth of the first child. *American Journal of Orthopsychiatry* 39:402, 1969.
8. Menninger, W. The emotional factors in pregnancy. *Bulletin of the Menninger Clinic* 7:15, 1943.
9. Rubin, R. Cognitive style in pregnancy. *American Journal of Nursing* 70:502, 1970.
10. Shields, D. Psychology of childbirth. *The Canadian Nurse* 70:24, 1974.

13. Staging a Status Passage:
The Birth Event. Donna M. Dixon and Katherine A. Cavallari

The status passage of birth in many ways parallels that
of marriage as described in Chapter 7. A couple's decision to have a child and
their decision to marry are similar in that both decisions change the direction
of the couple's relationship. Marriage and parenthood both challenge a
couple's ability to assume new roles and to negotiate the guidelines according
to which these roles will develop.

This chapter explores the status passage of birth and the issues surrounding
it. It deals with the process by which a couple decides to deliver a child at
home and the meaning the couple individually and mutually attach to this
form of childbirth. Chapter 14, which follows, then examines how couples
who chose home delivery function as parents.

Childbirth had a special meaning for the couples who were interviewed
for this chapter. Because they chose to deliver their children in their homes
with only the assistance of physicians, they were able to plan for and participate in the birth in the same way that the couples interviewed for Chapter
7 were able to plan for and participate in their wedding ceremonies. The
former couples presided over the birth of their children; they, not their
physicians, delivered their infants.

Thirteen couples were interviewed intensively both jointly and individually
before and after their home deliveries. The first interview took place during
the third trimester of pregnancy and the last interview within two months
after the birth. The couples' names were supplied by two physicians in
practice together in the Chicago metropolitan area who assisted with all
the deliveries.

Ten couples were first-time parents. The other three couples had one or
two other children, most of whom also had been born at home. While
seven of the couples had conceived their first child during the first year of
marriage, five couples had conceived their first child after four to seven
years of marriage.

181

The women ranged in age from 22 to 33 and the men from 24 to 41, with a median age of 27 for both. The educations and occupations of the couples varied widely. All of the women either had worked or were working. Eighteen individuals had attended college, and eight had earned a bachelor's or master's degree. Two of the women were professionals, one a social worker and one a nurse-midwife. Most of the men were white-collar workers.

One-half of the sample, six couples, identified strongly with a religious affiliation. Four other couples were Catholic and defined themselves as having moderate identification. The remaining three couples claimed to practice no religion.

Eleven couples had successful births in their homes. Two were unable to deliver at home as a result of unusually long labors. Even in these cases, however, almost the entire labor took place in the home. All the couples made full use of natural childbirth methods. No medication was administered to the women during labor, and episiotomies were avoided when possible. Moreover, breast feeding was the rule.

The couples attended two types of childbirth classes in preparation for the births. Four couples either attended Lamaze instruction or read Lamaze literature [4]. Eight first-time parents attended classes developed by Margaret Gamper [3]. These classes stress abdominal breathing and exercise and incorporate principles from the Grantly Dick-Read method [2].

The interviews did not focus primarily on the issue of having a child at home or on natural childbirth per se. While open-ended questions were asked that pertained to these issues, the interview guide used also addressed the progress of the pregnancy, the couple's preparation for the child, and their attitudes on parenting. The last interviews concentrated on the experiences of birth and the subsequent adjustments necessary to incorporate the new family member (see Appendix).

Each couple described the birth in detail from the start of the labor contractions through the first day after the delivery. The excitement and joy with which each couple related the experience was immediately apparent. It was further apparent that many of these intense feelings stemmed primarily from one source: each couple felt in control of the entire situation from beginning to end. Having natural childbirth and being aware during the whole process was for the women a part of feeling in control. Participation was an important aspect of control for the men.

Control was a pervasive issue in the lives of the couples. Informed decision making, a means of gaining control, took place throughout the pregnancies. The actual decision to have a home delivery was the foremost factor in the control issue. Other means of gaining greater control followed.

FACTORS THAT INFLUENCED THE DECISION TO DELIVER THE CHILD AT HOME

At some point after a pregnancy is confirmed, couples begin to contemplate the nature of the birth experience. Friends, relatives, and the media supply information about prepared childbirth, breast feeding, and prenatal classes.

The father begins to think about whether he wants to witness the birth. The woman seeks out information from many sources about the physical aspects of pregnancy, delivery, and the postpartum period.

Today prepared childbirth classes and literature are widely available. The concept of family-centered nursing care has infiltrated many hospitals, and rooming-in is becoming more popular. Moreover, husband participation is high, and the return to natural childbirth methods is on the rise.

How then do the couples interviewed differ from other couples experiencing birth for the first time? First we must examine what factors led these thirteen couples to choose to deliver at home. The data indicate four major influences on the decision making process: (1) the couples' commitment to experiencing natural childbirth and breast feeding; (2) their opinions about hospitals and physicians; (3) their finances; and (4) the role of significant others.

The first influence had the most effect on the couples' decision, yet in no case was it the only consideration. Most often, four influences combined motivated a couple to settle on a home birth.

Attitudes on Natural Childbirth and Breast Feeding

Natural childbirth was the goal of each couple interviewed. It was their strong belief in these ideas that motivated the couples to decide on birth at home. One woman's remarks are representative:

I like it [natural childbirth] because I don't like the idea of drugs. I like it because I want to be aware of what's going on. I just like the whole idea of it. I think it's easier on the mother and the baby.

Such attitudes stemmed from three sources: (1) personal background, (2) the attitudes of friends and relatives, and (3) reading and childbirth classes.

Four individuals had been exposed to the concept of natural childbirth while growing up. One couple commented:

She: His mother had all of her children by natural childbirth, and all of them at home, except one.

He: This natural childbirth sort of "runs in the family."

This man admitted that his parents were the most important influence in his decision to have a home delivery.

Three couples displayed a history of contact with a "natural" orientation to life and were in general very health-conscious. One man remarked:

My parents believe in eating naturally. . . . not a lot of refined foods that are so common in the rest of America. They educated me to think naturally. And we had some friends that had natural childbirth. To me, I equated the two.

183. The Birth Event

Another woman said:

You really haven't heard of natural childbirth until just recently, the last few years or so. But with me, I was raised more health-minded, and so it's just kind of an automatic thing with me.

Throughout the interviews this woman and her husband frequently mentioned their ideas on nutrition. They are members of a religious group, the Seventh-Day Adventists, who advocate a more natural way of life.

Other couples' contacts with natural childbirth came from friends and relatives. One woman admitted:

I wanted home delivery only because it seemed like the "in" thing to do, because I knew quite a few people who were doing it.

Books and other literature on the subject of natural childbirth also influenced the couples. In fact, one woman finally decided to deliver naturally at home because she had read a certain book:

Int: Since you have chosen home delivery, can you tell me how you arrived at that decision?

She: I think that I was a big influence . . . because when I first got pregnant I was going to a clinic . . . and I changed my mind after I read a book called The Immaculate Deception *[1]. I read my husband one chapter, and I said, "Look, this is it, regardless."*

Two other women also admitted being greatly influenced by this book, which examines the childbirth process in the United States and strongly recommends home delivery as an alternative to hospitals.

One woman was greatly influenced by another book she read prior to choosing home delivery. She said:

The biggest thing that I'm concerned about, the reason I'm going the home delivery route and so forth is Dr. Leboyer who wrote a book Birth Without Violence *[5], and it really goes into the psychological aspects that the ordeal of birth has on the child, and, to me, it makes a lot of sense.*

This woman explored the possibility of using this childbirth method in a hospital but later changed her mind.

In most cases, the couples were interested in natural childbirth before their reading and such material served mostly to reinforce their inclinations. For example, one man commented:

We've always wanted to have natural childbirth delivery, and we just learned more and more from Gamper classes as to why we should, and it's really reinforced our feelings.

Another woman stated:

*I think that natural childbirth is the only way to go because I read books about
it, how much better it is for the baby and you too.*

Some couples identified each of the three sources cited as having influenced
their decision to deliver their children naturally while others reported that
one of the three sources was particularly salient in determining the decision
to deliver their child at home.

Opinions About Hospitals and Physicians
Just as each of the thirteen couples felt strongly committed to natural childbirth methods, they each expressed negative opinions about hospitals and
doctors in general. Yet only two individuals told of a traumatic personal
experience with the hospital system. The remainder, although they admitted
that they had never been in a hospital as a patient, said they simply did not
like them.
Some of these opinions arose in part from the couples' attitudes about natural childbirth. Eleven couples felt that childbirth is not an illness but is treated
as such by the health care system. For instance, one woman explained:

*I felt having a baby is not a sickness: a hospital is for sick people. It's a natural
thing. . . . The doctor is there to assist and help when the baby comes
out. . . . So I felt I could be at home just as easily, as long as you have the
proper preparation.*

This woman believes that birth need not take place in a hospital. She also
cited another reason for her decision:

*I heard [from various people] how nurses treat the mother, and they're away
from their babies so long. A lot of those people had a child in the hospital,
and they said they wouldn't do it again.*

Eleven other respondents also related negative stories they had heard about
childbirth in a hospital setting.
One woman referred to a birth she had seen on television:

*It's ridiculous what they do in hospitals. They strap your legs and your arms
down, and the baby is born, and they hold it up, and your first impulse
is to reach out and touch it, but you've got these leather straps around your
wrists. . . . A baby doesn't have to be protected from its own mother.*

This woman had to have her child in the hospital due to a breech presentation
and an unusually long labor. When the couple decided to go to the hospital,
she immediately was frightened that she would be strapped down. She was
not, much to her relief. Yet her fear is not unjustified because the practice
is common in hospitals.

185. The Birth Event

In general, the thought of having a child in a hospital elicited fear among the couples interviewed. Seven respondents made comments using the word "fear" or the phrase "don't have control" when answering questions regarding their decision. For example, one man commented:

She [wife] would be more relaxed at home than in a hospital because of the psychological effects on any person who walks into the hospital: Right off the bat he is paranoid; he has fear in him. Because he is walking into this place where there are white rooms, lights, people walk around in white, you know, automatically, well, you think of life and death.

Another man said:

You don't have the control of what's going on in the hospital even though I know they are not out to kill you. Hospitals are fine, but on a general thing about childbirth, I think they're poor concerning the subject.

His wife added:

When you're at home you have the control over the delivery; it's your thing.

Yet these individuals admitted that they personally had never had a bad experience at a hospital.

Of course, the two individuals who had had upsetting experiences in a hospital had an even greater sense of fear and loss of control. One woman explained:

I have a very strong fear of hospitals. My fear of hospitals is stronger than my fear of anything, I think. I really fear to be in a hospital, so I think that had a lot to do with the decision because I hate them so badly. . . . I'd have to be on my deathbed, and then maybe you could get me in there.

This woman's husband also described what for him was a traumatic hospital experience.

Two people directed their negative opinions primarily at the medical profession. In an excited tone, one woman remarked:

Doctors have really inflated themselves into little gods, when actually all they are is a baby-catcher. The baby is going to come out whether there is a doctor there or not. And the doctors try to have too much part in childbirth. That is good for their ego but is very poor on the mother's ego.

Similarly, another man stated:

I think doctors are overrated in our society. Society in general has turned to the medical profession and sort of holds it in very high esteem and feels that

there's some things that cannot be done without the men in white and the
stainless steel hospital equipment around. And we don't feel that way. We
feel that we're made to have babies.

Interestingly, two health care professionals, one a registered nurse and the
other a nurse-midwife, also expressed negative opinions about hospitals.
They said:

R.N.: I don't feel that a hospital is security, you know. In fact, a lot more things
can happen in hospitals due to negligence than at home because you have
control over the situation in your home. Hospitals are notorious for making
mistakes, although I've never had a bad experience with any.

Midwife: I have worked in a lot of different hospitals . . . and I have never seen
one that I would like to go to.

Even the health care professionals readily admit that hospitals as they now
function ignore human needs. Such dehumanization breeds fear and forces
people to seek alternative forms of health care.

Finances
  The fact that the economic pinch resulting from rising medical costs contributed to the couples' decisions to have their children at home was an
interesting discovery. Couples soon found out that it is expensive to have a
child in a hospital. Recent estimates indicate that a couple with a moderate
income will spend $3,000 on a baby from conception to the first birthday.
An obstetrician's fees are estimated at $400 and a hospital bill at $1,800 "for
a four day stay in a semi-private room, as well as fees for the delivery room,
anesthetist, nursery, routine nursing, and medication and so on" [6].
  Couples can save a considerable amount of money by having their babies
at home. The only expense is the doctor's fee during pregnancy and a standard fee for the delivery and postpartum checkups. In all, the total cost
from conception to the first birthday is reduced by approximately a third.
  Financial concerns of the couples interviewed were the result of a number
of factors. In six cases the cost of a hospital delivery was cited as one reason
for deciding on the home delivery. In most of these cases the problem
centered on having no insurance or poor insurance coverage. One of the wives
described some of her husband's concerns thus:

He's also, he probably won't mention it, but he's also worried about the delivery
financially. It seems that I got pregnant just in the middle when B. was
changing jobs, and the insurance and stuff — we're going to have problems
with that. If I have a home delivery, it won't cost as much, you know, but
it's still going to cost money.

Finances also became a problem for some of the couples when the wife had to stop working. The problem was critical when the husbands were students. One of the husbands replied thus when asked:

Int: Well, what have you been thinking about since you found out your wife was pregnant?

He: Financial problems. Wondering whether . . . I know I'm going to have to take out a government loan, wondering when, when that should be done, and also thinking about part-time employment, which I haven't had to encounter up until this time because she's been working.

Many men took on a second job when the pregnancy created financial problems for the couple. For some, the second job created a financial cushion, allowing them to turn their energies to other things.

Seven couples saw the low cost as enhancing their choice to deliver at home but not as a contributing factor to the decision. One couple's remarks were typical:

Int: Is there anything else that influenced your decision to have a home delivery?

He: The price.

She: It's expensive [to have a baby in the hospital]. But I think that was just a benefit that came along with it that really didn't have anything to do with it.

Role of Significant Others

The fourth factor that influenced the couples' home delivery decisions was their degree of contact with others who also had had home deliveries. The role friends and relatives can play was considered briefly in regard to the respondents' attitudes on natural childbirth. Many of the same individuals who had recommended natural childbirth to the couples also had had home deliveries.

While they were in the process of deciding, eleven couples sought out friends or acquaintances who had had a home delivery. One man who attended school full-time knew many classmates who had had home deliveries. He described their influence:

Int: Was there any influence or opinions or advice from your school friends concerning the home delivery?

He: Yes, they were all fed into the hopper, and the decision was made. Some of them had their first in the hospital, and some had their next child as a home delivery, and they, every one of them, said I'll have the home delivery from now on. I mean there was no equivocation there — that was it. So if they were that positive, that reassured me that if I did want a home delivery, it was the right decision. . . . Sure, they did influence me.

One woman did not mention the word "influence," but she indicated that her friends' experiences played an important role in her own decision. She replied:

Int: How did you hear about Dr. F. doing home deliveries?

She: A lot of my friends had him, [including] my one girlfriend. I had just been to a shower, and my one girlfriend already had a baby by him, and the other one was pregnant and was going to him. My father's stepdaughter, she had her first one already by him, and a friend of hers had had two by him; so it kind of led into one another.

Because of her close relationship with her girlfriends, this woman respected their views and took them into account in reaching a final decision.

Eleven couples identified friends as an influence in their decision to have a home delivery. In only one instance did a respondent reach this decision without first discussing it with someone who had actually delivered at home.

While couples sought out friends to support their decision to have a home delivery, they avoided input from their families while in the process of reaching a decision. They anticipated and received a negative reaction when they announced their decision. Coping with these negative reactions added another dimension to the couples' attempt to maintain control of this aspect of their lives.

Four couples coped by not telling their families until after the baby had been born. This couple commented:

Int: What kinds of reactions have you received from family and friends?

He: We haven't told anyone.

She: I'm kind of not looking forward to it. I don't think it will be well received. I plan to tell them as little as possible.

He: We know what the reaction will be like.

This woman did deliver in the hospital; so she never told her family that labor had occurred at home with the doctor in attendance.

The other nine couples stood their ground. After some opposition, their families usually accepted the decision. The following remark is typical:

Our families frequently don't agree with things that we do, so it doesn't make too much difference. They know they wouldn't get anywhere by trying to talk us out of it; so they just finally accepted — well, they accepted it right away because they know that's what we were going to do.

By standing firm in their original decision, this couple maintained control of the situation throughout. By the time they delivered the child, the couples had support from either friends or family, or both, whom they had told about the decision.

Our data indicate that couples spend a great deal of time in making their decision to deliver their children at home. Four factors work together to lead a couple to a final decision. First, the couple is well-informed about natural childbirth. Then the couple's opinions about hospitals and physicians, finances, and contact with similar others are influential. Primarily, it is their strong commitment to and belief in natural childbirth methods that permit them to stand firm against inevitable opposition to unconventional home delivery.

THE BIRTH ITSELF

Anticipation of the birth is high in the last few weeks of pregnancy. Childbirth classes have ended, the baby's room is prepared, and the items needed for the delivery are near at hand. When labor begins, the husband is called home. He begins to time contractions for his wife. When they are regular, the doctor is called. The couples' descriptions of the rest of the process refer always to control and relaxation. One woman's comment is typical:

I was like in control of everything. Well, first of all, I was in my own house, and I didn't have anyone ordering me around, or I could do anything to make myself comfortable. I felt as though I was in command of the situation. I was in my own house, and it was just a good feeling. Everything was right there, anything I wanted, anything I needed.

Implicit in this statement is a negative opinion of hospital procedure. Many couples cited as their reason for feeling in control the fact they were delivering their children in their own homes. One woman's description expresses her concern that childbirth be both a controlled and a relaxed experience:

I was actually in the process of labor. I was absolutely thrilled that I was at home and not at the hospital. It made all the difference in the world. . . . The fact that I had the baby here at the house was a very relaxing thing for me . . . I had the confidence of knowing he [her husband] was there and that the situation was under control. I felt good being in my own home. I didn't have to be afraid of what was coming next and, as far as my surroundings, who was going to be coming in and what was going to happen to me.

The involvement of the husband was an important part of each couple's feeling of control and relaxation.

Natural childbirth was equated with husband participation. All the men took an active part in the labor and delivery process. The husband's most important function was providing support and encouragement to his wife. His presence alone served some very important purposes. The wife was comforted and reassured by the husband's presence during the labor and delivery. One of the women described how helpful it was to have her husband with her during the birth:

You [husband] helped as far as when my labor got to the point where I was pushing. You helped me with my legs. He [husband] helped by holding his hands up so I could push against his hands and that was really a big help. I thought for sure his back would kill him, and it did the next day. But that was helpful. And what I enjoyed was after each contraction when I would push, I'd say, "Did you see anything, was there any change, could you see the head?" And he'd give me a description of everything that was happening. . . . You know it was nice. You were more help than you think.

This woman's husband described his role and feeling of participation thus:

I would try and help her, you know. She was rocking back and forth; I would rock her, things like that. I tried to encourage her, and I imagine I did fairly well, I don't know.

This man and others mentioned that one of their contributions to labor was to coach their wives with breathing techniques. They identified this coaching as a way to help the woman maintain her control of the situation. Not surprisingly, this aspect was more pronounced in those couples with Lamaze training, since this method stresses the importance of breathing techniques.

The partners reported that sharing the birth experience brought them closer together as a couple and as a family. Many men mentioned that they felt especially close to those children in whose births they had participated. One of the men explained:

All you feel is peacefulness and harmony, which I think helps out a lot. It brings you closer and brings a stronger bond between everybody involved.

This early formation of bonds between mother and father and child may positively affect their later relationships.

Many couples described the birth as very exhilarating. One of the men said:

I felt very proud. I mean I felt, you know, like I was the most important person in the world. That was my feeling, you know. He was born at 5:04 (A.M.), and I went outside at 5:06, and I took this snow glosh from behind a tree and I wrote on the window, "It's a boy, 9-5." You know, it was so overjoyous. Fantastic, and ah, I'm ready to have another one. [Laugh] . . . I love children.

One woman's remarks also emphasized the new father's reaction and the importance of his positive reaction. With evident excitement, this woman said:

191. The Birth Event

Just because of the wonder of it, M. had all those feelings and elation. We were
able to get some slides taken at that point, and the look on his face was some-
thing that I'll just never forget. . . . I just could live the whole experience
through him. He was just so thrilled and so excited, and it just showed all
over, and it was just like something I'll treasure for a long time.

All the couples planned to have more children and were fully committed to
delivering all subsequent children at home. All also expressed complete
satisfaction with their management of the birth event. None mentioned any
aspect of the delivery they would have liked to change.

Since all the couples worked with a physician, his role also was discussed.
The physician's role was elusive throughout the pregnancy. He could be
identified as a major source of support or information for the couple. For
instance, one woman noted:

Well, I'm sure he would have given me information, but I didn't ask for it.

The general consensus among the couples was that the physician was available
and willing to help during the pregnancy but that he was not really needed
at this time.

The physician also maintained a low profile during the actual birth. In most
instances, the couple and the doctor were the only ones present at the birth
event. Typically, the doctor stayed in the background, letting the couple
manage the birth as they saw fit. One man who was struck by the doctor's
calm commented:

The funny thing about it was that in between 1:30 (A.M.) and 5:04 (A.M.),
when the baby was born, the doctor left one time; he went somewhere and
he came back, but during the labor itself, he was reading a book out in the
living room. Nonchalantly sitting around.

This man remained with his wife in the bedroom during the entire labor and
was her primary assistant. Another couple, experiencing their second home
delivery, described their physician's low profile thus:

The doctor got here, and he said things were progressing so it would happen
sooner or later, and he had gotten out of bed and everything. He took a
nap, and then about the time the baby's head was crowning, I called him and
he came in.

In a birth that was progressing normally, the physician was not needed until
the end of the second stage of labor. However, the physician took a more
active part in complicated deliveries. The physician spent an enormous
amount of time with one of the women, who had a long labor and eventually
delivered in the hospital. This woman and her husband said:

She: The doctor came at 5:00 (P.M.) Thursday evening.

He: Thursday night he stayed overnight. . . . Thursday night he got up every two hours and checked her, and Friday came. He kept checking her. He stayed all day Friday.

This fluctuating role of the physician was fully consistent with the respondents' views of what his level of participation should be.

THE IMPORTANCE OF LEVELS OF CONTROL

All couples begin the status passage of childbirth at conception. Each couple is united by the fact that in approximately ten months they will also have experienced the birth of their child. Between these two events is a matrix of pathways open to the couple. Once pregnancy is suspected and confirmed, decisions must be made. These decisions involve such things as finding an obstetrician and deciding whether to breast-feed or bottle-feed. Each decision closes some avenues and opens others. By the end of pregnancy, couples can be divided into groups defined by the type of birth experience they desire.

For example, a conscious decision may be made to give birth with the assistance of medication or anesthesia. Couples who make such a decision then must decide what medication they prefer or if they will let the doctor decide for them. Those couples who chose natural childbirth rejected this option.

Decisions are made on the basis of control. That is, each couple defines the degree of control they desire during this status passage. Planning the timing of the pregnancy and choosing a physician may be the extent of control desired by one couple. Another may want to plan the child, select a doctor, and learn breathing techniques to maintain control during labor.

The couples interviewed for this chapter made preliminary decisions that led them to elect home delivery. Early in the pregnancy the decisions of these couples were similar to those of other couples who want natural childbirth and attend childbirth classes. Yet at some choice point these couples decided to have a home delivery for one or more of the four reasons cited. These couples sought a high degree of control by which they could decide where the birth would take place and take charge when labor began.

When the couples achieved the level of control they had defined for themselves, the status passage of birth was an experience to savor and remember. This fact has wide implications for nurses. Every couple who enters a hospital labor room will not require the same interventions. The nurse will need to assess not only the woman's progress in labor but also how much control she and her husband desire. It is left to the nurse to discover the anticipated role of the father during labor, the couple's feelings regarding medication during labor, and the degree to which they have prepared for the event.

The couples interviewed had minimal need for a nurse or a doctor. The couples were well-informed and had prepared themselves extensively to take control at various points in the status passage. After assessing such a couple, and determining that they are well prepared, a nurse may decide she need only monitor the woman's progress while the husband will provide the major support and comfort. By accurately determining the couple's needs, the nurse contributes to the joy that can be experienced in childbirth.

REFERENCES

1. Arms, S. *The Immaculate Deception*. Boston: Houghton Mifflin, 1975.
2. Dick-Read, G. *Childbirth Without Fear* (2nd ed.). New York: Harper & Row, 1959.
3. Gamper, M. *Preparation for the Heir-Minded*. Glenview, Ill.: Midwest Parentcraft Center, 1971. (Pamphlet used in Gamper Childbirth Education Classes.)
4. Lamaze, F. *Painless Childbirth*. New York: Regnery, 1970.
5. Leboyer, F. *Birth Without Violence*. New York: Knopf, 1975.
6. Williams, C. How much does a baby cost? *Redbook*, April 1976. p. 6.

14. Parenthood as a Profession.

Katherine A. Cavallari and Donna M. Dixon

Our study of couples who chose to deliver their children at home indicates that this group was dedicated to traditional child rearing values. The women planned to dedicate themselves full-time to child care; they intended to stay at home and thus postpone or abandon their career plans. The men looked forward to being involved with their children. They expected that their roles in the beginning would be relegated to helping their wives but that as their children grew older they would devote more time and energy to re-sponsibilities ranging from teaching and discipline to play activities. Both parents expected to make heavy investments of time and energy in the care and raising of the child. This highly dedicated group of parents might be con-sidered "professional parents" because parenting was the primary role in their lives. They expected that matters involving their children would have priority over any and all other matters. This chapter explores the nature of these couples' dedication to parenting, examining how they came to be thus committed and how they expected to function as parents in the first few weeks after their children were born.

The attitudes and values of all these couples had developed along similar lines. Three themes emerged during interviews with the couples: (1) the deci-sion to have a child, (2) the various support systems that influenced the cou-ples' ideas about parenting and child rearing, and (3) the level of involvement in and commitment to the new parenting roles.

THE DECISION TO HAVE A CHILD

Control, which played such an important part in the couples' decisions to have a home delivery and in their handling of the actual birth, is integral to the very decision to conceive a child. This decision was made consciously and deliberately by all but two of the couples interviewed. When the pregnancy was first suspected and then confirmed, each of these couples expressed happiness and excitement about the coming event. Most had controlled the decision making process and as a result were happy with the outcome, conception.

The issue of control underlay many of the early decisions made by these couples. When they were able to exercise control, their levels of satisfaction were high, and they experienced little or no ambivalence about their decisions.

In general, these couples conceived their children at two points in their marriages — the first or after the fourth year. Seven couples conceived for the first time in the first year of marriage while the remainder conceived four to five years after marriage. The individuals cited the woman's age as a prime factor in the decision to have a child. One woman remarked:

I don't want to be 65 by the time my children grow up. I'll be 25½ by the time my child is born, which I think is more than late enough.

Another woman said:

Well, when I got married, I expected that I would probably have children. So, you know, I expected to get pregnant. I'm 33 years old, so I thought, well, if we have a child as soon as we're married that will be all right with me.

Another woman, who waited four years to get pregnant, cited age and social pressures as factors influencing the decision to have a child. She stated:

Society forces you to think about it. . . . So I found myself thinking about it. Well, do I want to have one or don't I? I figured I should think about it. . . . Then I figured, I'm 25; why not do it now?

The women linked the decision to conceive to their maternal feelings. One woman, who could not identify these feelings precisely, said:

I met N.; it seemed like he offered all the security I wanted, and somehow or another I got this idea in my head that I wanted a baby. . . . To this day I haven't figured out why I wanted a family. I wanted more than just myself and N.

Another woman explained:

I've always wanted a baby. I've always been around children. I think B. and I are both at our best when we're around kids.

In these cases, the woman's desire to conceive started the decision making process.

The couples who had planned their pregnancies expressed no feelings of ambivalence about them. Most of the couples had married expecting to have children soon thereafter. One woman who had lived with her husband prior to marriage stated that their decision to marry was based on their desire for children:

Well, you know, our relationship was such that we could get married. The relationship hasn't really changed, but we wanted to have a child in a stable relationship. You know, if you're not married either of you can get up and leave at any time. . . . I don't think we would have gotten married if we didn't have any children. I don't think I would get married if I didn't want children, because we can have the same thing without marriage.

This woman had stopped taking birth control pills one month before she got married and had conceived within the first six months of her marriage. This couple married specifically because they had decided they wanted children.

Although the majority of couples decided prior to marrying that they wanted children, two couples did not reach this decision until after marriage. These couples described their decision to have children as evolving gradually, flowing out of discussion and the quality of their relationship. One of the women described this gradual decision process thus:

Let's see, that started happening back in October [wanting a baby]. We were married in September, and by October I decided that would be kind of neat. But I wanted to make sure; so we talked about it until January. We didn't really even have the idea until March. We wanted to leave ourselves enough time. We talked about all kinds of things, our ideas of how to raise children, what to do in this situation. Every conversation was about a child. So we really discussed it a great deal before we had him, and I just all of a sudden felt secure enough and I wanted it . . . I just wanted this child. I wanted to be home and stay home and clean and take care of the baby and my husband.

Like the couples who assumed from the outset that they would have children, those who had reached a decision gradually felt little ambivalence once the decision was made.

The two couples who had not planned the pregnancies evidenced varying amounts of ambivalence. In one instance, the pregnancy was the result of a contraceptive failure. This couple had two other children and were very involved in their church. The ambivalence they expressed was related to the expected curtailment of their activities. This couple stated:

She: I had mixed emotions about it. Our schedules, with the type of work we do and everything, are pretty completely filled, and so the thought of having another baby at first was like, "Oh no, how are we going to do it?"

He: I felt about the same way, a little bit unsure because of the fact that we are very busy and don't have a lot of time. Mostly, being afraid that we wouldn't have enough time for the baby or else we would have to give up some other things, which is difficult to do.

197. Parenthood as a Profession

The deep religious convictions of this couple contributed to the resolution of their ambivalence about the pregnancy. The woman explained:

It's a gift from God, and we can't complain. . . . I've accepted the fact that we're going to have a baby now, and I'm looking forward to it.

Thus their uncertainty was resolved rather quickly.

The second couple's unplanned pregnancy occurred during the transition between two contraceptive methods, within the second month of marriage. This couple's ambivalence centered on their fear that they were neither financially nor emotionally prepared for parenthood. They replied:

Int: How did you feel when you first suspected you were pregnant?

She: Oh, I cried. I was neurotic, psychotic.

He: I was very emotional. I said, "Should we?"

She: He didn't want it.

He: Yeah, I didn't want it 'cause I didn't know what to do.

She: I think that's the biggest thing, the finances, when you're not ready. We weren't even ready psychologically because we had only been married two months.

In both these cases of accidental pregnancy, the couples experienced ambivalence based on their loss of control of the timing of the pregnancy. But both couples were able to quickly resolve the ambivalence and move on to other concerns.

In every case the decision to have a child resulted in the postponement, curtailment, or abandonment of the woman's career. In all but one case, the woman planned to remain home after the birth and care for the child on a full-time basis. Yet these women willingly put aside career plans and jobs. Their willingness to be full-time mothers relates to their need for control: they and their husbands were unwilling to permit anyone else to care for their children. Thus, the woman's plans had to be postponed so that she could be the primary caretaker.

One woman explained her feelings about staying at home and not working thus:

She: I want to be there with the children when they come home and try to be a good mother that's interested and maybe do some things that they want to do that I think will be good for the children.

Int: So this means that you don't plan to work?

She: No. I may work in the home or do something that wouldn't interfere with being a good mother. What I consider a good mother — not neglect the children or let someone else baby-sit or train them. They wouldn't train them the way I would want them trained.

Another couple voiced similar sentiments:

He: I think that's a primary responsibility that a parent has . . . to spend time with the children and to teach them how to act and how to respond and how to behave. How to do or learn things. . . . But I think there's also a requirement on the woman's part to be interested and willing to spend the time during the day, instead of going off and seeking a profession or satisfaction in business or industry or some other area. V. was a teacher before we got married, and she could go back to teaching, but she doesn't really want to.

She: I'm happy here.

One woman was very happy to give up her job and felt that working and raising a child were generally incompatible. She said:

No, I don't plan to go to work. You can't go to work and provide for a baby successfully, and besides that, we aren't in that much dire need of money. I don't like to work, and I don't want someone else raising my child.

These women easily postponed or dropped career plans in order to maintain control over child rearing. None experienced any ambivalence over the decision.

Many of the couples felt that the only reason that would justify a woman's returning to work soon after having a baby was extreme financial need. For three couples, the pregnancy created financial problems, but the woman still planned to remain at home while the husband sought extra income.

Only one woman planned to return to work after the birth. This woman was a professional and could leave her child with her mother, a caretaker whom she trusted and who previously had looked after the woman's older child.

Another woman planned to continue her involvement in community affairs after the child's birth. She and her husband lived in a religiously oriented commune. The communal relationships permitted the sharing of certain responsibilities; so the woman could continue to pursue these interests. However, in spite of her professional training, she did not intend to return to work until the child was in school. She stated:

I would like to see myself back in professional work after the children are back in school. That's a future goal — say, you know, in five years or so.

For this woman, too, child rearing took precedence over her career.

These responses illustrate the importance of the underlying issue of control. The decision to have a child exerted its influence on many of the decisions these couples made in planning for the child. The couples who did not plan for the woman's pregnancy experienced ambivalence that had its basis in the loss of control over an important event. Even the woman's decision to remain at home and assume a relatively traditional mothering role was based on the desire to remain in control of the child rearing process. Because they exerted control over the entire decision making process, these couples were content and satisfied with their chosen life course.

SUPPORT SYSTEMS THAT INFLUENCED IDEAS ABOUT PARENTING AND CHILD REARING

The views of the couples interviewed were amazingly similar in regard to the qualities they thought were needed to be good parents. Moreover, their ideas about child rearing in general were quite similar. Certain support systems influenced and reinforced these couples' views on parenting and child rearing. As they decided how they intended to function as parents, the couples selected the qualities and characteristics of certain support systems.

When questioned about parenting and child rearing, these couples repeatedly referred to five sources of support. These included religion, educational literature, the La Leche League (an international organization of nursing mothers), friends and relatives, and each other. By drawing from one or all of these sources of support, the couples developed definite ideas about how they would function as parents and how they wanted to raise their children. These supports also promoted the couples' development of confidence in their ability to function as parents and to carry out their chosen roles. In other words, the couples' ideas on parenting were based on these systems, a fact that gave the couples confidence in themselves.

Religion

One especially strong support system for over half the couples was religion. Seven couples had strong ties to fundamentalist religions. Their lives were guided by the Bible, and they drew their ideas about marriage and parenting roles from it. For these couples, the Bible defined the essence of their roles, and was the basis for their confidence in their ability to carry out these roles.

The Bible's influence is aptly illustrated in the following statements made by one couple as they described how the Bible changed their lives:

He: It's been gradual for the last four years because of the fact that we have been making realizations and learning more about our life. We study the Bible in great detail and what the Bible says, of course. The Bible teaches that the man is the head of the household and the one who makes the decisions, and it's helped us to change how we manage certain things.

She: I think I rebelled a little bit too. . . . I was saying wait a minute, I'm tired of thinking for two people. We sat down and talked about it, and I said, "I'm just tired of living, you know, responsibilities for two people, and I want to share them." And at the same time, like he said, we were studying the Bible, and he realized that a lot of the things I was taking the major worrying and mental responsibilities for should really be his rightful duty, and so that's when we really started to divide and say, "Now this is the area I'm going to have control over, and you're going to do this and that."

This man is a full-time Jehovah's Witnesses minister. His wife is also deeply involved in the religion. Because of the man's profession, we might expect their reliance on the Bible, but six other couples expressed a similar level of involvement and reliance. One of these six couples explained the importance of religion in their lives thus:

He: *Other than ourselves, the love we have for each other, I would say it [the church] would be next.*

She: *It's very important to us. It's something that as we raise the child, of course, it's something that he'll experience himself, but we believe in it very strongly, what the church teaches, and you could almost consider it like our life revolves around the church.*

He: *I would say it is a part of our relationship.*

This couple placed their religion second only to their marital relationship in importance.

Religion or the Bible also played an important part in determining how these couples expected to raise their children. Some accepted the need to follow very specific guidelines about what they should be doing as parents. One man remarked:

We try to base our life on the Bible and on the things that it teaches, and we feel that it has definite things to say about child rearing and the way a child should be taught and brought up, and it goes back to what I said about obedience or respect for parents and others in authority. And we think that's very important.

This man, citing the Bible, identified obedience and respect as two values he planned to instill in his children. Because they based their lives on the Bible, it is natural that these couples used this source in structuring their parenting roles. Another man stated his case even more strongly:

The Bible gives us quite clear indications as to how we should take care of our children, what kind of responsibilities we should have for them. So in that way we want to be constantly improving our ability or improving our attitudes toward our children. Of course, this implies a definite diligence in our studying of the Bible, learning more about how to take care of the children. So in that way we feel successful; we're allowing God to raise our children.

For this man, reliance on the Bible meant that God was raising his children. In other words, he thought he and his wife were simply instruments of God.

The couples who identified strongly with religious groups also drew heavily from these groups when they developed their friendship networks. In some cases, these religious friendship ties had greater importance for and impact on the couples than did their kinship networks. This fact reflected the high level of these couples' involvement in their religions. Out of one support system, religion, they developed a second support system, a religious friendship network.

201. Parenthood as a Profession

The strong religious identifications of these couples were frequently cited as one reason for deciding on a home delivery. Their religions emphasized natural methods and the avoidance of drugs. Choosing a home delivery was one way to avoid drugs being administered during the delivery.

Certainly, not all of the couples interviewed displayed the intense religious involvement of these seven couples. Of the remaining six couples, three were Catholic, and three mentioned no religious affiliation. The Catholic couples expressed a moderate level of identification with their religion. Two Catholic couples increased their religious involvement after the birth of their babies. In both these cases, the decision to increase religious involvement was based on the belief that religion and a parochial school education are essential parts of child rearing. One of these couples said:

He: I don't know, I have always had the schizoid idea that it's good to be brought up in a faith of some sort. . . . It's part of that bit I was talking about childhood. I walked around when I was a kid believing in devils and gods and angels and everything. . . . And I thought it was pretty good. You know, I kind of grew out of it after a time. I don't think it hurt me.

Int: So you want to give that same sort of thing to your child?

He: Yeah. I want to maintain it for the child, and we'll go back to church regularly, right?

She: Yes.

He: As soon as she's aware, maybe about 3, we'll start taking her to church. No, I think it's a good thing.

She: Yeah, I think so too.

This couple felt that they had to become more involved in their religion in order to set an example for the child. The man felt that his previous religious training had exerted a positive influence on his life, and he wanted to provide this same influence for his daughter.

Educational Literature

A second major support system for these couples was educational literature on such topics as pregnancy, natural childbirth, child care, and child rearing. The reading was done primarily by the women, and they would usually communicate some of this information to their husbands. All of the women read at least two books, and some read numerous books. The reading began early in the pregnancy and continued on a more limited basis after the child was born. All the women had read the La Leche League's book entitled *The Womanly Art of Breast Feeding* [7] and *Emergency Childbirth* [9], by Gregory White, M.D. The nine women that took the Gamper childbirth preparation classes read the accompanying book entitled *Preparation for the Heir-Minded* [5], which describes the Gamper method of childbirth. Other sources were varied, but all were aimed primarily at the approaching birth experience and subsequent events.

In at least two cases, the literature was the basis upon which the couples made certain decisions. One couple made the decision to have a home delivery after having read *The Immaculate Deception* [1]. Another couple decided that they could continue having sexual relations late in the pregnancy because they had read of this possibility in *Husband-Coached Childbirth*, by Robert Bradley, M.D. [2]. The woman remarked:

We read it before the baby was born, and I thought it was great, and there are kind of unconventional things in there. You know, things that contradict what other doctors say. I thought, well, if he says so, it must be okay. Like he even says there's no reason not to have sexual relations unless your doctor says so. So we just continued having it right up until the week the baby was born.

This same couple also made the decision to resume sexual relations prior to the wife's postpartum exam because of what they had read in a book. The woman added:

This other book, by Gutmacher [6], says that conventionally you're supposed to wait until the six-week checkup, but if you feel okay, it's no big deal; so we didn't wait until the six-week checkup.

This couple made many other decisions based on information they had read.

In some cases, the literature so impressed a couple that they searched out more information on a subject. In several cases, this process precipitated the decision to have the home delivery. One woman explained how an aversion to hospitals, together with her reading, led her to have a home delivery. She said:

I just don't like hospitals. Then all of a sudden I started reading things in the paper, first about the Chicago Maternity Center, and then I hunted desperately for information about them and called them up, and they gave me Dr. F.'s name, and it was a real coincidence. I mean this was way before we even planned to have a child. And then I read articles about Dr. F. and people like him. So it just kind of fell together.

In these instances, decisions were made as a direct result of what was read.

Literature often reinforced the decisions or ideas of the couples. Some of the couples sought out literature that would support their decision to have home delivery. One woman describes how she found literature that supported her belief that an episiotomy was not always a necessary procedure. She remarked:

I'm telling you what I read. They say in some of the books I've read that the

*episiotomy is not always necessary but they just do it as a matter of course
because they figure, well, five times out of ten or whatever, it will be necessary; so we'll do it because it's easier to stitch a straight line than a jagged line
if the woman should tear.*

One woman whose mother-in-law alerted her to the benefits of natural childbirth turned to educational literature to confirm and support her decision to
use it. She stated:

*Oh yeah, well, I must admit she [her mother-in-law] did influence me on that
[natural childbirth]. I didn't really know that much about childbirth, and I
heard all these stories and things like that, and then I started reading. I think
I read every book there is to read on it.*

Literature reinforced a couple's ideas and gave them a strong base of
support.
   In most cases, the reading enhanced the couple's knowledge and understanding of the birth event, of breast feeding, and of child rearing. By reading
the literature, the couples could better prepare for coming events. One couple
described the type of literature they sought:

He: We read books on being parents.

*She: That's right. After I became pregnant, we did a lot of reading on different
kinds of books about preparing for childbirth itself and also about parenting,
and we're still reading those sorts of things. How to be a good parent or whatever.*

Preparation is an important aspect of home delivery, and reading was an
important means by which the couples interviewed prepared.
   The couples also found solutions in these books to problems they encountered. The books served as a ready reference when new situations created
problems and elicited questions. One woman described how she was helped
by reading about breast feeding:

I had the handbook The Womanly Art of Breast Feeding *[7], plus I had another
book that N. bought me,* A Complete Book of Breast Feeding *[4], and although I didn't read those too much till right after he was born, boy did they
come in handy after he was born.*

Another woman reported a similar experience:

I got a copy of The Womanly Art of Breast Feeding *[7] from La Leche League,
and I'm reading through it 'cause it's useful. They have little tips on things.*

The couples viewed books as important sources of advice.

204. The Expanding Family

These comments demonstrate how strong a support system educational literature was for these couples. All of the women interviewed relied heavily on such literature for information and support. In a number of cases, certain decisions made by a couple triggered a search for support for these decisions. Frequently this search was satisfied by information found in the literature. The couples also used educational literature to prepare for and learn about the new roles they were assuming. Most of the men did very little actual reading; they received information through discussions with their wives.

The La Leche League

The third major support system used by these couples was the La Leche League. Because this organization is primarily set up to offer support and information to mothers about breast feeding, few of the men were involved in it. The men were encouraged to attend the meetings with their wives, but only a few went and then they went to only one or two meetings. Of the thirteen women interviewed, all but two had attended at least one La Leche League meeting. But all of the women had read the La Leche League's book, *The Womanly Art of Breast Feeding* [7]. Seven of the women who reported a high level of involvement in the League had joined the League and had attended meetings on a regular basis.

The La Leche League provided these women with a wide range of services. Many of the women commented on the helpfulness of the breast-feeding manual published by the League. In addition, the highly involved women reported that they had found the meetings extremely helpful as they began breast-feeding their babies. One of the women reported that she would highly recommend the organization to anyone planning to breast-feed. She also described her experience at the meetings and how the organization helped her move into the role of nursing mother. She stated:

Anyone that wants to breast-feed really needs help and encouragement because it's not such a common thing. The women do bring their babies with them, a lot of them already have babies, and you see people nursing their babies. They share their experiences, and they make you feel comfortable, that it's a normal thing to do. By the time she [baby] came, I think I was fairly well prepared for it. I'd never been around little children or nursing mothers, and I was kind of hesitant. But I know I wanted to do it, and they made you feel comfortable doing it.

Another woman described her involvement in the organization:

I belong to the League, and I still go to their meetings and stuff like that. In fact, I find them even more beneficial now than they were when I was pregnant, for two reasons. One, I get more ideas now, and I can relate to their experiences, plus I feel that by my going and saying what I have felt from nursing and the problems I have encountered nursing, I may be able to help somebody else out.

205. Parenthood as a Profession

This woman not only got information and support from the organization but felt she was providing the same to other women.

The League did provide support and information for its members. Its members were available day and night to answer questions and help solve problems. One of the women explained how the organization provided this help:

They let you call if you have any problems. They gave you two numbers of leaders in the area; people you could call day or night. You could call in the middle of the night when you had problems, if your nipples were sore, or the baby wouldn't nurse, or the baby was spitting up, or anything. They say call them. They reassure you or tell you what to do.

Although this service was not used by all the women, it was a source of security and comfort for those who belonged to the League.

Only three women reported having severe problems nursing. One woman sought help from Dr. F. A second woman, not a member of the La Leche League, sought help from her mother-in-law, a cofounder of the League. This woman never felt a need to join the organization since her mother-in-law gave her all the information she needed. The third woman sought help from the La Leche League because of her inverted nipples. She stated:

I had gone to two meetings before he was born, the second and the fourth meetings. I called the League when I couldn't get him to nurse, and I had gotten engorged [breasts] and everything; so they were extremely helpful. I probably would have given up if it hadn't been for the support of him [her husband], Dr. F., and the League.

The woman's area representative supplied her with breast shields that eventually solved the problem and also visited her every day until the problem disappeared.

The League also offered help concerning child rearing. One woman who was expecting her second child reported that she planned to attend League meetings that would focus on topics other than nursing. She commented:

That's one reason I want to go to them [the meetings], too; they have a program of lectures. One of them is related to getting older children or the last nursing baby to accept the newcomer, and I do plan to go to those. Also they cover that sort of thing. They consider children and family-oriented type things.

Several of the women sought out the League for information about matters other than breast feeding.

The women who had joined the League and were highly involved in it also found it helpful and supportive in matters other than breast feeding. Many of them developed new friendships through the meetings. The League offered information about parenting and child rearing. In some cases, the League had had such a great impact on the women that they felt it had changed the course of their lives. The majority of the women used the League for support, and they appreciated very much the information they received there.

Friends and Relatives

The fourth major support system used by these couples in the development of their ideas on parenting and child rearing was their network of friends and relatives. This system was used in one of two ways. First, friends or relatives were viewed as either positive or negative role models for the couple. Second, the relatives or friends were used as advisors by the couple. When the couples encountered problems or new situations, relatives or friends could be sought out for counsel.

All the couples used this support system to some degree. Some used only friends while others used only relatives; the majority of the couples used a combination of the two. The life-style of the couple frequently determined the person who was sought out or modeled. Couples who were deeply involved in a religion usually had developed a strong friendship network with other church members. These couples turned to this network for role models and advice. In a similar fashion, women who were strongly committed to the La Leche League used this network of friends most frequently. All the couples cited parents as important role models and advice-givers.

In most cases, relatives and friends were positive role models. A number of couples mentioned that they had gotten many of their ideas on parenting and child rearing from their parents. One husband pointed this out as follows:

Where I got most of my ideas on how to raise children . . . I suppose a lot of them come from my parents. As I got older, my parents discussed a lot with me about some of the ways they were raised, some of the ways they raised me, and a lot of the reasoning behind the ways they raised me. . . . I could see how they've changed their techniques for raising children through a generation spread from my sister who is 27 to my younger brother who is 8. . . . I had twenty years to observe.

This man watched his parents raise him and his siblings and assimilated many of the ideas and techniques that they had used.

One woman also pointed out that many of her ideas about parenting had come from her own parents. She stated:

You get ideas on how to be a parent from your own parents and what they've given you.

Another woman got the idea that she wanted to breast-feed her child from watching her stepmother do so with her children. She said:

I did because my stepmother had breast-fed her children, and I thought it was a beautiful thing. I really did. I felt she was closer to the children.

207. Parenthood as a Profession

These couples assumed the child rearing style of their parents.

Several of the couples viewed their parents as negative role models. Three women came from broken or unhappy homes and felt that they would work to see that a similar situation did not develop to affect their own children. These women tended to seek out friends rather than relatives as role models. In most cases, however, only certain parental characteristics or child rearing ideas were rejected. For example, one woman said:

One big thing I can think of right offhand is I would not want to raise my child to be overly conscious of social amenities. My mother was always worried about the effect of what you did: what will the neighbors say, or what's the right thing to do?

Another woman expressed a similar sentiment as she explained why she and her husband were seeking outside role models for parenting. She remarked:

We are looking outside of ourselves for good role models because although M. [her husband] had a happy family, there were areas that he has expressed that he'd like to do a little different for ours.

Although many parental ideas on child rearing were rejected, many were also accepted.

When couples encountered a problem or needed information, they often turned to others for advice. When asked to whom she turns, one woman replied:

I think basically the people around us. That's where we get our perspective from. . . . I turn to V. [a friend] for a perspective on whether or not that would be something suitable to do with my baby. . . . so, within our peer group in the community.

This woman lived in a communal, religious network with several other couples. She found advice and support within this community.

Friends and relatives were valued for the experience and information they could impart to the couples. One woman reported that she turned to her friends and the La Leche League for any advice she needs. She stated:

I know I'll call her [a friend] a lot of times for moral support. B., you know, what do they need; what type of things does an infant need; what type of handling; is it possible that I'm handling him too much? Am I going to get him so geared to just me that he won't go to anyone else? . . . She's read a great deal on child rearing, and she usually has my answers. . . . I would avoid asking older generation people. I stick to the younger generation or the League.

This woman had a history of problems in her relations with her parents, so she found that friends and League members were her best source of support and advice.

Another couple reported that they also seek out friends for advice; they had no close relatives nearby. This couple stated:

She: In general, I think you just talk to friends about things.

He: We have enough friends that are both old and young enough that they have been through everything and have faced the problems before and can tell us what to expect.

Couples were selective about the information they sought. One woman explained that she would seek out her mother-in-law for advice in certain areas and not in others. She said:

I'd, well, with my pregnancy go to his mother. But ideas on babies are a little bit different. So I don't think that I would turn to her that much after the baby is born.

These couples sought advice and information from people with whom they basically agreed. In some cases, they agreed with relatives and in other cases they agreed with friends.

These examples illustrate how the couples used parents and friends as sources of support. They demonstrated a high degree of selectivity about whom they chose to rely on. By watching friends and relatives, they developed ideas about how they would like to function in their new roles and who they could go to for advice that would be compatible with their own ideas on parenting and child rearing.

Husband and Wife in Support of Each Other
The last and probably most important source of support for these couples was each other. All but one of the couples had especially close relationships. These couples spent most of their free time together. Their relationship was the basis of many of the important decisions they made. It is easier to understand the supportive role that each spouse assumed in view of this closeness. Each partner drew support, encouragement, and information from the other.

One partner often influenced the thoughts or positions of the other. For example, one partner would bring certain information to the other's attention and as a result change the other's position or thoughts. This was the case for several of the couples when they made the decision to have a home delivery. One of the women described how she influenced her husband in this regard. She said:

I changed my mind after I read a book called The Immaculate Deception *[1]. . . . And it totally changed my mind. I read T. one chapter, and I said, "Look, this is it, regardless." . . . I said, "Well, I think that, you know, having it at home would be best," and T. said, "Well, if you think that's it, then I'm all for it." . . . He was very receptive, and when I had told him my feelings both ways, you know, he thought it was a good idea.*

In another case the man influenced his wife's decision about home delivery and natural childbirth. She stated:

Joint decision. He was stronger on it. He grew up with the [natural] food and then the idea of thinking naturally at the beginning. He educated me. I knew a little bit about it, but I wasn't as strong with it. But by the time we had a child or were ready to have a child, we were both in full agreement that it was the best way to go.

Situations in which one spouse changed the mind of the other were frequent among these couples.

During the pregnancy, the women often discussed reading material with their husbands. Because many of the latter spent long hours at work or school, they were unable to read the educational literature about pregnancy, labor, delivery, and child rearing. Sharing the information allowed the partners to jointly make decisions or adopt new attitudes or ideas.

The partners also sought out each other as sources of expertise in certain areas. For example, the man would frequently seek out the wife for help in learning certain child care skills. One wife describes how her husband sought her help in learning how to put an undershirt on the child. This couple exchanged these comments:

She: "I'll change him," he says, "and we're all out of the undershirts that snap. It has to go over his head." I said, "I'll put it on him," but no, he says, "I'll do it," and all of a sudden I hear him [the baby] screaming, and he goes, "How do you get this over his head?"

He: There are some techniques that I forgot about.

The men tended to seek out the wives for information on many aspects of child care. They also learned most of their child care skills from their wives, who were usually more experienced and skilled than they.

These couples tended to depend upon each other a great deal. In addition to being called upon to give information and teach skills, one partner might be called on to provide support for the other. Such support is best illustrated by the role the husband assumed during the labor and delivery. Although the husband was unaware of having assumed this role, the wife was very much aware.

This support system is particularly important when we realize the depth and strength of these couples' relationships. They tended to place heavy reliance on each other and to make all decisions jointly. This interdependence made each partner the most important source of support for the other.

INVOLVEMENT IN AND COMMITMENT TO PARENTING ROLES

The couples who chose to have their children delivered at home appeared to make the transition to parenthood with relative ease. In most cases, anticipated problems failed to materialize. The problems that did arise concerned the delivery, breast feeding, rest, or scheduling of activities. One factor that distinguishes these couples is their confidence in performing the role of parents. In addition, each couple had very definite ideas about the characteristics they would need to function successfully in their parenting roles.

The Father's Role

The man began preparing for his new role as father early in the pregnancy. In all but one case, the husbands had a relatively high level of involvement prior to the birth. This was the case even in the five instances in which the husband worked two jobs or was going to school and had a job. Although their time at home was limited, these five men became involved either by assisting their wives with household chores, by providing moral support for wives attending Gampers or Lamaze childbirth preparation classes, or by helping with the physical preparations for the baby.

One woman whose husband held two jobs described at length how her husband helped out while she was pregnant:

I think he took on a little more than he did before, although it's hard to compare because we got married in September, and I got pregnant in March. So we didn't have that long of a time to spend when I wasn't pregnant. I know in the beginning of the pregnancy he took over the cooking, he took over everything, because I would come home from work, and I would be sick. I didn't do anything. I would just sleep at night. I fell asleep at 8:00 [P.M.] in the evenings lots of times. Then in the middle again when I was feeling better, I started to do most of the cooking, and toward the end he took over again because physically I wasn't able to get to a lot of things.

To some degree all the men assumed some of the wife's chores at different times during the pregnancy. In some cases, like that of the couple cited above, these responsibilities were assumed because the wife was ill in the beginning of the pregnancy or unable to perform certain tasks in the latter part of the pregnancy.

In two cases, the husband insisted on assuming more responsibilities in order to relieve the wife of the burden of the chores and to make her feel better. One man stated:

Well, I do more of the dishes now, and when she has things to be done, I try and do them immediately. I try and do nice things, like the first thing in the morning, you know, I will like rub her feet and wake her up. Oh, I'll turn the heat on when it's cold, you know, 'cause we usually have the window open for fresh air in the evening and the room's cold. So I'll usually get up and I'll turn the heat up so the oven will warm up the place sooner. Things like that, you know, that I can make life a little bit easier for her.

The men were very conscientious about helping their pregnant wives.

The men also became involved in many of the activities associated with preparing for childbirth. All of the first-time fathers and one of the men who already had a child attended childbirth preparation classes with their wives. The men's reactions to these classes varied widely. One couple felt that the information given in the early classes was not worthwhile since they already were familiar with it. They stated:

He: It's a long time to sit for nothing.

She: Yeah, the first class was just lecture, and most of it B. and I had already known.

Another man felt that there was too much socializing at the classes. He remarked:

Initially it starts out, well, any group situation starts out with how are you? Which is fine if you're in the group of people. Different people find different satisfactions at different levels, and to them, a lot of them, I imagine, this is a big thing in their lives, and this is a support function of the group. To me and for D., we like to go there and get information and take our information and go home. And I'm not going to say it's not good, but it could have, you know, it could be set up for people like us who just want to come and go and not . . .

She: Socialize.

Later, however, this man did admit that the classes were helpful because of the information they imparted.

The value of the information imparted at these classes was a theme consistently voiced by all but one of the men. They found that the classes increased their knowledge and understanding of the delivery process and, in so doing, made them feel a part of that process. They felt that the classes were a valuable experience. For example, when asked how the classes were going, one couple replied:

She: We finished them but they were good. They weren't as helpful as I thought they would be, but I think for my husband. . .

He: For me it was helpful.

She: It was probably more beneficial.

He: I learned and I understand. I have a better understanding of childbirth at home.

212. The Expanding Family

She: Men are very much in the dark. They say, you know, you're going to have a baby, and it comes out, and this is it.

He: I walked in there, and all I knew was we were going to have a baby, and that's it. But when they got down to details, you know, there was more to it. I understood, you know.

As these comments illustrate, many of the men felt they had benefited more from these classes than their wives had.

The husbands also became involved in many of the physical preparations for the baby, such as getting baby furniture and fixing up the baby's room. The amount of involvement in these activities varied; some men helped out only when their wives requested help, others initiated involvement themselves.

The men also provided support for their wives during the pregnancy although they never directly mentioned their role in this regard. This support usually took the form of physical help, encouragement, and maintenance of a stable emotional environment for the wife. Many of the men reported that their relationships with their wives had changed because of the pregnancy. Some reported that they were getting along better since the wife had gotten pregnant. One man said:

Before she was pregnant we used to fight like cats and dogs, and now we don't fight at all.

This same man reported going out of his way to avoid arguments with his wife. The avoidance of arguments frequently required special effort by the men since many described their wives as being more irritable during the pregnancy. Other husbands described the change in their relationship as an increased "closeness" brought on by working together toward a common goal.

The men did begin doing more things for their wives during the pregnancy. They also reported that when they were asked to do something by their wives, they got it done immediately whereas prior to the pregnancy they would have put it off. One husband said:

You know, when she says go right now, I jump and go.

The women were very much aware of this increased level of cooperation. One woman remarked:

Well, he does do more for me now, but he's been that way, you know, like if I say, "Will you do it?", he does it. I don't have to ask him two or three times now, where before I used to have to say, "J., will you please do this," you know, two or three times, but now he'll do it. Like once and he'll do it.

In effect, the men's increased level of cooperation helped maintain a stable emotional environment.

213. Parenthood as a Profession

All the men played an active role in the labor and delivery. Since the previous chapter examined the home delivery in detail, we will not dwell on it here. It is sufficient to say that the men were highly involved in the delivery process and felt that they played an extremely important role in their child's birth.

In the first few weeks after birth, most of the men became as involved with the child as possible. Obviously, because the breast feedings were frequent during the first few weeks and the men were away from the home at work for a large part of the day, their contact with the child was somewhat limited. The women assumed the primary responsibility for the care of the child. The men assisted their wives by helping with the household chores and relieving them of child care for varying periods at night, during which the men held and played with the child or baby-sat while the mothers went out on some errand.

Only a few of the men admitted that they participated in child care tasks such as diapering or bathing. All said they felt capable of performing these tasks, but only a few reported that they had actually done them. In a majority of the cases, this lack of participation was the result of the limited time the men spent at home. The men regretted not performing these tasks, and they felt that as the child grew, they would be assuming more of the child care responsibilities. One couple commented:

He: I only changed him once 'cause I'm never around. See, that's the problem with two jobs. I'm never around. I hold him as much as I can so, you know, he becomes aware of me.

She: You did take a bath with him.

He: Right, I gave him a bath last Sunday, but as far as changing his clothes goes, I'm never around, which is a shame. And when I am around, I'm either sleeping or else he's sleeping, one of the two. In fact, I don't like to change him; I really don't. I will, though; I'm going to have to make a start.

This same sentiment was voiced by other men who held two jobs or had a job and were going to school. They all expressed regret that they could not spend more time with their children. Another man stated:

I act the father role. I tell everybody I know. But I guess I won't be his father until he recognizes me more. He knows D. more than he knows me because of the fact that he's with her all day and he sees me for maybe I'd say six or seven hours at the most. That's not very long. I mean it ain't bad, but when I'm with him I feel very fondly. I pick him up, and I hold him and talk to him, pull on him, and dance with him.

This father's comment, "I guess I won't be his father until he recognizes me more," illustrates the initial difficulty that some men had in beginning to move into the role of father. In the beginning, a child responds only minimally to a father's stimulations. As the child grows older and becomes more responsive, fathers can anticipate taking a more active role.

The men also reported they were surprised that the physical size of the child did not present a barrier to their first attempts at child care. In the past, when they were confronted with a small child, they had experienced nervousness when holding the child or had just refused to hold the child. All the men reported that they were able to hold their own children without experiencing the anxiety that had been present when confronted with other people's children. When asked if he felt comfortable holding and taking care of the baby from the beginning, one man replied:

Un huh. I had no problems adjusting to it. I think I adapted to him just fine. Because I didn't feel awkward holding him.

When asked if he had any feelings about handling such a small child, another man admitted:

I'm petrified. I would never hold anybody else's child. I would be afraid that if something happened to him, I would be responsible, you know. Like when you're a little boy, you happen to handle something and you break it, boy you're in trouble. Him [his child], he came naturally. I would not hold anybody else's child. . . . As far as holding him, I have no problems, you know. I'll hold him whenever I can.

This man's nervousness diminished because the child was his.

All of the fathers were asked to project ahead and discuss some of the responsibilities they thought they would be assuming as the child grew older. Few were able to respond to this question. Most admitted that they had not thought that far ahead because they were so concerned with what was going on now. Two of the men responded in general terms about the probability of increasing financial responsibilities as the child grew older. Two men with other children cited authority and discipline as important responsibilities they would be assuming as the child grew older. One man stated:

I think every child, boy or girl, needs a strong masculine influence in his life. Somebody that can lay down the law and be respected.

The fact that the first-time fathers seldom responded to questions about increasing responsibilities may be due to the fact that the questions were asked within six to eight weeks after the birth. These men may still have been so involved in the passage to the new role of father that they were not yet able to project this role into the future.

All the men moved into the fathering role slowly and cautiously. Their early explorations of this new role were somewhat tentative as they learned the skills they would need for child care. Although they tended to become involved with the child soon after birth, they hesitated somewhat at assuming total responsibility for the child. This hesitancy was frequently mentioned when the couples talked about the first time the men were left alone with the child. Nevertheless, the men all reported that they had made a successful transition to their new role, and all expressed satisfaction and delight at being fathers.

The Mother's Role

In contrast to the men's fatherhood, the women's motherhood profoundly affected almost every aspect of their lives. Careers or jobs were suspended or abandoned. Freedom to travel, shop, or visit was frequently curtailed or at least limited more than it had been before the child was born. Household chores such as cleaning and cooking were no longer high priority tasks. Even the women's relationships with their husbands were described as different.

All the women interviewed made the transition to the mothering role with relative ease. Their preparation for their new role was usually much greater than that of their husband's in that they usually had had broader experience in child care, had read more, and had discussed the coming event and future responsibilities with many more people. Thus they approached the whole experience well-informed and with a fairly clear idea of the responsibilities they would be expected to assume.

All the women were enthusiastic about assuming the role of mother. The experience of having the first child evoked intense maternal feelings in these women. They viewed this experience as a life-changing event, and most felt like mothers from the moment they delivered their children. One woman stated:

As he was born, during the labor and afterward, I kind of felt like I had changed, and I kind of felt an inside feeling of womanhood come on. I don't know what it is, and I don't know how to explain it to you.

Another woman expressed similar sentiments:

I never used to think it was something special, but when you have a child, it is; I mean that's something that you created, and it's very overpowering.

All the women referred to these special feelings and felt that they had changed in some way. This change had begun when they first saw, held, or cared for the new baby. When asked what made her feel like a mother, one woman replied:

Her [her daughter]. Having her, holding her, feeding her, just generally taking care of her. . . . I didn't feel it as soon as she was born; I felt it as soon as she was put in my room.

This woman, because her labor was prolonged, had her child in the hospital, and it was not until the child was brought into her room that she experienced these feelings of mothering.

Despite strong maternal feelings in the first hours or days after the birth, these mothers never described their initial explorations of the mothering role as an easy process. The preparations they had made never totally prepared them for the realities of the child. Their primary problem in the first few weeks was their overwhelming feeling of responsibility for another human being. Whereas their specific child care problems were minimal, they feared being unable to competently assume the general responsibility. One woman admitted:

Since he's been born, all of a sudden I feel like the whole world is on my shoulders, you know? Like, isn't there anybody that's going to help me, you know, take him off my hands and change him for me, do something? For once let me be the person who sits back and watches this somebody else take care of him. But that's my role. I should be doing it anyway.

Although she expressed an overwhelming sense of responsibility, the woman pointed out that assuming the responsibility is a part of her role. Other women expressed similar feelings about assuming the responsibilities of the new role, but their feelings seemed to be based on uncertainty about their ability to perceive and satisfy the child's needs. One woman remarked:

There are times when I feel awkward, or I guess it's more frustration, when she's crying and I can't do anything about it.

Another woman commented:

I thought it was all me, and then, of course, it did upset him [her child] because I was upset. Because I didn't figure out why he wouldn't accept me, you know, and it was kind of, why did I just get him to sleep and he's been fed, he's burped, he's dry. He'd be so asleep, and I'd just leave, and he'd wake up screaming, and I'd think it was kind of a stab at me. I guess it's the blues you get. I don't know but at three months he's just starting to calm down. I'm more on my feet now.

These women experienced frustration when they were unable to interpret the child's cries.

Adjusting to the new baby, getting to know his needs and how he expresses these needs, was an important issue for these new mothers. Such adjustment was the first obstacle they encountered as they began to assume the new responsibilities of their role. For some, the adjustment and acceptance of the responsibilities of mothering occurred very rapidly; for others, such as the last-quoted respondent, the process was much slower. The speed of acceptance was related to the woman's previous experience with children. Women who had had previous experience made the adjustment to the child with greater speed and ease than did women who had had very little experience.

In either case, in the process of accepting the new responsibilities and adjusting to the baby, the women began to develop confidence in their ability to function as mothers. One woman described her movement from uncertainty to confidence thus:

As of right now I can say, yes, I feel like a mother. Before I didn't think so. I felt more like a slave, you know . . . the first couple of months. Yeah, it was really hard because it was more of an adjustment for me, I think, than a lot of women have because I'd never grown up wanting to have a baby. In fact, we hadn't planned on having any kids until last year; so this was quite an adjustment. And so now I'm starting to really feel like a little mother and really beginning to fill [the child's] needs and wants.

This woman attributed her adjustment problems to her lack of preparation for the role. Her refusal to consider motherhood prior to her decision to get pregnant contributed to her slow adjustment to the child and her new role. Initially, the woman experienced difficulty in adapting to the child and his needs. But as she cared for the child, she became more experienced at being a mother. With this growing body of experience, the woman developed confidence in her abilities and began to feel like a real mother.

Breast feeding was a very important part of the mothering role for all the women interviewed. All successfully breast-fed their babies, but three did have severe problems initially. All the women viewed breast feeding as one of the primary tasks of the mothering role. They felt it established a special relationship between the mother and the child. One woman explained her feelings about this special relationship thus:

I feel close to the baby. I don't know if I feel any closer than I would if I was bottle-feeding him. But I know that he likes the warmth, you know. I mean because there are times when all he has to do is lay next to my breast and he's asleep, which is the security, you know.

Other respondents expressed similar sentiments. One woman said:

I think your relationship with your child is better. I think they're healthier children, and I think it's better all the way around. I really do.

Another woman linked breast feeding to being a better mother and spending more time with the child. She stated:

I think breast feeding . . . it makes me more of a mother to him, and it makes me stay home rather than say, "Hey wait, I've had enough of this," and take him to a neighbor's and be gone for three or four hours or the whole afternoon. It makes you be a little more of a mother to him.

All the women considered breast feeding an integral part of mothering.

These comments touch on several important characteristics of mothering, one of which is the close relationship that develops between the mother and the child. That this relationship existed between these women and their children is not surprising in view of the time the women spent breast feeding. Each woman interviewed expressed a very high level of commitment to breast feeding. All intended to breast-feed without any supplemental feedings for at least four to six months. This dedication to total breast feeding also meant a commitment of time needed for the task. One reason the women were willing to expend such time was their belief that breast milk was the best thing they could give their children. One woman said:

I've done enough reading to know that for the first five or six months mother's milk is the best thing for them.

This knowledge was reinforced and supported by the physician, members of the La Leche League, and frequently by the women's husbands. As a result, these mothers planned to provide the total nutrition for their children for the first few months. It was a task that only they could perform. They could not solicit help from others unless their milk was expressed into bottles. This option was taken on occasion by several women, but all the women felt that they would exercise this option only in special situations. None wanted to express milk on a regular basis.

Although breast feeding was time-consuming and placed special demands on the mothers, all of them regarded the experience as a positive one. For example, when asked how breast feeding had fit into her routine, one woman replied:

Wonderfully, marvelously. Sometimes I get a little frustrated, and it's taxing because it's not like putting a material object in the baby's mouth; it's you. It takes your time, but there are so many advantages.

All the women interviewed were happy about and successful at breast feeding their babies, undoubtedly because of the strong support and encouragement they received from their physicians, the La Leche League members, and relatives and/or spouses. Breast feeding enhanced the women's maternal feelings. Being successful at such feeding made them feel successful as mothers since they believed breast feeding was a fundamental part of the mothering role.

Another characteristic of mothering is provision of love and stimulation to the child. Providing such by holding, cuddling, and talking to the child was another fundamental part of the mothering role for these women. For example, one woman said:

Well, he [her child] needs a lot of physical contact, touching, fondling, and I think what is important is talking to him. 'Cause I think that makes a big difference.

219. Parenthood as a Profession

Unlike breast feeding, this responsibility could be shared with the father and others. In fact, the fathers viewed this as one of the most important parts of their role in the early months.

During the first few weeks after delivery, some of the women displayed somewhat possessive behavior. They would hold the baby for prolonged periods of time and allow their husbands to relieve them only briefly. This behavior might be a manifestation of the woman's need to control the child, or it may just be a result of the woman's wonder at having a child of her own.

The women were asked if they had left their babies at any time since birth. The majority reported that they had not left the child with anyone, the reason being that breast feedings were so frequent. In the few cases in which the mother had left the child, the father or a close relative had cared for him or her. Most of the women were quite hesitant to leave the child with anyone. For instance, one woman said:

You know, before I ever had a baby, I thought, oh, so you want to call a baby-sitter, you know, big deal. You can still do what you want. Now I won't leave her with just anyone. . . . I guess it would have to be a relative or L. [a friend] and nobody else. . . . You do feel bad about leaving her. It's funny, I never thought, I used to think, oh, that's for real fanatics; I'll never feel that way.

These women were not looking forward to leaving their babies. They did not want to leave the infants with baby-sitters unless someone they trusted, such as their husbands, close relatives, or friends acted in this role.

After assuming the mothering role, major changes occurred in the lives of all of the women. These changes were precipitated by the child's taking priority over all other things. The women placed their children's needs above all their other responsibilities. One woman reported:

I don't keep up with the house like I used to, and I really don't care because, like she's more important than the house any day. . . . I don't have petty things on my mind any more, little things, you know, like am I going to get dinner ready by 5:00 (P.M.) or, you know, I just get it ready when I get it ready. She comes before dinner.

Placing the child's needs first was a consistent theme voiced by all the women. One woman stated:

So I think that there are two elements that I'm most in touch with, the increased tiredness with everything I'm doing, and then the added responsibilities of the baby changing the focus of my responsibilities. So that she has to come first. . . . I feel a little pressure to center more of myself around the child.

All the women had expected their lives to change after the child's arrival, so none of them expressed surprise over the changes. The changes were simply accepted.

For these women, the mothering role had many facets. We have focused on only their major concerns or responsibilities in the first few weeks after the birth. At this time they had to accept the maternal role and develop confidence in their ability to perform that role.

CONTROL, PACING, AND ADJUSTMENT

The couples who chose to deliver their children at home can be characterized as a group of dedicated parents whose attitudes about parenting were relatively traditional. The parenting roles they assumed were those in which the woman devotes full time to the mothering role and her husband assists her and assumes more responsibilities as the child grows older. Underlying their commitment to parenting was the couple's need to exert a high level of control over their own lives and those of their newborn children. This control generally was exercised from the very beginning, when the couple made the decision to have a child, and continued throughout the pregnancy, labor, delivery, and afterward. At every point in this course of events, the couple's decisions were aimed at maintaining control of the situation.

When developing their ideas and attitudes about parenting and child rearing, the couples continued to maintain control by using support systems selectively. The couples made use of five major support systems: religion, the La Leche League, educational literature, friends and relatives, and each other. The first four sources of support were filtered through the primary support system, the couple, who thus ultimately remained in control of the whole process. From the five major sources of support the couple selected the characteristics and attitudes they felt they needed to function in the roles of mother and father.

The pace at which the partners assumed these parenting roles was quite different. The woman's transition into the mothering role occurred quite rapidly, as she began to breast-feed the child immediately after birth and assumed almost all the child care responsibilities shortly thereafter. In contrast, the man generally had to explore the fathering role at a slower pace. The men interviewed began their preparation for the fathering role during the pregnancy. They took an active part in preparing for the birth event and the child and considered themselves to be major participants in the birth event. Their involvement continued after the child's birth but was limited by the woman's involvement in breast feeding. Initially, the men assisted their wives and offered them relief for brief periods of time. Thus the men were able to move into their new role gradually. Considering the usually limited preparation they had for the fathering role, their slower pace seems quite appropriate.

The women faced a major obstacle in making the rapid transition to their new role: the need to accept the responsibilities of this role and to adapt to the child. Soon after the birth the women interviewed began adjusting to their children. During this time, they accepted the responsibilities implicit in having a child and began to develop confidence in their ability to interpret and meet a child's needs. Once they were confident that they could perform in the mothering role, they were able to gain satisfaction from that role.

The couples interviewed appeared to be enthusiastic about and highly committed to their new roles. The birth experience and the child appeared to strengthen their relationships as couples. From this strengthened relationship they gained the support they needed to begin their new roles as parents.

The results of our study take on greater significance in light of the emphasis on family-centered care in maternal-child nursing. In attempting to understand the family, we must increase our knowledge of the critical events in the family life cycle. Having a child and becoming parents is one such critical event. Because this event precipitates changes in life-style, it is important that we nurses understand the meaning the event has for couples and the process they use to adapt to these changes. When we have thus increased our base of information, we will be better able to assess a couple's progress in making the transition into parenting roles. If problems arise as they are making this passage, we may be in a position to identify the problem and offer assistance in overcoming it. In addition, understanding how a couple goes about gathering the information upon which they base their decisions may allow us at some appropriate time to offer information that they might find useful.

Although the sample of couples studied in this chapter is unique, many of the conclusions drawn from their comments are relevant to other couples who display similar characteristics, such as a high degree of control over the birth event and a deep commitment to parenting. The sources of support and methods of adaptation used by these couples may not be unique to them. Further investigation and observation may reveal that these are common sources and methods of adaptation that are used by many other types of couples. If this is the case, then the information contained herein has broad implications for nurses as they learn about the beginnings of parenting roles.

REFERENCES

1. Arms, S. *The Immaculate Deception.* Boston: Houghton Mifflin, 1975.
2,3. Bradley, R.A. *Husband-Coached Childbirth.* New York: Harper & Row, 1965.
4. Eiger, M.S., and Olds, S.W. *A Complete Book of Breast Feeding.* New York: Workman Publishing, 1972.
5. Gamper, M. *Preparation for the Heir-Minded.* Glenview, Ill.: Midwest Parentcraft Center, 1971 (pamphlet used in Gamper's childbirth education classes).
6. Gutmacher, A.F. *Pregnancy, Birth and Family Planning: A Guide for Expectant Parents in the 1970's.* New York: Viking, 1973.
7. La Leche League International. *The Womanly Art of Breast Feeding.* Franklin Park, Ill.: La Leche League International, 1958.
8. Pryor, K. *Nursing Your Baby.* New York: Pocket Books, 1973.
9. White, G.J. *Emergency Childbirth: A Manual.* Franklin Park, Ill.: Police Training Foundation, 1958.

15. Creating a New Role: The Professional Woman and Motherhood. Norma Traub Cox

This chapter, like most of the others in this book, considers processes associated with assuming a new role. The focus here, however, is on the interplay between the mothering role and already established roles, on the realignment of professional and marital roles that must accompany development of the mothering role.

In contrast to those women who are committed to a full-time mothering role and who willingly restructure their lives around their children, the women interviewed for this chapter were attempting to integrate mothering into previously established life patterns that they wished to maintain. Given the diversity of these role demands, it is no surprise that such women were most concerned about managing and controlling their lives.

The professional woman who becomes a mother is not unlike the circus juggler. She must keep the components of her varying roles in motion, balanced, and complementary. While she may temporarily focus on one role, she cannot totally ignore all the others. For example, the woman lawyer who becomes a mother may take a leave of absence from her work, but she still maintains contact with her place of employment. Her clients and ongoing responsibilities do not disappear. Particularly if the professional woman anticipates reentering her work role, she must maintain her place so that her career remains viable.

A professional woman may be assumed to have established a certain self-image related to competence in her chosen work. As she enters motherhood, her standards of excellence and expectations for role performance as a new mother are likely to be as high as those she established for her professional life. Given these sets of role expectations, what problems does the professional woman who becomes a mother experience and how does she manage her complicated life?

The ten professional women interviewed for this chapter were selected from the rosters of Lamaze classes conducted in the Chicago area. Each respondent was interviewed twice. The first interview was conducted two to four weeks post partum and the second took place when the infant was approximately 3 months old. All the women were first-time mothers. The group included five teachers, two psychologists, one attorney, one editor, and one actuarial assistant. Six of the ten had completed courses beyond the baccalaureate degree. All had worked in their professional fields at least two years following completion of their degrees. They ranged in age from 24 to 36. All led active professional and social lives. Housework was not of great concern to these women. They did what they could and accepted living in a less ordered environment. Several had household help; others shared tasks with their husbands. Six returned to work immediately following the birth of their babies; the others planned to resume their professional lives after a leave of absence. All expressed feelings that their work was essential to their personal contentment. Management of their busy lives was a common concern.

MANAGEMENT AND CONTROL

As individuals experience shifts and realignments of social roles, they must more tightly manage and control their lives. Professionals in particular have to exercise a high degree of self-discipline to achieve professional goals. Each of the women interviewed had led a carefully planned life with clear-cut goals in mind. Each had completed an extensive educational program; each had managed an active professional life. All had practiced birth control, and for them the birth of a child was but another carefully planned event.

Their accounts of their attempts to become pregnant further illustrate their efforts to control their lives. Three women had attempted to conceive for some time before becoming pregnant. Two women had had spontaneous abortions. These women said they had felt increasing anxiety over their inability to conceive and carry a child as they had planned. One woman had begun psychotherapy in response to her frustration, and another had seriously considered psychotherapy. Yet another woman had enrolled in graduate school in an attempt to take her mind off her frustration. These women viewed not being able to have a child when planned as a thwarting of their ability to maintain control over their lives. Timing of birth was another important control issue. One woman did not wish to be pregnant during the summer. If she had not conceived by a particular time, she planned to resume birth control until the following year, when she would try again.

The women's enrollment in Lamaze classes reflects their desire to have control over the birth process. The women recalled their labor in terms of the amount of self-control they were able to exert. One woman said that although her labor occurred during the day and she had slept well the night before, she slept between each contraction. She described the birth process:

I had the urge to push. The contractions were very intense, and I couldn't even stay awake during them. I couldn't keep my eyes open. I think I must have psyched myself up so much that I would fall asleep before the contraction ended. While I was having a hard contraction, my husband would tell me to relax an arm, and I would just go limp.

Most women received no medication and took pride in being able to manage without it. In this respect, these women are similar to those interviewed for Chapter 14, who regarded mothering as an all-consuming role, but the reasons underlying the similar behavior differ. For the professional woman, success-fully managing the birth process is a further affirmation of herself as a com-petent individual. For the home delivery mothers, natural childbirth is more closely tied to the welfare of the child.

Limiting or governing visitors was a common problem for the women. Some absolutely restricted visitors for up to two weeks after the child was brought home. Others had big parties to welcome the new baby and celebrate the birth event. One woman expressed her concern by stating:

I feel that I should stand at the door and sell tickets to the relatives. They came by the carload the first week.

While sometimes viewing the number of visitors as a problem, these profes-sional women seemed relatively powerless to simply tell people that their presence was not desired. Instead of directly confronting the problem of too many visitors, one woman, for example, kept people away on the grounds that they would bring germs into the environment.

Scheduling of activities was a matter of some concern to these women. The unpredictability of the child's behavior and the women's resultant inability to control it caused problems. These problems were further complicated when these new mothers attempted, often unsuccessfully, to "follow the doctor's orders," a somewhat ironic development in that these women were highly competent in their professional roles and were used to making their own decisions. Yet knowing how to respond to a baby's cries was not some-thing they trusted to their own judgment. Rather, they deferred to the doctor's directions. Their pediatricians commonly advocated feeding every four hours although their babies did not necessarily follow this pattern. Even though their infants might appear hungry after three hours, these mothers hesitated to feed them and were intimidated by the pediatricians' instruc-tions. One woman compromised by feeding her baby every three and a half hours but expressed a great deal of concern over whether she was doing the right thing. Again, this pattern is in sharp contrast to the home delivery mothers, who fed babies on demand. Perhaps the professional woman who spends much of her time ordering other peoples' lives is more inclined to follow orders than to trust her own judgment in an area in which she is not yet an expert.

Two of the ten women had twins, which created special problems. One woman operated without a schedule because she found it impossible with twins. The other woman said she could not manage unless everything was carefully scheduled. The less rigidly scheduled mother received almost continuous assistance and support from her husband, which perhaps allowed her the greater degree of flexibility.

Scheduling became especially crucial as these professional women returned to work. The situation became very complicated for women who were breast feeding. One woman likened the contrast between her professional and personal worlds to that between a quiet mountain stream and a traffic jam. In trying to adjust all roles at one time, some women became frustrated as behaviors appropriate to one role were inappropriate in another. For example, a mother must be sensitive to the child's cues and respond accordingly; the child is the initiator. In her work world, however, a professional woman must be self-initiating; if she waits to be told what to do, she is relatively unproductive. For this reason, scheduling becomes important to the professional woman because it serves as a means by which she can impose some controls on her child.

The women also had difficulty establishing satisfactory baby-sitting arrangements. They expressed great concern over the qualifications of an acceptable baby-sitter. After making a selection, most women felt the need to be present during the first few times the baby-sitter was in charge. One mother of twins explained that she wished to observe the interaction; another woman wanted to be sure the schedule was maintained. While these women did use baby-sitters to assist them in child care, they monitored them very carefully in order to maintain control.

The birth of a child not only necessitates adjustments in professional roles and the learning of new mothering behavior but requires readjustment of marital roles. All the women expressed concern about their inability to resume the sexual relations they had established before pregnancy. One woman was worried because her constant concern for the new baby had affected her ability to relax and therefore to achieve orgasm. Most women were surprised and dismayed at the amount of discomfort accompanying intercourse at this time. Some used their physical condition, such as breast tenderness, as a barrier to sexual relations (e.g., "My breasts belong to my baby"). The child and his or her needs were frequently used to keep husbands at a distance, to control husbands who placed demands on the wife for resumption of usual marital roles. One woman remarked:

We haven't gotten back to our pre-baby sex life. I've been too tired, and there is always that feeling that the baby is going to wake up and need me.

In some instances, marked competition between the partners over the child was apparent.

In summary, the conflicts that accompanied the women's role shifts increased their need to control the situation. The many new physical and emotional demands placed on the women caused them to depend on their own resources or to rely on external supports. They controlled their world by scheduling, limiting visitors, and refraining or withdrawing from physical and emotional intimacy with their husbands. If the women felt in partnership with their husbands, they shared the role negotiation process consciously with them.

AMBIVALENCE

The professional women who became mothers expressed considerable ambivalence about their multiple roles. Some were ambivalent about having a child in the first place. One woman stated:

I would not have had a child had I not felt that my husband would be at least as responsible for the child as me. There are too many other things I want to do with my life.

Another woman avoided having a child for some time because she feared the "trapped mother syndrome." This woman said:

I have become the epitome of all that I held in disdain. I can stay at home and not read, not write, maybe watch some TV, and play with the baby. That consumes my day, and I love it. I suppose if it weren't time-limited, I wouldn't like it so much.

This woman's realization that she would return to her professional role allowed her to find pleasure in temporarily assuming a full-time mothering role.

All the women interviewed had decided prior to conception to return to work. Even though they had previously decided to resume their careers, when the time came, their return to work was fraught with ambivalence. One woman admitted:

I never expected to feel as conflicted as I have about leaving him. I never thought it would be like that at all. I didn't believe that it would happen to me. . . . that I could be so bound up in such a mundane thing.

The women attempted to make acceptable compromises in response to this ambivalence. One mother, a psychologist who had always been heavily involved in her work, noted:

I could be just as happy working part-time, but I like my job so that I get more involved than I should for part-time, so I might as well work and get paid for it. It's a real dilemma, and I've thought a lot about if things will always be this way.

That this woman is torn between a job that is enjoyable and mothering is clearly apparent.

Another woman, a lawyer and mother of twins, not only wished to resume her profession but also wished to develop as an artist. She arranged to work three days a week in the office and spend the rest of the time at home dividing her time between child care and her artistic endeavors. She stated:

I'm committed to the idea of having my own career in the sense of earning my own money, having a life of my own that relates to the outside world. . . . I'm also committed to my art, getting a tremendous amount of satisfaction out of it and thinking in some ways it's the most important thing in my life.

This woman's response to conflicting pulls was to carefully balance and allocate portions of time to the various activities she valued.

Like control, ambivalence was pervasive in the lives of these women. Although every woman had planned her child, its actual birth caused conflicting feelings. One woman admitted:

I was a little afraid I might even resent her when she was born, even though I wanted her and she was planned. I'm very much career-oriented, and I'm independence-oriented. I know she's going to take time. I was a little afraid that I was going to find her imposing upon me.

All these women had experienced a high degree of independence in their lives; the birth of a child placed a new set of demands on them that conflicted with their freedom.

Generally, independent people find it difficult to accept help from others. These women had problems accepting help from relatives and husbands in caring for their children. While they appreciated any help, they also felt a certain urgency to manage on their own. For example, one woman said:

We had a nurse for a week. I was very happy to see her go. She was very good and helpful, and she showed me lots of things. I'd watch her so I'd know what to do. The night before she left I made sure I bathed the baby. I was terrified of that. But by the end of the week I was feeling good, and I wanted to take care of my baby.

Several women arranged for their own mothers to stay with them, but most asked them to leave after a short while because they wanted to be alone with their husbands and children. Fear of arguing with family members over child care was a common concern. One woman remarked:

They could help, but it would be more difficult to correct them if they did something I didn't like.

Here, again, the woman who had experienced a high degree of independence had difficulties assuming help and direction from others.

The women were similarly ambivalent about receiving help from their husbands. On the one hand, they wanted support and help in caring for the infants; on the other, they thought that the men were not capable, needed too much direction, and were not really interested in this activity. One woman described having left the baby at home with her husband and returning to find the baby asleep in his swing. She was upset that her husband had not put the tired baby to bed as she would have. Obviously, women who have pursued professional careers set high standards for themselves, and these standards extend to those on whom they must rely for child care if they are to continue their professional careers.

Ambivalence over social activities was also universal. All the women felt that maintaining social contacts was important to them and to their husbands. However, very often the effort required was perceived as greater than the anticipated rewards. The women cited such reasons as the difficulty of engaging a sitter, the worry about what is happening in their absence, the effort to take the child along, concern about whether the baby is disturbing others, and the time spent in preparation and in settling down upon return. One mother of twins was planning a vacation trip and was both excited and worried. She felt that a change of scene would be good for her and her husband but that the requirements of daily living might make her life harder in a new setting where she would not have access to all the equipment she had at home and where the twins' schedule would be disrupted. Several women said that they would rather stay at home with their babies than go out socially. One went so far as to say that she planned to stay at home until the child was at least six months old, at which time she would begin to go out for short periods. In the meantime, her husband would maintain the couple's social interests alone.

Ambivalent feelings were manifest before pregnancy, during gestation, and after the child was born. Expressions of contradictory feelings were directed not only toward the child but toward the husband, the work situation, visitors, social situations, relatives, and breast feeding. One woman described spending alternate half hours marveling at her child and wondering what she had done to her life. In short, ambivalence was a part of the everyday lives of these women and resulted in their marked concern for the future.

CONCERN FOR THE FUTURE

Both this group of professional women and the women interviewed for Chapter 14, who regarded motherhood as a full-time profession, expressed concern for the future. The nature of their concerns differed, however. While the women described in the previous chapter wondered if they would adequately fulfill their mothering role, the professional women questioned their ability to successfully integrate two roles. As the day of returning to work approached, the women questioned their ability to resume their professional roles. Those who had returned to work prior to being interviewed found that they were received by their co-workers in a party spirit. These women were also surprised that they did not miss their children as much as they had anticipated.

Most women expressed concerns about being both mothers and women and fulfilling the expectations of both of these roles. One woman stated:

It's hard to feel like a woman when you're so wrapped up in being a mother.

In defining, formulating, and experiencing the mother role, the energy available to a woman for other roles is diminished. All but one of the women interviewed expressed concern for their future relationships with their husbands. All thought their relationships with their husbands had changed. While they were not sure if the relationship had improved, all felt that having gone through the pregnancy, labor, and delivery together was a positive experience.

However, this intimacy was soon lost when the excitement wore off and the period of adjustment began. One man was very busy with work and social activities; prior to the birth, the wife had shared these interests, but now she spent her time at home with the baby.

These professional woman mothers expressed a great deal of concern over the psychological development of their children. One mother of twins was concerned about the long-range psychological consequences of her approach to each child. She feared that if she thinks of either child as aggressive or easy-going, for example, her thoughts will become self-fulfilling prophecies. She and her husband also disagreed about the way he acted toward the twins. As a result, she quarreled with him more than before the birth. On the other hand, one husband complained:

I haven't gained a son; I've lost a wife.

His wife spent her entire day holding the baby.

The high expectations these women set for their children, as for themselves, were apparent in their concern for their infants' developmental achievements. Several women even discussed college plans for their children. Their soft voices, qualified statements, and sometimes questioning expressions reflected the difficulties they were having identifying their mothering roles in the same way they identify with professional roles.

Some women had not thought about having other children; others knew exactly when subsequent births, if any, were planned. The mothers of twins stated that they had all the children they wanted and that, in fact, having twins seemed an efficient way for a professional woman to complete her child-bearing tasks. Other mothers felt that a two- to four-year interval between children is optimal family planning.

The concerns expressed by these mothers were many. Some stemmed from their fears of resuming a professional role. Others focused on their relationships with their husbands. Still others related to the satisfactory development of the child. The high achievement orientation of these women carried over to their children and to their families and was expressed in their conviction that "it will all work out over time."

EXPERIENCES IN THE HOSPITAL SETTING

Accustomed to having a high degree of control over their lives, the women found themselves reduced, when hospitalized, to the common denominator of patient and therefore not entitled to basic information about themselves or their babies. When questioned about the nurse's role in prenatal, delivery, and postpartum care, the women's perceptions of the ability and interest of nurses to help them were limited. One woman described the nurses she had met:

They were nice — at least the ones who waited on me.

Another woman stated:

The only time the nurses came in was on the first day after delivery and then only to push stool softeners. They didn't encourage me, but they didn't discourage me either.

Another woman said of nurses:

They would answer my questions and bring me whatever I needed.

Certainly these women did not perceive nurses to be actively involved with them.

Most women saw their obstetricians at least once a month before delivery. Although many nurses work in obstetricians' offices and theoretically could offer assistance, no respondent mentioned any nurse who was helpful during their visits. The obstetrician and the Lamaze instructors were the only people they identified as helpful to them in assuming the new role of mother.

One of the women who had twins said that when the presence of two babies was confirmed by x-ray, she was excitedly greeted by her doctor and staff while her own feelings of ambivalence, fear, and being overwhelmed were ignored. She remarked:

I brought back the x-ray, and he said there were twins there for sure. He was overjoyed. I know that he loves children, and the nurse was overjoyed. I wasn't. I felt like they expected me to be more overjoyed, and I wasn't sure. I wasn't prepared for it.

Neither mother of twins considered anyone to be particularly helpful or interested in their feelings. The twins were greeted by the hospital staff with such comments as, "Aren't they adorable?", "Isn't it exciting?", and "Do they look alike?" It was as though having twins and the natural excitement about them resulted in the mother's being even more ignored than usual.

Being identified as a woman who has gone through Lamaze preparation for childbirth was an asset or a liability for the women depending on the nursing staff's perceptions and feelings about this mode of preparation. Upon admission, one woman was told: "Oh, we love you Lamaze people." In contrast, others were obviously degraded by the nursing staff with such comments as, "Oh, you Lamaze people, you think you are so smart." Another woman was greeted with the comment:

Well, you can try it [Lamaze], but don't expect it to work. When the pain comes, it won't work.

It was almost as if the women's preparation in Lamaze classes was part of a power struggle between the nurses and themselves, as if the nurses expected that in the pain of birth the women would be forced to need what the nurses had to offer and could not be self-sufficient.

The postpartum period in the hospital setting was equally troublesome. Either the women's questions were unanswered, or the women were instructed to ask their doctors about the health of their babies. With only one exception, the women were helped with breast feeding only if they requested help. They were offered no unsolicited instructions on rotating the baby or length of time to feed or any practical advice on breast feeding.

Several of the newborns had jaundice, which was particularly upsetting to their mothers. When questioned, nurses refused to provide the women with information and referred them to their pediatricians. For these mothers, with their high expectations for themselves and for their babies, any indication of imperfection was particularly threatening. One mother described her feelings:

There was a moment of alarm. I would have welcomed a little support during that. A few nurses, when badgered, would give a little information, but nobody came in and made an effort to discuss the problem and how frequently it happened.

When one set of twins was judged too small to go home from the hospital, no hospital staff member provided support or showed an understanding of the mother's distress at leaving her babies behind. When she returned to visit, she was allowed to view them only as a stranger behind a glass partition.

Several women mentioned crying frequently in the postpartum period, but only one reported that a nurse noted her state or responded to her tears. While the hospital staff's failure to respond to psychological needs may be no surprise, we would expect that the practical aspects of caring for a baby would be addressed by the hospital staff. Yet most women reported that they were not taught such basic skills as how to give a bath or change a diaper. Perhaps the staff failed to perceive the particular needs of women who are highly educated professionals and assumed that such women would know such basic things, but our study indicates that this assumption is not warranted.

The professional woman who becomes a mother must add another role to an already complex set of interlocking roles. The addition requires that the woman maintain a tight control over all of her roles to adequately meet multiple role expectations. The professional woman views motherhood as another role to be managed at the same high level of competence as she manages her other roles. Unlike the mothers described in Chapter 14, who surrender all other roles to focus solely upon mothering, these women try to reach a compromise between multiple and sometimes conflicting role demands. Their lives are hectic and fraught with concerns about themselves, their marriages, their children, and their futures as professional women. They receive little help from friends, relatives, husbands, or health professionals, who apparently anticipate that such highly competent people have the capability to manage almost anything and therefore do not need outside support. Ironically, these professional women, perhaps more than other women, need assistance in sorting through their very complicated, demanding lives and specific guidance in learning child care techniques.

V. The Child Rearing and Child Launching Family. The parenting

years offer a rich variety of experiences. Once the initial newness and excitement of becoming a parent has passed, individuals begin the ongoing adjustment to the everyday tasks of parenting. Above all, parenting is regarded by those engaged in it as a profound responsibility requiring much effort if it is to be successful. Moreover, it is regarded as somewhat of a gamble in that there is no guarantee that any amount of hard work and dedication will necessarily culminate in the kind of person the parents had hoped to raise. Thus, while parents speak at length about the heavy responsibilities of their role, they attribute a sizable portion of their ultimate success or failure to luck. This theme is especially apparent in Chapter 20, where we see empty-nest parents often referring to themselves as "lucky" that their children have become reasonably happy and responsible adults who have gone on to establish families of their own.

Parenthood brings about interesting changes in the individual's perception of the couple relationship. The couples in Chapter 16 credit the parenting experience for bringing an added depth of meaning to their marital bond. They view parenthood as both contributing to the quality of the marital relationship and providing an important motivation to keep that relationship viable. Interestingly, at the same time these parents were reporting the positive impact of children on their relationship, empty-nest couples were noting how no longer having children at home had enhanced their relationship to one another. Thus one of the more interesting and surprising findings brought out in this part is that couples interpret both the advent and departure of children as positive factors in their lives.

While Chapters 16 and 20 look at parenting from the perspective of the mother-father unit, two other chapters consider these roles separately. Chapter 17 discusses fathering and how men who are fathers view and enact that role. Chapter 18 addresses the situation of women who simultaneously maintain family and professional role commitments. Finally, since the individuals interviewed either identified or experienced or anticipated adolescence as especially difficult years for parenting, we present here a dual perspective on this situation. Chapters 16 and 20 include data on the parents' views about dealing with teenagers, and Chapter 19 presents the young person's perspective on the situation. In the end, adolescence emerges as a difficult, often painful, but also rewarding period for all involved. Taken together, these chapters address some of the key issues associated with enacting parenting roles. By looking at parenthood from the perspective of those actually engaged in it, we have been able to portray it as a role that is neither overly idealized nor unnecessarily grim.

235

16. Parenthood: Mother-Father Interaction.

Dorothy D. Camilleri and Mary M. Glenn

In this chapter, our attention turns to the matter of what it is like being a parent. Parenthood is generally acknowledged to be a major phase of life, one that most adults eventually experience. Its place in the institution of the family has been debated in recent years, as has the position of the family itself as a social institution. A common argument asserts that parenthood is an essential ingredient of the family and that the family is an essential means for society to perpetuate itself. This view emphasizes the family's role as a source of the nurturance and socialization that must be provided to each succeeding generation if society is to continue. Parenting thus is the role set through which socialization is carried out, the social cement without which the family would not be able to perform the functions it has been assigned by society.

Other viewpoints consider the family to consist of primary relationships that are strong enough to maintain the viability of the family even though no offspring are produced and nurtured. From this point of view, parenthood is one of several relationships that are equally important to the concept of family. The family stands as the epitome of committed, intimate, holistic relations even when procreation and parenthood are not among its tasks.

In the past parenthood has been regarded from a number of points of view, which have shed little light on the realities or significance of the parenting roles for the people engaged in them. Parenthood has been romanticized as a joyous, fulfilling experience, moralized about as a duty to one's God or social order, and despaired over as a thankless, dreary task. It has been cautioned against as courting ecologically disastrous overpopulation and has been regarded as simply the result of an automatic, biologically determined drive. Clearly, it has been neither well documented nor well understood in terms of the variety of its performance or its effects on the lives of the people it involves.

The research reported in this chapter is intended as a step toward remedying this situation. Our inquiry into parenting is from the perspective of the people now performing as parents. Our focus is that period of time after the initial adjustments to parenthood have been made and before the empty-nest syndrome sets in. More specifically, all the parents interviewed for this chapter had had at least twenty months as parents, and all of them had at least one child who was still living at home and was not older than the early teens.

These particular limits grew out of the purpose of our inquiry. Our goal was to discover as much as we could about the place and significance of parenthood in the lives of those acting as parents. Our interest in capturing these experiences while they were still current led us to eliminate parents who were just entering or just exiting that role. It is a well-known fact that our assessment of any specific experience is not constant; our view changes as our milieu or developmental stage changes. It has been said that memory organizes past experience in the service of present needs, fears, and interests [1]. Thus we might assume that reports of parenting would vary depending on whether the parent was anticipating, actually engaged in, or looking back on his or her parenting career. Our goal was to understand the realities of parenting for those currently engaged in it.

We sought to discover what being a parent meant to the parents interviewed and, specifically, what kinds of changes parenthood had caused in any and all aspects of their lives. We wanted to know whether the realities of parenting were congruent with their expectations and what those expectations were. We asked what they thought parenting required of them, how they had learned it, and how they had negotiated the mothering and fathering roles they played with their children and with one another. No attempt has been made here to judge the quality of the parenting involved or to include the viewpoint of the children.

A discussion of the method we used in collecting data and a description of the kind of people we interviewed precedes our discussion because parenthood viewed by parents from backgrounds different from those we interviewed could yield quite different results. The data are discussed in three parts: attitudes about parenthood, values and commitment, and parenting style. Each focuses on content — what the parents do in the setting within which their parenting occurs — and mechanics — *how* their parenting is performed. The first two parts focus more on content and the third part more on mechanics.

THE PARENT SAMPLE

The data reported in this chapter were collected during unstructured interviews with a total of 34 individual parents who constituted 18 parenting units; that is, two of the parenting units consisted of the mother alone. One of those mothers had never been married to or established a household with the father of her child; the other had been widowed for about eighteen months before the interview. The remaining 16 parenting units consisted of a married mother and father. Interviews with the two mothers were, of course, conducted individually; interviews with the remaining 16 parenting units were conducted with both parents present.

There were both advantages and disadvantages in interviewing parents together. The presence of a partner may sometimes improve the accuracy of the reporting, but at other times it will cause omissions to occur. There is always the possibility that one partner will fail to report some piece of information because he or she does not want the other partner to hear. On the other hand, exaggerated or one-sided accounts are discouraged since the partner is there to correct gross distortions. Ideally, we would have attempted to maximize the advantages and minimize the disadvantages by conducting three interviews per parenting couple: one with the mother, one with the father, and one with both parents present. But because of the lack of time these parents had, particularly the fathers, we opted for one joint interview, a decision we felt would encourage participation in the study.

During the interview, care was taken to secure input from both parents on each topic. In instances when one parent seemed to be doing most of the talking about a particular topic, the reticent partner was asked directly about how close his or her own thoughts were to the view being expressed. The latter was asked to identify differences and to add any other thoughts he or she had on the subject.

The interview itself was structured only in identifying key areas that the respondents were to address. Sometimes the interviewer introduced a topic using a lead question from the interview guide; frequently, however, respondents spontaneously discussed a topic without being directly stimulated to do so by the interviewer. Some of the topics discussed were identified earlier in this chapter. A copy of the interview guide appears in the Appendix. In general, the respondents were encouraged to talk about the topics from their own unique perspectives, based on their own experience, without regard for what they thought would be true for most other persons.

In addition to the topics already mentioned, the parents were questioned concerning their goals for marriage, ideas about good parenting, opinions about the advantages and disadvantages of having children, and the kinds of parenting models they had available before they had their first child. They were then asked to talk about these same topics as they saw them at present. They were asked to talk about their relationships with friends and family members before and after the birth of children. They were also asked about the conflicts they had with their children or one another as parents and how they negotiated these conflicts.

The parents in this study were more representative of middle-class suburban America than of any other group. Incomes for the group were all above poverty level, and most families had comfortable, middle-class incomes and living quarters. None of the families were from rural areas. All were from the suburbs of Chicago except two, who lived in the city itself. One family lived in an apartment, and the rest had their own homes. As is the case

nationally, the one-parent families headed by women were the least economically secure.

The educational levels of the parents interviewed were higher than would
be expected in the population at large. One of the women, the oldest, had
not completed high school, and three other individuals had had no formal
education beyond high school. But the remaining thirty had had at least
some college education, and some had more than one degree. In only one
of the two-parent families did neither parent have at least a bachelor's degree.

In addition to having more education than the population at large, this
sample was probably older than a comparable sample of parents with children not older than mid-teens would be. Most of the parents were in their
30s and 40s, with some in their 50s. One mother was 29. While most child-
bearing in the United States is completed while the mother is in her 20s,
five of our couples did not begin having children until the mother was at least
30. The number of children in these families ranged from one to ten. The
greatest age spread for children in one family was, not unexpectedly, in the
family with ten children; the oldest child was 33, and the youngest were
twins of 11. Most of the parents had four or fewer children. The exceptions,
in addition to the ten-child family already noted, were one family of seven
children and another of six children.

It was not the intent of this study to inquire into the issue of employment
of mothers outside the home, but the subject came up frequently, with varying degrees of primacy. All the fathers were employed and regarded their
economic contribution to their families as an important part of their role. The
situation was much more variable for the mothers. The mothers ran the gamut
of involvement in outside employment from very career-oriented, full-time
workers to women who had no interest in such work. At the time of the
interview, seven of the women were employed full-time, and eleven were not
working.

Some of these nonworking women had been engaged in pursuing a career
at an earlier point in their lives and had stopped when their first child was
born. Others had never had an occupational identity or work career. It was
common for these unemployed women and their partners to define the
women's homemaking and mothering activities as constituting a full-time
work load that would not permit an outside work commitment, but there
were exceptions to this view. One woman was at a disappointing and frustrating plateau in her career before her child was born and now finds her involvement in home and hearth to be an exhilarating experience. She plans to rein-
vest in her career if and when her assessment of staying at home changes.

The absorption of the unemployed group of women in homemaking and
mothering activities did not have the same meaning for all the women. Some
thought that such activities provided sufficient bedrock from which to
build a complete and satisfying identity as a woman. Others did not find
them a sufficiently nourishing basis for a complete identity and looked
forward to adding new dimensions or renewing old interests as their children
grew older. One of these latter women had a pair of pedigreed dogs and

planned to develop a business of breeding and selling dogs as her family grew older. Similarly, a woman who had run a church-connected music program before her children, of elementary school age, had been born lamented the fact that she had neglected her musical career over the years. She felt that her abilities had withered beyond repair because of the lack of attention and practice and that she had lost her professional standing and identity in the field. She identified this area as the one in her life that she would change if she could repeat her parenting career.

At least some of these women who planned to return to work were influenced by their wish to be able to let go of their children in comfort when the time for their children's independence came. They felt they would need something to replace the mothering busyness, and their thinking along this line can well be considered as anticipating the next stage of their lives. It is noteworthy that what would serve as replacement varied. An occupational involvement was desired by some women; others desired a community interest or hobby.

Some of the women who were basically disinterested in outside employment had worked on occasion since they became mothers in order to supplement the family income. The mothers of the larger families were in this category, and part-time clerking in stores was the kind of work they had done. This work seemed to serve a useful economic function for these families but added little to the basic identity of the women involved.

Perhaps the crucial difference between the group of women who were employed and the group who were currently unemployed lies in the way the two groups regarded the relative importance of the two segments of their lives: mothering-homemaking and professional-occupational. The unemployed women tended to view the mothering-homemaking aspects of their lives as having a top priority and a justified claim on their total allegiance; when present, their occupational aspirations were secondary and were to be acted on only when the more important mothering-homemaking responsibilities allowed for it. The employed mothers accorded a more central position to the professional-occupational segments of their lives. They regarded such endeavors as important parts of themselves as persons and as worthy of the required adjustments in other aspects of their living situations. This difference in emphasis did not necessarily entail their willingness to abrogate their mothering; it meant that they believed that with some juggling, families and occupations could both be reasonably well tended.

The position the employed women accorded their occupational identities and careers varied. The occupational endeavors of three women were just as strong as has traditionally been the case for men. Just as the men took for granted their work role outside their families, so did these three women. While our data include no information about the source of this orientation for the women involved, they do verify that each woman's occupational intentions were a matter of negotiation or disclosure before marriage. The partners of these women supported their wives' occupational commitments.

For example, when discussing their marriage, one couple said:

He: We had advanced considerably in the, you know, meeting of the minds, becoming more compatible, working toward [career] goals. She was working toward the things she was interested in; I was working toward the things that I was interested in.

She: I don't think either of us felt that we were so tied that we couldn't just do things without one another; so he had his career kinds of things, and I had mine, and we supported each other in them.

Some of these women regarded working as a welcome restorative break from the daily home routine and as a chance to vary their contacts. Working was particularly tension-reducing for one woman, whose small children were close in age and whose husband traveled a great deal. In general, however, knowledge of a woman's occupational status was not particularly helpful in predicting other characteristics about the parenting couple.

ATTITUDES ABOUT PARENTHOOD

For the parents interviewed, parenthood was a natural and desirable part of their life pattern. For some, it was the culmination of the purpose of their lives. For all, it was a most serious and absorbing undertaking, one that became a primary focus for the organization of their activities. The fact that parenthood was a chosen status, viewed positively by the overwhelming number of persons interviewed, made it no less a serious undertaking. Two men stated:

The test, you know, it's almost like death, the finished product; you're going to be 73 years old [before you know] if it turned out all right. That's something that you just wonder every day whether you're doing the right thing in molding these six people around here so they are going to make some sort of contribution to society. And you don't know. You know, they could all turn out to be rummies. That's true.

The character traits that we'd like to see developed — that's a lifelong struggle. We won't have any clues until well after the fact whether we've created these qualities.

Even when the desired qualities were displayed by children, the parents remained watchful lest subsequent influences change those qualities or other undesirable qualities develop. Two men noted:

About the time we think we've got it made, we stumble.

If they can learn the good things, they can learn the bad things. If they got in with the wrong group. . . .

The behavior of the child was an indicator to parents of the success of their

parenting. This rather stringent criterion held true in spite of acknowl-
edgments that parents can make all the correct moves and still have a child
who does not turn out well. One woman admitted:

We have friends whose kids . . . have consistently made very, very bad choices
in spite of what their parents have tried to teach and are now having real
problems. So in our case we might be able to evaluate [how good our
parenting is] according to L.'s behavior. But for somebody else, that
might be very bad, you know.

Parents tended to consider deviations from the desirable as indications of
poor parenting on their part. One woman's comment is representative:

When the oldest ones were little, and if I had known I was going to have six,
I think I would have been more consistent in punishment with them, or
something. Because now, I find it's a real battle getting them to do something.

The parents also thought that the child's behavior, whether desirable or not,
could be a reflection of qualities harbored by the parents. One man said:

The truth hurts, you know. The truth hurts. And your children are a mirror
of you. And so I look at them, and I see my qualities in them, and I don't
like it sometimes. Sometimes I do.

All these elements combined to heighten the parents' concern about the characteristics and abilities developed by their children throughout childhood,
and, particularly, as they left adolescence. Clearly, the characteristics
displayed by the children were considered a measure of the degree of success
the parents had had in discharging their responsibility. The characteristics
identified as having this significance were so broad as to include any possible
area of growth and development. Traditional academic skills, such as reading
and school achievement were mentioned, but so were social skills, such
as the acquisition of manners, the ability to make friends and to fit into
social groups, and cultural achievements, such as music and art. One man
said proudly:

It was easy for us to go to a restaurant with five or six kids, and sit down
and watch all the heads turn, and everybody enjoyed themselves. The kids
ate with knives and forks, and they didn't stick them in their ears and most
of the food stayed on the plates. Just a thoroughly enjoyable experience.

Perhaps most important to parents, however, was the inculcation of values,
this having considerable overlap with the related area of guiding children so
that they acquired personality traits reflecting the virtues required to succeed
in society. Evidences of the latter were considered good and were eagerly
looked for by parents. Obedience, independence, and responsibility or
reliability were commonly mentioned in this regard, and parents frequently

arranged tasks so that these good character traits would be stimulated. These tasks included household maintenance tasks, care of pets, and faithful participation in extracurricular activities.

Providing discipline for children was the single most commonly mentioned function or concern of parenting. Usually introduced by the father, it was typically discussed as a necessary part of the structure children needed to develop desired qualities. While parents endorsed its need, they were often displeased with the issue of discipline in their families, finding it difficult to recognize and maintain a middle ground between too strict and too lenient. For some families, discipline was an interesting joint accommodation. Often the mother would ask a child to perform some task or obey some family regulation and be more or less ignored. The father would then either discover this for himself or be told by the mother and bring some greater force to bear on the child, thus getting some action. In so doing, he was defining himself and being defined by the others as the disciplinarian. This behavior was actually in response to an either explicit or implicit signal for help from the mother.

Parents emphasized the importance of imparting a sound value system and character traits that they saw as particularly needed by the child because of the great number of potential dangers in society. They felt children are exposed to more stimulation and freedom now than was the case formerly, and face a more complex social era. One couple stated:

She: Anticipating high school has got me.

He: There are a lot of problems that weren't even around when we were in school. You know, the sexual revolution. These are all things these kids are going to have to cope with.

She: The kids are so much smarter, and they are freer.

One man said:

I feel sorry for the things, the problems, that these children are going to face. They are much more serious than we're facing in our generation.

As we examined parental statements about the task of parenting, particularly those about what must be learned by the children, it became clear that the goal of parenting for most of these parents was to produce young adults who are essentially like the parent — that is, they hold the same value system, attitudes, and character traits as do the parents but do not have the traits the parents consider unfavorable in themselves. When unfavorable traits appeared in the children, the parents tried to eliminate them. Keeping children on a suitable path was viewed as the primary responsibility of parenthood, and the respondents defined potential threats to this endeavor as a problem.

It was this concern about the desirable outcome for children that led to the parents' designation of adolescence as the most difficult **age**. For some parents, the concern was anticipatory, based on what they had heard; for others, it had been experienced. All parents who had children near or in adolescence noted the growing independence of their children. While some nurtured and enjoyed this development, they still noted the lessened influence they had on their children, the greater the propensity for them to side with opposing values of peers against the values of the parents, and the greater the likelihood of defiant behavior. While the moodiness and changeability of the adolescent were mentioned, it was not the major problem that parents experienced at the stage. The lessened control parents had over their children's behavior was the real difficulty.

One father, who felt the world was not a good place into which to introduce a new life, identified child rearing as growing worse at each succeeding phase of a child's life. He identified his teenage daughter's present stage as the worst because she was facing more of the world than she had previously. This man stated:

I think it [this stage] is much more difficult than when she was not a teenager. . . . she has to start dealing with her peers on a more adult level, and my own estimation of the peer group is that it's a wretched lot at best. [Laugh] The more I see of them, the more disgusted I get. So it's a − I vacillate between being appalled and despairing.

This man's position is extreme, but many of the parents interviewed would have some sympathy for his discomfort with his daughter's peers and did feel a sense of trepidation about the influence of peer groups on their children.

The adolescent age is difficult not only because children can be more defiant and influenced more by peers than by parents but also because the parents cannot protect the children through their supervision the way they could during earlier stages. One man remarked:

It's hard to stand by and watch them stumble when you know it's coming; when you know he's going to perform poorly at the next day's match [wrestling] because he's watching late TV instead of getting to bed like he knows he's supposed to; it's hard not to take over. But you just hope these small falls now will prevent really big ones later on. Because they really won't listen to you; they've got to find out themselves.

While most parents identified adolescence as the bête noire of parenting, many with experience acknowledged it was a time when their children could be particularly gratifying to them, since they were now interesting companions with whom stimulating exchanges of ideas could take place. When this stimulating exchange did not proceed to the child's abandoning or violating the parents' value system, it was viewed positively.

Another age identified by some as troublesome and by others as simply not interesting was infancy. Some parents had difficulty in knowing just what infants were needing, feeling, or wanting. For these individuals, the infant's signals were not easily interpretable, and these parents experienced more helplessness in caring for their babies than they were comfortable with. More men than women reported this discomfort, but some mothers did identify it as a problem. These parents' enjoyment of their children grew as verbal abilities increased and language communication was possible. A substantial minority of parents, particularly fathers, identified the infancy period as simply less interesting than subsequent ones.

The few individuals who identified themselves as not wanting children before their children were born cited the overwhelming responsibilities of bringing a life into this world as the principal source for their feeling that the infant stage was troublesome or uninteresting. One man stated:

He: I did not want children. I felt that the world was a very bad place to bring any life to.

Int: And what, for you, would be the disadvantages?

He: The responsibility that naturally ensues.

VALUES AND COMMITMENT

The parents interviewed possessed a set of related ideas concerning the nature of the family and the meaning of that concept in their lives. These ideas reflected a general commitment to having children. Before they married, the overwhelming majority of these parents had harbored ideas about the desirability of having children. Although before marriage many had not made detailed plans about having children, they indicated that the subject of having children had come up prior to marriage and had been endorsed by both partners at least in a general way. Intentionally or not, they evaluated each other's willingness or suitability to be a parent.

Most couples could not recall how this evaluation took place or even that they went through such a process. Yet evidence of the process occurred frequently enough to suggest that it was the rule, not the exception, and that it was not limited to suitability as a parent. The couples in this study seemed to have measured each other in relation to many issues and to have satisfied themselves that sufficient similarity or compatibility existed on key issues. Whether to have children was one of the key issues. The couples who did not have becoming parents in mind when they got married had also managed to communicate this information before marriage and were just as vague as the children-oriented couples about how they did it.

Two methods were used to evaluate the partners' commitment to having children. First, conversations took place that on an overt level were somewhat casual and not to be taken as serious negotiation. On a covert level, however, these conversations transmitted needed information about the partners' positions on relevant topics and allowed them to make judgments about the distance between them. Second, behavioral cues were noted and processed in a similar fashion. One woman said:

My little sister was only 5, and I remember him [husband] telling me what
a little stinker she could be. And B. [husband] was very good with her already
and didn't mind her teasing us.

Most parents verbalized the intentions they had to have children before their
first child was conceived, and even though the timing was not planned in
many cases (no particular attempt was made to conceive a child), the birth of
most of their children could hardly be considered to be accidental. Some
of these intentions were so nebulous that they would be better classified
as general predispositions. The woman whose child was born out of wedlock
said:

I had never really thought about it before, except that I thought I wanted some
children at some time. . . . I guess every girl grows up that way, with this
thought, you know — for a meaningful life you have to have some children.

This woman, who held no convictions against abortion, never considered
abortion for herself when she became pregnant, although other people did
suggest that option to her at the time.

Other couples' intentions to have children were more definite. One woman
stated:

I can remember discussing the number and sexes we wanted before we ever
got married.

Perhaps the feeling of almost all parents can best be captured in these words
of one woman:

I didn't really see having life without children, growing older and just having
ourselves.

The exceptions to this general feeling were very few. One couple at the time
of marriage were concerned lest children be too much of an encumbrance
on them. They became positively disposed toward children only after three
or four years of freedom, during which they came to define their life-style
as not being sufficiently goal-directed and meaningful.

These favorable dispositions toward having children seemed to be an out-
growth of the parents' views about the desirable or "good" life. The family
was their means of achieving the good life, and for most, children were an
essential ingredient for the establishment of a family. One man stated:

I didn't have a family, see? A family to me was constructed when you have
brothers and sisters. Parents have nothing to do with it. . . . I'm serious. I
didn't have a family when I was a little kid as far as I was concerned because
there was only me.

While no one else was willing to discount parents as "family," a number of individuals indicated that having more than one child in a family enhanced its ability to generate closeness.

The family was the matrix through which the parents satisfied their own needs for sharing warm, caring, and safe relations with other people, and it gave the major direction and meaning to their lives. They usually married for a sense of family, and when asked what they had hoped for from marriage, they typically mentioned goals that can be regarded as part of an affectively positive, secure interpersonal relationship. Goals such as "companionship," "partner," and "someone to share with" were common. The data on this point certainly support the view of man as a social animal, highly motivated to avoid loneliness. The family itself was seen as a sheltering citadel for all its members, one that enabled them to function comfortably in the larger society.

Families gave these parents a sense of continuity with the past. They continued in their own families those aspects of their past that they considered valuable and felt they were contributing to a heritage that would carry on through future generations. In general, the importance of the family is perhaps best expressed in the words of one man:

You stop to analyze what it's all about, when it comes right down to it, you can probably name fifty or a hundred different things that people might have in mind as their goals for life. But nothing really is permanent except a family. You have a family forever. Unless some tragedy occurs or something like that, you know. But family is what it's all about. And so, some people choose not to get married, and I try to think of myself in those positions at say 60 or 65, and there's nothing there, you know.

Although parents talked about recapturing a warmth or closeness they had experienced or witnessed in other families when they themselves were children, they did not maintain particularly close ties with members of their families of origin. More often than not, it was the nuclear family of their creation, and not other relatives in a more extended network, that they felt to be the successor to this closeness. Relationships with relatives were individualized, depending on feelings about the particular relative. The mobility that characterizes modern society certainly reinforces these tendencies. The fact that the parents' families of origin were usually scattered over a wide geographic area made frequent physical contact impossible.

One final note about commitment to family and children: the early experiences of these parents with their own parents did not seem to make much difference in their level of commitment to being a parent. When the parents interviewed disapproved of the kind of parenting they had experienced, they simply resolved to behave differently when they had their own children.

PARENTING STYLES

This section focuses more on the structure or mechanics of parenting than on its substance or content. Here, too, there is ample evidence of an evaluation process between the parents that more often than not went unnoticed by them. The parents typically reported their division of labor was an unplanned state of affairs that had evolved rather than a system they had negotiated. They discussed their roles as though those roles had evolved independently of the persons occupying them. Some acknowledged the fact that their division of labor was strongly influenced by the partners' availability (depending on demands of job, student status, number of children) to perform the various tasks to be done. But even adjustments based on such factors were most often handled on a nonverbal level. Task allocation became a matter of discussion when one partner felt that the prevailing arrangement was unduly burdensome and the other partner had failed to notice the nonverbal cues given and to adjust his or her behavior accordingly. Even then, the individuals did not recognize their negotiation of roles and tasks openly. Generally, the parents' descriptions of how their roles evolved reflected the attitude of one man, who said:

But you can't explain these things. I mean, you can't, you can't give a reason for it or a scientific principle or anything else.

This lack of clarity about the manner in which role decisions were made was an almost unanimous characteristic, although some of the parents reported more conscious awareness than others. The most thoughtful reports came from a family in which the role allocations had come to be associated with conflict and in which the parents had had to engage in a sorting out process regarding their priorities and needs. The following exchange illustrates a rather typical description of the manner in which roles were determined:

Int: Well, who did the diapering?

She: Well, we both did. I did it 90 percent of the time, but the 10 percent I wasn't around, H. was glad to lend a hand.

Int: But if you were around, is that something that you always did?

She: Yes, I just automatically did it, unless I was busy, or if I was busy doing something else and . . .

Int: But that was something you never discussed; it just sort of happened?

She: Right.

Int: I'm interested in how these roles get negotiated. Did you ever discuss what everyone was going to do, or did it just sort of happen that way?

249. Mother-Father Interaction

She: I assumed — I assumed the responsibility. I felt like it was my task. Like it was a woman's job. You know. And I assumed he would help me whenever I needed help with any of my tasks — Children, anything in the household. If I need help, he's always willing to help. And I try to help him, you know, with anything that I could help him with.

Int: [to him] So there are no areas that you feel that you take care of as opposed to your wife taking care of?

He: Well, no. No. I found it fun, you know, messing with the kids, giving them a bath once in a while. We never talked about it.

This example also illustrates other important facets of role arrangements, in addition to their amorphous character. First, even though it was not negotiated, there was a very definite structure to the task allocation in all the families studied. This does not imply that the roles were rigid; they were usually far from rigid. But they were definite. Parents really knew which one of them (or, in some instances, which child) would take out the garbage, fold the laundry, or supervise the children, even though they had no formalized plan for the accomplishment of each task.

Second, the role arrangements reflected the parents' notions of the proper functioning of a family, whatever those notions might be. These notions had been validated between them earlier by the evaluation process already described, with varying degrees of accuracy. When they drew reasonably accurate conclusions about each other's notions of child rearing, the parents could develop a common frame of reference and make adjustments to one another and to their situation fairly readily. In the example cited above, the woman stated that she automatically did the diapering, assuming it was the woman's role. Since she had never had cause to alter this assumption, her husband must have found it acceptable and molded his role to complement it. In many cases, parents said their similar backgrounds had provided them with common values so that they held similar views in such matters.

Because this system of role differentiation generally worked well for the parents interviewed, they hardly noticed the process of establishing roles at all. Many of the respondents thought the question rather peculiar in view of the automatic nature of roles. But process it is, a fact that can be illustrated by an example in which the partners' expectations did not prove to be accurate. One man said:

So, I found times like, again I was sitting in the home in California and I wouldn't hear R. [child] for awhile, you know. And I remember a time when I said, "Why in hell doesn't J. [wife] respond to this silence?" Here's R., she's out playing, she's 2 or 3, and we haven't heard any noise or anything, you know, . . . and I wondered. I found again and again, I was the one with the big motivation to get up and go find out what was going on, and at that point I realized that something innate within me said that if J. doesn't take up the ball — which, you know, nothing negative or any-

thing — but if she just doesn't, . . . then I have to. And not only that, I realized that I wanted to.

In this instance, tasks were reallocated as the husband came to take on some of the child care he had originally expected his wife to do.

Another factor about role negotiation was described by the parents interviewed. There are two kinds, or levels, of negotiation taking place. We have been discussing the initial, more basic one, which deals with the partners' all-encompassing but very generalized points of view that reflect basic values and sense of family. There is also the secondary and less emotionally involved negotiation based more on the particular abilities or likes of the negotiators than on the sense of what is proper for the particular role. For instance, once the partners agreed that daily household maintenance should be a joint enterprise, they could openly and easily negotiate specific jobs. One woman stated:

Well, we had to negotiate certain things, like he'll do the floors and wax them because he does that well. He doesn't like doing bathrooms; that's still my job. And because I do bathrooms, I think he can change the cat box . . . whoever has time does the vacuuming.

For most of the families studied, role arrangements were a flexible matter that reflected a team orientation to living together as a family. There was just one exception to this generalization; here male and female roles were very separate and had definite boundaries. A widow believed that the running of the house is woman's work and definitely not masculine, except in cases involving a woman's temporary incapacity. She stated:

He's got a purpose in life, he's the man, you know. When I used to go by my sister's, and her husband had an apron on, he'd be doing the dishes, he looked like a fairy to me.

The couples did not express this point of view, although their task allocation tended — by mutual agreement and because it was considered functional — to be somewhat traditional. The men were the breadwinners, a duty that kept them out of the home to some extent, and the women were the major child-rearers and home-makers. In those instances in which women shared the breadwinning role, a more even distribution of tasks involving running the home and caring for the children occurred. When the men were home, they assumed definite roles within their families and in maintaining their homes.

The team orientation was as striking a feature of the family organization as was the basically traditional task allocation. Many references were made to the family as a team, with everyone pitching in. For example, one woman said:

*Whatever had to be done, it got done. If [one] was busy, the other guy did
it . . . we work as a team.*

All members of the family were part of the team, and a significant portion
of parental socializing efforts were directed to getting their children to care
about that team and to regard their individual tasks as necessary to the
team's proper functioning. The children's tasks were assigned by their
parents, usually on the basis of promoting those characteristics that the
child had to acquire for success as an adult in our society.

The team orientation was quite consistent with the expectation of role
flexibility and balancing of the work load, at least between mother and
father. They started out with their own somewhat traditional roles, but
they expected each other to modify traditional roles and to take on each
other's work quite frequently. Basically, each partner was responsible for all
the tasks that needed doing in the family, and this feeling of responsibility
for the total functioning of the family unit resulted in some periodic shifting
of tasks from one partner to the other and some sharing of tasks between
partners as a balance was maintained in the amount of work each person
did. This sense of balance, rather than sex role typing, was sometimes the
determining factor in specific task allocation. For example, one woman said:

*He was working very hard. He was going to school, and he was holding down a
part-time job. And when he did come home, he was tired. And, you know,
you don't ask people then, when they're working very hard like that, to take
on extra things, you know. So everybody works hard, and you pull your
share of the load.*

Another woman remarked:

*Well, really, so many times, we haven't had specific roles. Now like if you
needed help painting the outside of the house, I was there to help, but if I
was bogged down by housework, J. [her husband] will take the mop and
mop the floor, you know.*

Rather than having to be asked to help, one partner frequently assessed the
situation and then stepped out of his or her usual role to help the other
partner with whatever job had to be done. One man stated:

*I probably don't do the dishes once a week, but there are times where I can
see she could just use the help; so I do the dishes.*

This flexibility is both a product and a reinforcement of the family as a team
and the sense of family solidarity that the majority of respondents had.

Conflict between parents about parenting, when it occurred, was usually
handled by discussing the problem until consensus was reached. In some
instances, a parent who felt less strongly about a particular issue would

give in, in which case it would be acknowledged that the issue was being handled in a certain way because of the strong feelings of one parent about it. Parents recalled very little conflict about important parenting issues; this consensus may reflect inaccurate recall of earlier experiences or establishment of a broad common frame of reference, and thus few conflicts. The parents themselves attributed the lack of major conflict to their similar backgrounds and value systems and to long-term knowledge of one another.

Yet not all couples were conflict-free. One couple admitted disagreeing about 90 percent of the time on discipline and other parenting matters. This couple was plagued by an inability to arrive at a consensus on issues other than those involving their children; indeed, they seemed much less disposed to fit their behavior one to another than did most of the parents interviewed. They attributed some of their difficulty to not having had sufficient time together as a couple before embarking on parenthood.

The majority of parents, while not considering their parenting careers to be without fault or failure, could identify no major changes they would make if they could begin their parenting careers again. Most of the changes that had occurred over time in their thinking about the ideal parent represented a softening, a more accepting attitude toward their children's behavior and their own.

In conclusion, the parents interviewed for this chapter addressed the meaning of parenthood in their lives by relating to the interviewers (1) their definitions of the task to be accomplished, (2) their values and definitions of family, which provided the context for the task, and (3) the particular arrangements and task allocation they instituted in carrying out their parenting. These parents defined parenting as a serious, engrossing task, one that results in the transformation of a helpless infant into a responsible adult — they hope, in their image. Their belief in the strength and worth of the family contributed to their feeling that parenting is a desirable, worthwhile occupation.

They saw their children as unifying assets, not as encumbrances that ruin the marital relationship. Their children became the focus of their joint commitment as they shared the task of parenting, and, when minimal conflict occurred about how that commitment should be carried out, the parents described themselves as being closer to one another because of the commitment. In essence, parenthood was a heavy but rewarding responsibility, one that was essential to their sense of family and gave them a feeling of goal direction and fulfillment. Many of the parents interviewed might have wondered, as one parent did, "how marriages stay together if they don't have children after a period of time."

The admonition to health care workers to consider or include the whole family when dealing with only one of its members has become a cliché that nurses hear so frequently it now conveys little meaning. Perhaps this chapter can help illuminate why that advice is given and can provide some clues about the kind of intervention that is useful for a family.

The parents studied did not seem to notice the everyday transactions and communications that occurred between them and seemed unaware that they had established any particular system for their families. They thought their roles grew out of the natural order of things, without any particular help from them. The data indicate, however, that their roles grew out of a continuous process in which some minimal common understandings were developed and an allocation of tasks in keeping with those understandings occurred. Several ramifications of this fact may be useful to nurses.

Nurses with knowledge of the underlying process can intervene at any or all of its steps, reinforcing its useful elements and helping to remedy its deficiencies. The whole matter of information exchange is open to intervention. For instance, we know that signals — information — are passed back and forth between individuals but that some individuals do not recognize the signals they send to others and some individuals cannot identify the signals to which they respond. Other individuals may signal incorrectly on purpose, because they do not want another person to know their true feeling for fear that person will not like that feeling. While the goal and result of this incorrect signaling may well be avoidance of conflict, people who use this technique habitually in managing their relationships often feel overburdened by the arrangement that they themselves have negotiated, and then the relationship they had tried to simplify becomes instead conflict-ridden. The experience of some mothers when setting limits for their children may fall in this category. These mothers may have stated a limit for a child that was largely ignored by the child, and the mother's subsequent behavior may have signaled that the child really did not have to obey the limit. The mothers may have expected obedience but grew concerned about being too harsh, and so did not follow through on the original task requirement. The upshot may be a feeling of resentment on the mothers' part and an inaccurate assessment of her true feelings on the child's part. The frequent use of incorrect — or mixed — signaling usually causes rather than eliminates problems.

In order to foster accurate information exchange, nurses could help individuals develop a high degree of accuracy in assessing others' positions on relevant issues. These assessments are an essential aspect of a couple's developing a common frame of reference. Those couples who have a common frame of reference have a much easier time with role negotiation and experience less conflict.

One ramification of the interdependence of roles concerns the changes in roles that health care workers may witness or attempt to induce. A change in one person will alter, to a greater or lesser degree, the roles played by everyone in the system, and a nurse's anticipatory guidance with families may help individuals to identify just what these alterations are likely to be and to predict their probable effect. Planning about how to restore a satisfactory balance in the system can then proceed.

Nurses interested in anticipatory guidance may well note the difficulty with adolescent children reported by the parents studied. Two elements of this difficulty may serve as foci for interaction between nurses and parents about this stage of development. The first has to do with the loss of control parents feel over how their children think, act, and feel about issues that have been important to the parents. The second concerns the independence of their children. These difficulties cannot be avoided; they seem to be a part of the "letting-go" process. Those parents who have limited outside interests can be encouraged to invest themselves in other endeavors in order to minimize some of the stress. In general, parents at this stage of their children's development need to have faith in their children's ability to learn from their own mistakes. Parents who seem unduly concerned may need help in viewing their children as essentially separate individuals who are responsible for themselves and their behavior and who are influenced by many things and people in addition to their parents.

Finally, it is important for nurses, who are in contact with people from a wide social, economic, and cultural spectrum, to note that the information presented here represents primarily an urban, educated, middle-class view of the matter of parenthood, which may not be congruent with the views of other groups. For example, when economic deprivation is an overriding concern, matters of money may be the basis for many of the values and decision making arrangements in the family. In any given situation, it is perhaps wise to determine what the individuals being cared for feel to be true of parenthood or of any other relevant values and life-styles. Doing so will enable the nurse to avoid one of the most common pitfalls in health care: recommending courses of action that cannot be followed because they violate a patient's ingrained principles or everyday practices.

REFERENCE

1. Elkin, F., and Handel, G. *The Child in Society: The Process of Socialization* (2nd ed.). New York: Random House, 1972.

17. How Fathers Perceive the Fathering Role. Constance Ritzman and Dorothy D. Camilleri

Until very recently there has been an obvious imbalance
in the literature on parenting. Compared with the profusion of books and
articles for and about mothering, there has been a dearth of material on
fatherhood. Traditionally, women have assumed the major responsibility for
the routine tasks of child rearing. Fathers, on the other hand, have been assigned the task of major breadwinner and final disciplinarian. In recent years,
as men and women have begun to embrace more flexible definitions of appropriate role behaviors, both popular and scholarly literature on parenting has
given more attention to fatherhood. Books on fathering have begun to appear
on the market as clinicians and scholars alike seek to share their views on the
role with those men engaged in it.

Such books are often prescriptive in nature, advising fathers on the "best"
way to fulfill their role. While such treatments are meant to be helpful, they
too often neglect the father's view of the situation. Intended to help remedy
this situation, this chapter examines fathering from the viewpoint of the
father himself.

The data on which this examination is based were gathered during intensive
interviews with thirty well-educated, middle-class men who were fathers. All
had bachelor's degrees, and nineteen graduate or professional degrees. Their
employment reflected their educational background. They were all pursuing
careers in either a profession, business, or academia. At the time of the interview they were between 25 and 36 years of age and were comfortably situ-
ated financially. The children of the men interviewed ranged in age from 1 to
12. All the men were part of intact families; no divorcés or widowers were
interviewed. Each man was interviewed alone in either his home or his office.
The interviews were tape-recorded, processed, and analyzed in the manner
described in Chapter 3.

This chapter discusses several key topics that emerged during the interviews. It begins with a brief description of the fathers' reactions to the pregnancy and birth experiences. The bulk of the chapter deals with how these men view the fathering role and themselves as fathers. Since all the men were part of two-parent families, this chapter also examines how these men interact with their wives in rearing children. An effort is made to document these men's experiences with health care personnel and to identify how such personnel can help fathers such as these carry out their fathering role.

ANTICIPATING FATHERHOOD DURING THE PREGNANCY

To a surprising extent, the men generally took their wife's pregnancy in stride as an expected occurrence. One man's statement is representative:

I think it's one of those things where you make a decision when you get married, that at a certain point in time you will have children. It's sort of anticipated. Maybe it's something you sort of float into, but you really don't consider the consequences.

In other words, all the men interviewed had always assumed that they would one day be fathers. While they greeted their wife's announcement of a pregnancy with varying degrees of enthusiasm, the news was predictable and certainly not overwhelming. Clearly, the popular image of the astonished young man who immediately begins to pamper his wife and look for a better paying job simply does not hold.

While the fathers acknowledged the financial responsibilities of fatherhood, they did not focus on these. Rather, they assumed they would be able to meet the financial burdens of parenthood and that to do so would not cause an inordinate number of problems.

In reflecting on their reaction to becoming fathers, these men emphasized the symbolic importance of this status passage. They defined becoming a parent as the final confirmation of their adulthood. For instance, one man stated:

It was a matter of pride and a sense of growing up. All of a sudden you're 21 years old and you are supposed to be an adult, but you are really not until this, because that is probably the biggest responsibility you'll have. You can take on a big financial burden, but as for an actual responsibility that is heartfelt, you don't have it unless you have a child or take care of somebody that you are responsible for.

These men viewed fatherhood as a normal adult developmental task. At this stage, they did not discuss it as a crisis or as presenting them with insurmountable actual or anticipated problems.

In addition to regarding fatherhood as a move toward full adult status, the men talked at some length about the changed life-style they had anticipated as a direct result of becoming fathers. One man remarked:

*Having a child really changes one's life; you realize you are no longer free to do
some of the things you want to do. In one case it meant postponing a lot of
things we wanted to do for about five years until the child was old enough.
There are hardships involved in terms of baby-sitters and sickness. But mainly
it's an inconvenience; you want to hurry up and get somewhere [but] you
have to drag him.*

Not only did the men have a fairly realistic picture of the various constraints
imposed on their life-styles by children, but they accepted these as simply
"part of the bargain."

The men stressed the normal, nontraumatic nature of becoming a father.
They did not paint an overly idyllic picture or imply that fatherhood was
problem free. Yet they also did not cast the adjustments of parenthood in a
crisis framework. Certainly, they anticipated encountering difficulties, but
they also anticipated being able to deal effectively with these in much the
same way they had dealt with difficult situations in the past.

THE BIRTH EVENT: LABOR AND DELIVERY

Considerable variation was evident in the men's experiences with their wives'
labor and delivery. Nonetheless, certain patterns were apparent. The men had
one of two basic orientations to the birth of their child. The first orientation
we shall call traditional, that is, the pregnancy and birth were conducted in
the prevailing, medically prescribed manner: both parents had a somewhat
passive role, a doctor supervised the course of the pregnancy and delivery, and
the delivery itself was managed by health care professionals who took charge
of mother and child. The second orientation we shall call participatory to
focus attention on the one difference between it and the traditional approach:
both parents assumed an active role. These parents sought to manage the
course of events during labor and delivery themselves rather than relying
entirely on health care personnel to direct the process. They tended to regard
health care personnel as assisting with the process rather than as taking it
over completely. This orientation involved — to varying degrees — the man's
participation in his wife's preparation for labor and delivery (such as childbirth education classes) so that he could coach her and give her moral support
during the labor and delivery, his learning about the physiological processes
and chain of events that constitute the birth event, and his learning something about newborn babies. The fathers who assumed the traditional, more
passive role were, in contrast, outside the main arena of activity as far as
giving birth was concerned. When they were in the labor room, they were simply
witnesses, not helpmates. The actively participating fathers had a more vital
role, which tended to give them a more central position. Of course, variations
occurred. Not all these latter men participated to the same degree, but all did
feel a basic sense of participation. One characteristic of the participating fathers
was that they wanted to and usually did see their babies being born — an
exhilarating experience indeed, according to the fathers' reports.

Some of the fathers in the traditional group would have preferred greater involvement in their wife's labor and delivery. The experiences of this third group of fathers underscored another fact apparent in the data. This third group had some of the same intent as the participatory group — they were interested in being a part of the scene and, particularly, in being present at the delivery of the child — but they had had difficulty in realizing these goals. This was seen when some of them contrasted their experiences with the first child with subsequent births. These men were discouraged from participating with early children but finally made their way to the delivery room during later deliveries. As a group, they highlight the way in which health care professionals can influence the fathering experience.

About half the men interviewed fell into the traditional category. For one reason or another, these men had a passive, nonparticipatory role in the birth process. As a group, they were the most likely to have little to say about the event. When asked whether they had ever considered Lamaze or natural childbirth, a good portion of these men either said, "What's that?" or " That was never an issue," particularly when their children had been born ten or more years ago. Another subgroup, however, replied in the following manner:

We had considered it, but the doctor my wife had didn't buy it at all.

The doctor's stance seemed sufficient grounds for these couples to abandon their inclinations toward natural childbirth.

Because of either personal inclination or professional discouragement, the traditional group of fathers had little involvement in the birth process. These men were characterized by a strong feeling that giving birth was an ordeal, a painful piece of work to be gotten over with as much dispatch as possible. They indicated that giving birth essentially involved the mother, the doctor, and the hospital personnel and that the father's role was to wait for word of the proceedings, since he could not help, and to hope and pray that mother and child were all right. Birth to them seemed in some ways to be an unpredictable, alien affair, requiring a kind of help that they, the fathers, could not provide but that medical people could. One father said:

I've been in labor rooms, and that is very painful, not an easy thing. . . . It's really tough on the gal — it knocks the hell out of her.

One traditional father described his wife as having wanted natural childbirth and as having prepared herself by reading a book on the subject. He felt that the effort would be doomed to failure because of his experience with watching childbirth in the movies and his knowledge of his wife's propensity to "jump with this pain business." His description of the actual event included the elements mentioned by the other men in this group. He first described his wife's being taken upstairs for an enema while he spent an hour filling out forms downstairs. He continued:

I went up and the girl said, "Your wife is over in Room 2," and I walked into this
room, and I see this lady, crazy lady, screaming and banging on the walls by
the bed, and I came out of there. I'm looking for my wife, and the girl said,
"Mr. Z, that is your wife!" She screamed, "Kill me!" and I said, "Honey, you
will be all right — just 6 more hours." That's something you just have to
understand — how women can take this! If you can stand pain, and somebody
has a shot for you, and it will be over in 5 minutes, maybe you'll have some-
thing to live for . . . and the doctor told us "She's doing fine; she'll be ready
at about 2 or 3 in the morning, and this is about 8 o'clock at night, and she's
screaming, "Kill me!"

Mr. Z.'s experience contrasted with the experience of one of the participatory
fathers as described below:

He: Yes, we did Lamaze and that was fantastic!

Int: I take it you'd do it again if you had another one?

He: Oh, definitely! The experience was like extremely intimate — we both really
felt close — when the baby was born, I was holding her shoulders up; we both
watched the baby get born, and we were both literally crying with joy!

Int: So she felt the same.

He: Yeah — right after the baby was born and S. was sewn up, we were in a
little room right off the side taking pictures of each other with the baby,
while other women were off in the recovery room, throwing up.

Even allowing for a dramatic flair on Mr. Z.'s part, there is a marked difference in the meaning of the birth experience for these two men.

The positive feelings described above were common among fathers in the
participatory group. They tended to describe the Lamaze method in very
favorable, even glowing terms, feeling that this method allowed them to have
a happy, productive experience with childbirth. Some fathers expressed the
belief that this form of birth strengthened their relationships with their wives,
identifying the intimacy and the shared effort toward their common goal as
drawing them closer. It was clear that these fathers felt they benefited from
their active roles; they cited advantages such as not having to wait and worry
about what was going on and feeling close to the baby right away. Overall,
the Lamaze or other self-help methods these couples used for natural childbirth seemed to give father and mother a sense of control over what was happening and a sense of success in managing one of the most important events
in their lives. This sense of control and mastery most accounted for the enthusiastic response of parents to natural childbirth. For the most part, the
participating fathers were very immersed in their helping roles and felt cut off
when those roles had to be terminated prematurely. One man said with regret:

*She was just about to deliver when her contractions stopped, and they had to do
a cesarean section. And so I didn't get to participate in the birth, which was
disappointing. You know, you go through this whole thing, and then you get
shut off at the end . . . but the baby was born anyway.*

The men and their wives' physicians had differing viewpoints about the
degree to which the father should participate in the birth. Reference has
already been made to certain of the traditional fathers, who unwillingly
adopted that approach because the physicians did not approve of natural
childbirth. A few other men were not so willing to settle for the sidelines during
the birth event; their reports of their efforts to resist being sidelined illustrate
the resistance of an established system to change. Now prospective parents
are able to find physicians and hospitals willing to allow the father a participatory role. But during the 1960s men were encouraged by professionals to
assume a more traditional role. It took considerable effort and determination
on a man's part to persist in the face of professionals' efforts to discourage
him. In some cases, even the wife had to be sold on the idea. One man described the change in his wife's attitude over time:

*For the first one, she didn't allow me to. For the second one, she was still a
little skeptical, but I was such a pain about it, she said okay and told the
doctor that I wanted to see it. And the third one, she insisted that I was
there; so it was a pretty good feeling.*

When asked if the physician had been willing to let him participate, this
man replied:

*Well, he didn't let me; I just plain old insisted. We'd known the man for a long
time then, and he knew me well — knew I wouldn't pass out, or something like
that. I wasn't actually in, but I was right outside the door, and he made a big
deal trying to make me sick with bringing over a bloody, sloppy baby and
bringing over the afterbirth — "What do you think of this afterbirth?" —
right?*

Another man documented changing policies as he noted changes from first
to second to third childbirth experience. The first time, even though the hospital was chosen because of its sympathy to natural childbirth, he and his
wife were not allowed to do Lamaze, and she was automatically given an
episiotomy and a spinal, apparently without her consultation. The man was
directed to a stool in the corner of the delivery room and told that he was
there because he'd hit his head if he fainted and that if he did, he'd just have
to lie there because no one would help him. When this man's third child was
born, even though the hospital now was accepting of fathers, he met resistance on the part of his particular obstetrician. He said:

I kept asking the OB, "Well, am I in here or not!" and he'd say, "We'll see," and finally I figured the hell with it, and I grabbed myself an intern and went and got a scrub outfit and put it on. I was absolutely unrestricted, and I wandered around. There was a resident that was working, and I watched him through-out the whole thing — but it was totally unrestricted and that was really good. It was a lot easier on me because I was right there.

Noteworthy is the resourcefulness of this particular father and the fact that the newer, still-in-training professionals had no difficulty in accepting the presence of the father while the established obstetrician had difficulty modifying his already set practices.

INFLUENCES ON AND PREPARATION FOR THE FATHERING ROLE

Two factors influenced the way the men arrived at their definitions of their fathering roles and their ideas about child development. The first concerns the wives' influence on the thinking of their husbands, and the second concerns the positive value the men placed on independence of thought or freedom from outside influence.

Defining parental roles was a joint enterprise for the men and their wives. All the couples had exchanged views on the manner in which their children should be reared. Although it was not clear how thorough such exchanges were, it was apparent that such exchanges led the parents to believe that they basically agreed about child rearing issues. However extensive the discussions, the partners had exchanged sufficient information and had agreed to the extent that the men used "we" instead of "I" when describing some matter of child rearing. These men claimed a common frame of reference for themselves and their wives about key aspects of parenting. The claim was stronger for basic child rearing policy, the "what should be done" aspect, than it was for specific roles, the "who should do it" aspect.

Difficulties resulting from unique frames of reference were rare and stemmed from two sources: inaccurate initial assessment and incomplete assessment. As an example of the former, one father talked about the fact that he had devoted most of his time to his selling career when his two older children were very young and therefore had very little involvement in their care. He had thought, then, that his wife had understood and agreed with his system of priorities, only to find out later that she had resented his devoting so much time to work and his lack of involvement with his family. This man's error was in thinking that an agreement had been made when in fact it had not. The second difficulty was more common and was reported by some of the fathers of infants as a manageable, time-limited conflict. The conflict focused on the fathers' unwillingness to involve themselves in the physical care, such as bathing and diapering, of relatively small babies (less than 5 months old). The mothers felt that the fathers ought to master such tasks. In this instance, the agreement that both parents would share in the tasks occasioned by the presence of a new baby was an agreement in principle, not in particular; the specifics of task sharing simply had not been discussed.

None of the men interviewed discussed in any detail the process of arriving at common understandings with his wife about parenting, although some commented that they and their wives "see things" pretty much the same way. The fathers who offered explanations for this similarity of viewpoint attributed it to the fact that they and their wives shared a common background. The men whose backgrounds were different from those of their wives offered no explanation for the similarity.

The common frame of reference concerned the basic orientation and values that the parents held about child rearing more than the specific skills or substantive knowledge about children required for adequate performance. While a few men identified themselves as having had a lot of contact with children before their own children were born, a contact that gave them a feeling of relative comfort and confidence in being around children, most men reported themselves as having very limited, if any, such contact. The men who did have some earlier contact with children seemed to have profited more in attitude than in skills since all the men interviewed placed themselves in the category of unskilled and unpracticed insofar as the physical care of children was concerned.

In all of the families studied, the mother was the parent primarily responsible for child care. The men assumed that the woman's femaleness endowed her with innate abilities or predispositions. Whatever knowledge or skill the woman did not already possess, the men thought the woman could and should acquire. The woman, then, occupied the role of child specialist in these families. While no man regarded his wife as being a strong determinant of his fathering role, it is quite clear that in fact the wives were important influences insofar as specific activities, knowledge, and skills were concerned. Given the previously mentioned common frame of reference about child rearing, it would seem that such influence occurred in an automatic fashion, not particularly noticed by the men. Throughout the majority of interviews, however, numerous references were made to the input of wives on fathering activities. Some fathers were aware of taking many cues from their wives. In fact, the man who was most definite about his freedom from influence and his independence in the creation of his fathering role paradoxically stated:

You pick up through your wife or through whatever other people you watch. N. [his wife] is a big help; in other words, I pick up on the good things, and then I add my own twist to it.

Evidently, many of the men did not regard taking cues from their wives as synonymous with being influenced by them.

The data suggest that the woman's influence was not simply a function of the degree of the man's involvement in the lives of his children (less involvement associated with more influence for the mother). Men who spent considerable time and energy on domestic roles, who shared much of the care of children, reported the same quality of influence that was reported by fathers who spent much more of their time pursuing their breadwinner roles. The mother's influence seemed to be the result of the division of labor — the fact that she filled the role of family child specialist.

If the woman's influence was frequently unnoticed, how did the men account for their being able to perform as fathers? Most men felt that they had learned through experience, although there were differences in just how that experience was described. Some men described how they reflected on and evaluated their transactions with their children. Others regarded the whole process as natural or instinctive. One man remarked:

You don't need any special preparation; you just work yourself into it. It's a natural thing.

The men's reluctance to admit that they underwent role preparation (notwithstanding their acknowledgement of experience as a major influence) seemed to be related to their very positive evaluation of independence of thought. These men tended to present themselves as having arrived at their definitions of both fathering and child development in an independent fashion, impervious to the popular and prevalent modes of the day. It is as though they thought that popular or recommended practices were nothing more than worthless fads and that to be influenced by them indicated a lack of character. This sentiment was particularly apparent when the fathers talked about any source of "expert" opinion. Only four or five of the men interviewed made some reference to having been influenced in their ideas about fathering or child care by reading or other recourse to "expert" opinion. The overwhelming number of men were negative about such sources. One man stated:

. . . all the child psychology and things being thrown about nowadays about how you will suppress your child's feelings, and he'll grow up with this problem or that problem. Well, you worry about that all the time and probably mess him up more than you would otherwise.

Many men echoed this man's devaluation of the input of specialists, although most men considered such input as unhelpful and irrelevant to their particular situation rather than as damaging. Pride of independence, reflected in the men's response to acquiring information from anyone, whether it be expert or friend, was expressed most strongly by one man, who stated:

I've got a thing about that — I don't think anybody can tell me how to do something that I want to do — I think I'm much better at it on my own. I don't think anybody could tell me how or where to buy a house, or how to get a good education, or how to solve a personal problem, or how to rear my kids. These are things that I do on my own, and I don't want to complicate it by listening to discussions and seeking out advice; that is such an abstract way of doing something that is so important. It's almost tragic, I think, that a person has to go and read something on how to be a father! Jesus, if you have to go read it, then forget it! Don't do it!

This man was more sensitive to suggestions about influence of any sort than were the other men who discussed the issue. But his statement does reflect their feeling that it is somehow better to work a particular role through for oneself than to rely on outside sources.

The men also thought themselves to be quite independent of peer group influence. For some, such freedom was a function of having been the first in their circle of friends to start a family. For others, it was a matter of principle. One man stated:

I decided not to be influenced by the opinions of any of my friends.

Many men reported that child rearing and fatherhood were rarely topics of discussion among their male friends even when those friends had children. The one exception cited was a child's involvement in sports. Because they never discussed fathering with their friends and peers, the men concluded that they were uninfluenced by this group in this regard. The male failure to discuss children or fatherhood was a typical enough characteristic of men in general to lead some fathers to conclude that they were more involved with their children than the typical father was because they either did talk to friends about their children or had photographs of them prominently displayed in their places of work.

It should be noted that the men's negative reaction to "expert" kinds of opinion was confined to child rearing and not to the matter of childbirth. The actual birth event was recognized by all the men interviewed as an occurrence of unusual dimensions, calling for the participation of experts. Those men who, with their wives, had chosen the more traditional, doctor-oriented mode of childbirth (as opposed to the self-help methods such as Lamaze) were most willing to rely on the direction of experts in staging the birth of their children. These men, however, were not willing to use experts as sources of guidance in the more mundane aspects of subsequent child rearing. Those men who had had more participatory roles in the birth also valued the use of experts for this event, tending to regard them as resources who could teach the parents how to participate effectively. Many of these participating fathers also saw the experts as useful only in this phase of their fatherhood. But four or five of these men reported that reading and consulting with expert friends were helpful to them. Yet it is quite possible that the help they refer to was in the category of giving birth as opposed to longer term child rearing.

INFLUENCE OF THE FATHER'S OWN PARENTS

The influence that the men's own parents had on the way they define and carry out their fathering roles is somewhat unclear. There is copious evidence that parents — both of the men and of their wives — do constitute a salient reference group, but it also seems probable that these parents determine the fathering role less than do other factors.

All the men were able to describe and evaluate the parenting performances of their own parents and to identify points of similarity or difference when comparing their parents to themselves. While the differences and similarities between the men and their own fathers will be described more fully in a later section, it can be said here that there was no direct connection between the kind of parenting a man had experienced and the way he structured his own fathering role. In other words, knowing that a man's own father had been very strict and uninvolved with the running of the home did not help us to predict the man's views about fathering. No reliable pattern of either modeling behavior after or rejecting and being different from parents was apparent. Some men considered themselves similar to their fathers in some ways, and some men felt that they hardly resembled their fathers. Generally, the men had established their own standards of fathering against which they measured their performance and that of their own fathers. As a result, the men's judgments in many cases were based on some standards other than ones acquired from their parents.

The men did use their parents as a reference. It was not uncommon for the men to behave in a certain way toward their children based on the experiences they had had as children when their fathers behaved similarly. They evaluated the end result of their parents' behavior and decided whether to adopt it based on how useful they thought that end result was. For instance, one man who considered his own father to have squelched his independence tried to behave quite differently from his father on matters involving his children's decision making. Another man who regarded the freedom-mixed-with-responsibility that he had experienced as a child as producing positive results for himself tried to make sure that his own children were exposed to that same combination. He had enrolled his children in a Montessori school because he approved of the approach used, in which each child has to make decisions and then live with those decisions.

All the men had progressed some distance from their own fathers in their definitions of fathering. In general, the men characterized their fathers as being much more concerned with the breadwinning aspects of the fathering role and leaving all domestic matters in the hands of their wives. They regarded their fathers as distant or at least as more unavailable than they would have liked them to be. When their own fathers were home, they shared very little in the running of the household, except to serve as the source of authority in the family. The men usually described their fathers as never having anything to do with the care of children, although a few described their fathers as kindly or patient. According to the men, the role allocation in that older generation was much more rigid and had less overlap. Many of the men identified parental traits that they admired (in one case, a father was admired for being strict; in another, for being democratic); many wished to emulate some personality characteristics and not others. But even when the men described themselves as similar to their own fathers in outlook, a change away from the patterns of the older generation was apparent.

ACTUAL PERFORMANCE IN THE FATHERING ROLE

In this section, we turn away from a concern with how definitions and skills required of fathers are developed and toward identifying the kinds of activities or goals that the men interviewed considered to be the key ingredients of their fathering roles.

In any event, the men tended to regard themselves as having worked through their own definitions and patterns of fathering relatively free of outside influences, their own experience being the teacher they most readily acknowledged. Although the men's fathering efforts differed in detail and in the relationships described, the efforts had an underlying similarity of purpose or goals. Without exception, the men felt that engaging their children in a meaningful, positive affective relationship was the sine qua non of fathering. Therefore, the men's statements describing the "nuts and bolts" of their fathering frequently concerned the conduct or management of their relationships with their children. While specific activities, expectations, and tasks changed according to the age and, to some degree, the sex of the child and to parental circumstances, the men always strove to be emotionally close to the child, to make the child feel that he or she was a central figure in the father's life, and to engender a feeling of security and of being loved. The men frequently talked about the concrete activities in which they engaged, but these activities served primarily as vehicles for forging the emotional bond between child and father.

The fact that the men engaged their children in this way was not simply a matter of responding to their children's overtures; it was a matter of active pursuit. The men sought to foster such relationships and to fit their behavior to the changing needs of their children. For example, one man had the habit of getting down on the floor with his 8-month-old daughter when she was placed on the floor to crawl around. He joined her on the floor because she enjoyed his company there and played with him. This man also had a 3-year-old son whom he took on walks around the neighborhood. These walks were a sharing time for them. The father imagined that as his boy gets older, he will want to be taught to play ball; the father looked forward to such a request. This man did not venture to guess what his daughter might want when she is 3 years old, but he is sure that he will be able to do something with her. This man's confidence about his ability to carry off such a relationship was typical. The men seemed to assume that they could and would succeed in their efforts, at least while their children were preadolescent. (None of the men had adolescent children. Four fathers projected ahead to that period of their children's development and registered some apprehension about the difficulties of parenting during that stage. They thought that adolescents sometimes become distant and different from their families and that such a development would be difficult to endure as a parent.)

The emotional bond that the men sought to achieve with their children was not an end in itself, although the men did get direct gratification from their relationships with their children. The bond was also regarded as a means to an end — as the necessary condition that would enable them to succeed in the most basic parenting task of all, that of socializing their young. The men thought the bond would allow them to inculcate in their children those qualities thought necessary for success as adults in our society. In other words, the men believed that children acquire those characteristics thought necessary by their father because of their close bond to him and through the interactions they have with him — and others. If the father were absent most of the time, thus not relating much to his children, he would have a minimal influence on them in spite of his love for them.

Although the men did not attempt to describe the type of persons they desired their children to be, many of the men talked about certain qualities or characteristics they hoped their children would acquire during their formative years and which of these they as fathers tried to promote in their fathering role. These included character traits, attitudes, and values rather than specific skills. The men wanted their children to feel good about themselves as individuals and to have a well developed sense of individuality, a trait they often associated with independence. They wanted their children to be confident and to be able to stand on their own two feet with ease. Some included responsibility as a desirable trait. No father identified physical or scholastic abilities as something he hoped for for his child although many fathers of sons mentioned their enjoyment of participating in physical activities with their sons (they felt much more constrained about this kind of participation with their daughters) and were pleased at any display of athletic ability.

THE EFFECT OF THE CHILD'S SEX AND AGE

The impact of the child's sex on the kind of fathering provided was difficult to assess. Very few daughters were in the later elementary school years; more often, the eldest child was a son, and when that was not the case, all the children were toddlers. One family that included school-age children consisted of three girls and no boys. It must be acknowledged, then, that this group of fathers was too skimpy on experience with daughters as girls rather than as infants for us to draw any conclusions.

Most of the men felt that sons would be easier than daughters to rear since sons would be more like them and therefore would share their experiences or activities more automatically. The fathers favored doing physical things and contact sports with their boys and, in a sense, were particularly pleased to have sons because the sons provided them with an opportunity to do what they wanted to do anyway. The biggest drawback to having daughters was that the men could not expect them to be interested in things like football. The men frequently envisioned that their wives would have a more active role with their daughters, teaching them feminine things.

On the other hand, the fathers who had daughters never had any difficulty in arriving at activities to share with them and usually commented that so far there had not been much real difference between their sons and daughters. The difficulty seemed to be one of anticipation rather than reality except for the matter of contact sports. It was clear that the fathers did feel some responsibility for appropriate role training and that they thought contact sports were not as appropriate for girls as was swimming. The fathers seemed able to organize a satisfying fathering role around their children of whatever sex, although their perspectives on the matter were influenced by the sex of their children. The father of three girls stated that boys would be too much trouble to raise, adding:

Well, everybody insists that I have a boy or try for another one, but three with us is fine. So maybe I missed a lot by not having a boy, but there is a heck of a lot of kids in the neighborhood to play with, and I like to play ball and all of this. Of course, I'm the neighborhood warrior. When they see me out there, it's "Come on, Mr. W., let's play" and I do . . . but my girls are as involved as any of the boys. Of course, now they are at the age when the boys are always over here. As far as being different, I don't know . . . boys, they're all "Let's go get the frogs and put them down the girls' backs" and this kind of stuff . . . and maybe I just don't have time for that or something, but I think I enjoy the girls more than I would the boys. They are a lot of fun, anyway.

Of all the factors that made a difference to the fathers studied, the age of the child was probably most important. No matter how proud and elated the men may have been at the birth of their children, it was the rare father who did not tend to "wait in the wings" until his child was a little older before assuming a significant share of parenting responsibility. Some men did share in the care of their small infants, some even willingly, but they usually did so to afford relief to the mother, who was generally regarded as the major care-taker. Some fathers also claimed to have very little to do with their children when they were infants, choosing to leave the infants to their wives. The men preferred the stages after the children developed language and other skills. They felt that more of an exchange was possible at that time and thus found the child much more interesting. Some men's feeling that the child was fragile and could easily be damaged added to their experience of awkwardness with infants.

If a contest were held to determine the single most unpopular child care task, diapering would win hands down, particularly when the diapering involved cleaning up after a bowel movement. With few exceptions, diapering was the task most often mentioned as objectionable and most likely to be shunted off to mothers, with varying degrees of apology. Bathing was also a task to be avoided, primarily because of the fathers' fear of handling the baby. The men's reluctance to attempt to master these tasks occasionally led to conflict between the parents.

DIVISION OF LABOR AND ROLE NEGOTIATION

The division of labor within the families of the men interviewed followed the traditional pattern, the father being primarily responsible for earning the family's living and the mother being primarily responsible for running the household and caring for the children. In the words of one of the fathers, the mother was the "architect of the family home life." Actually, the boundaries of the female homemaking role are now somewhat fuzzy; homemaking is more often shared with the males, while the male role remains intact but less single-minded. Mothers may contribute to income, not as a responsibility but as a matter of choice, but fathers are expected to share in child rearing and homemaking. The more traditional pattern, however, was present in the families of the men interviewed, whether or not the woman had a career she was interested in maintaining. When the woman wished to work, she did not relinquish her responsibility for running the home although she may have shared more of that responsibility. One woman who was employed full-time delegated much of her homemaking and several hours of child care per day to a housekeeper, but she retained the primary responsibility for seeing to it that the household ran smoothly (as determined by the fact that if the house-keeper was sick, the woman would be more likely to stay home than would her husband). The men whose wives had strong career interests were gener-ally accommodating, in the sense of approving of those interests and in sharing in the household maintenance tasks and child care. For example, the men would take care of the children for periods of time when the woman had to do the "homework" that their careers demanded.

Yet work outside the home had a different place in the role definitions of mothers and fathers. For mothers, working was a matter of choice or of self-expression. Fathers saw it as an integral part of the fathering responsibility. That breadwinning part of the fathering role has never changed. Worth no-ticing, however, is the fact that, for the men interviewed, the breadwinning role was a responsibility to be built upon and did not constitute the totality of fathering. Only two men mentioned providing the living for the family as an element of their fathering. Most of the men regarded fathering as referring largely to the emotional bond and influence that they established with their children.

Since fathers must be close to their children in order to fulfill the fathering role, this definition has certain consequences for the division of labor. Not all the men felt that they devoted the time they should to child rearing matters; the biggest competitor for their time was their work. A few men's work made unusual seasonal demands on their time; other men gave their careers a high priority as a matter of routine. These men did not feel entirely comfortable or justified in their emphasis on work. Some had plans to devote more time to their families.

For the most part, however, the men were inclined to share the many tasks required to maintain a family. It is probable that the major role negotiation between the father and the mother was predicated on such sharing, although the common frame of reference established between them assigned the mother the role of family child specialist primarily responsible for child rearing. Since the mothers had the major role, the fathers' role was usually the complement of it and rarely stood in opposition to it. It is as though the father chose things to do that fit into the family value system and allowed him to relate closely to each of his children. He was influenced by his wish to relieve his wife of some of her responsibility and to share her burden. Yet most facets of child care were absorbed by the mother. What the father chose not to do or could not be persuaded to do by the mother automatically became part of the mother's role.

Because they shared a frame of reference, the parents were, for the most part, in agreement about the major strategies of their parenting. The men identified only minor conflicts and usually said that by discussing the matter they and their wives could arrive at a reasonable resolution. According to the men, the women frequently felt more strongly about issues than they did, a fact they attributed to the women's greater exposure and vulnerability to the home scene and the behavior of children. The men described themselves as giving in to their wives in many conflicts, either because of their wives' emotional response or their own sense of fair play, i.e., if the wife must contend with the children, she should have the greater voice in deciding child rearing policy.

In conclusion, the accounts of the men's experiences during the births of their children point out the degree to which the men who wanted a participatory role had to buck the system. The health care system certainly was recalcitrant and unyielding in its opposition to the wishes of these fathers, although it was less so with the passage of time. When arranged sequentially from the earliest births to the latest, our data provide the chronology of an idea whose time had come. Many of us now take the reasonableness of the fathers' wishes for participation so much for granted that we fail to perceive the underlying dilemma.

The problem is, how can we arrive at reasonable solutions when consumers request one kind of service and in the judgment of professionals another kind of service is more appropriate. Accurate assessment of the validity of both positions is always difficult, especially when both sides are convinced of the rightness of their own and the error of the other side's point of view. The delivery room nurses who requested fathers to sit on stools in the corner undoubtedly were convinced of the dangers of fathers being present. Simply making changes in order to accommodate patients' requests is not a particularly viable alternative either. The real problem lies in knowing whose interests are being served by a particular course of action. We must muster the courage to ask ourselves that question even when it entails the possibility of giving up practices to which we are accustomed. For this reason, newcomers to a field are often the best hope of change.

The men interviewed for this chapter are not the same people as their own fathers, in spite of the similarities between them. They tend to define their fathering roles in a different way, and these differences have consequences for nursing care. These men are less committed to the breadwinner role that once absorbed a major share of their attention and now seem to invest more of their energies in domestic roles than they did formerly. Thus fathers are logical targets for inclusion in whatever family planning a health problem requires. Since the opinion of the father will be an important determinant in how well any health recommendation will be carried out, nurses would do well to ask about the consequences on the family system, father included, of any recommendation she makes.

The high value placed on independence of thought by the men interviewed suggests that professionals should proceed with caution. The men welcomed professional advice when they needed technical knowledge that only a professional could provide. They doubted the value of other "expert" opinion. This being the case, a nurse's inquiries and advice about growth and development matters should be handled more carefully than those about matters involving technical procedures. Men may respond better to material that they have had a chance to process and work through themselves, that provides them with an opportunity for choice, and that allows them to fit practices to their own situations.

18. How Professional Women Balance Careers and Motherhood. Hildy Heine Reiter and Norma Traub Cox

This chapter focuses on the concerns of married women who are pursuing professional careers while mothering young children. Although at present the number of women who balance careers and motherhood is relatively small, more and more women are opting to remain in the work force while simultaneously raising families. This chapter examines: (1) the importance of support systems to such women's multiple role management; (2) the strategies such women use to balance the three roles of wife, mother, and professional; and (3) the women's subsequent self-evaluation of their performance in each of these roles.

Twenty women were interviewed in an attempt to learn how women who combine family and career roles perceive and manage their lives. The women interviewed worked a minimum of twenty-four hours a week, had at least one child under the age of 12, and lived with their husbands. Table 1 summarizes the specific demographic characteristics of this sample.

THE SUPPORT SYSTEM

The women balanced their multiple roles with varying degrees of satisfaction. While some were comfortable managing their multiple roles, others viewed their situation as problematic and burdensome. Their perceptions of their situations hinged on the presence or absence of a functioning support system.

Fourteen women expressed general satisfaction with the way they were managing their roles. Although they had encountered problems, the presence of a supportive person had enabled them to squarely confront these problems. For twelve of the fourteen women, this supportive person was the husband.

Husbands were regarded as supportive when they encouraged the women in their pursuits and shared in enough tasks to make these pursuits possible. One woman described the crucial role her husband played:

Table 1. Demographic Characteristics of the Women Interviewed

Subject Number	Age	Years Married		Occupation	Husband's Occupation	Number of Children	Ages of Children	National Origin
1	38	14	D.D.S.	Professor of dentistry	University professor	3	8, 10, 12	Foreign
2	37	13	Ph.D.	Professor of microbiology	University professor	3	11, 11, 12	U.S.
3	36	16	Ph.D.	Professor of anatomy	Managerial	2	3, 7	U.S.
4	41	8	Ph.D.	Professor of biochemistry	University professor	1	4	U.S.
5	30	6	Ph.D.	Child psychologist	Psychologist	1	1	U.S.
6	42	14	Ph.D.	Professor of biochemistry	Pharmacist	1	9	Foreign
7	39	22	M.D.	Professor of psychiatry	Physician	3	5, 9, 14	U.S.
8	28	5	B.A.	Professor of medical records	Sales	1	1	U.S.
9	31	5	M.S.W.	Administrative social worker	Social worker	1	2	U.S.
10	42	16	Ph.D. candidate	Educational psychologist	Writer	1	1	U.S.
11	36	4	M.D.	Professor of pediatrics	Engineer	1	2	U.S.
						5*	14, 16, 17, 18, 20	
12	44	16	M.D.	Radiologist	Physician	3	6, 7, 9	U.S.
13	31	10	M.D.	Pediatrician	University professor	1	1	U.S.
14	42	16	M.D.	Pediatrician	Social worker	3	12, 14, 16	U.S.
15	36	17	A.M.L.S.	University librarian	University professor	4	9, 13, 14, 16	U.S.
16	34	13	Ph.D.	Psychologist	Physician	2	1, 5	Foreign
17	41	7	M.S.N.	Professor of public health nursing	Physician	2	3, 5	U.S.
18	29	2	M.S.N.	Instructor of general nursing	Medical student	1	1	U.S.
19	48	21	M.N.	Professor of medical-surgical nursing	Theology	4	9, 13, 14, 16	U.S.
20	29	8	M.S.	Instructor of maternal-child nursing	Counselor	1	7	U.S.

*Five children from husband's former marriage.

*I'm extremely grateful to him for his support. I know he's not happy when
I'm out two or three nights a week, but he accepts it as best he can. Back when
we were in graduate school together, he used to go out with me and help me
get frog eggs and select insects, and he's drawn drawings for me and prepared drafts for talks when I've been short on time. When I first started
teaching, he actually taught me how to make up exams. He's always very
interested. . . . My husband was really very supportive, extremely so, right
after the baby was born. He never, never said anything that was guilt producing. He always said things like, "Do you see anything wrong with the
baby? Isn't it a beautiful baby? It's smiling," and he would say, "I didn't
see my mother for the whole day. She was always in the office, and there's
nothing wrong with me, and I know who my mother is," because I was
crying and saying things like, "Maybe she won't know who I am. Maybe
this other woman will be more important to her."*

These husbands provided both emotional and practical supports. They not
only participated in household and child care tasks but urged their wives
to continue in their multiple role commitments. The women perceived such
support as an essential element in their being able to manage their various
roles in a satisfying way.

Parents and older children were also mentioned as important sources of
support. One professional woman whose parents lived on the first floor
of a shared two-family flat said that she would not have been able to proceed
in her career if her parents had not been nearby. She said:

*If I had had to leave the children with someone that wasn't close to me, I'm
not sure if I wouldn't have temporarily given up my profession and stayed
home. My mother has been extremely good with the children. We have never
had, really, in the 12½ years she's stayed with the children, a misunderstand-
ing as far as disciplining them or anything like that because she would
follow pretty much everything the way we would talk about it. That's the
biggest plus; not every professional woman can have this. My parents never
looked at my working in a profession as something fickle or that I'm
neglectful of my family. They thought that it was a very definite commitment I had made. I would say we always helped each other out, and they
were very much for it.*

One woman identified her baby-sitter as a key support person. She recognized that this woman met her own as well as her baby's needs. The woman
stated:

*I would say she's a great person for providing emotional support to me too.
She realized the guilt I had when I first was coming back to work. It was
very hard to leave my baby, who was only 3 months old at the time, and
everyday, when I would come home, she would tell me all the little things
that he had done, and we would just sit down, and we'd have a cup of coffee*

*and talk to each other. She was very observant, and she would pick up
little things about how he had liked this little toy or she had noticed that
he was just starting to get a little bit of a diaper rash — terribly supportive.
She met my needs as well as my baby's. So I would say she was a great
source of emotional support.*

Whether they were husbands, family members, or persons outside the
family, support persons made the women's lives manageable by providing
general encouragement and participating in household and child care tasks.
In short, the women interviewed attributed much of their comfort and
satisfaction with their multirole life-style to the presence of a central person
who shared tasks and provided emotional support.

The fourteen women who expressed relative comfort with the way in which
they were managing their various roles also drew on peripheral sources of
support. These peripheral persons provided support similar to that provided
by the central persons but on a less regular basis. For example, one woman
described an emergency during which her baby-sitter was unavailable. Her
mother, who lived 200 miles away, was able to provide temporary child
care. While such peripheral sources of support helped maintain the women's
sense of manageability, they were not essential to it.

Peripheral individuals were identified as sources of criticism as well as
support. Their criticisms were typically directed toward the women's
"unnecessary" career involvements that took them away from their "more
appropriate" maternal role. Such criticism either implicitly or explicitly
maintained that the children of professional women suffer as a result
of their mothers' careers. One woman described how her friends questioned
her child care arrangements. She remarked:

*I have picked up obliquely from personal friends very curious comments at
times. They are always interested to know how we manage this and that and
who takes care of what child at what time, and this sort of thing. No one
has ever said anything to me directly, but I can perceive that they sometimes
don't entirely approve of my having people look after my children while
I work. But that's just one of those things.*

Obviously, this woman has learned to ignore or discount her friends' subtle
disapproval.

The husbands of women who work also may be criticized. Several women
noted that others sometimes thought their working was a result of their
husbands' inadequate earning power. Such persons were unable or unwilling
to understand the women's commitment to their work.

None of the fourteen women who saw themselves as adequately managing
and balancing their multiple roles viewed their lives as problem-free. All
believed that being a professional-wife-mother was a difficult and at times
almost overwhelming combination of roles. All believed that the presence of

a central support person was absolutely essential to their being able to simultaneously undertake and sustain the three roles.

In light of the great importance these women attached to the presence of a central support person in their lives, it is hardly surprising that the six women who had no such support person reported extreme difficulties in managing their multiple roles. While these six women had persons to whom they could turn in times of acute need, they did not have a reliable, ongoing support person. These women conveyed a sense of sadness and disappointment when discussing their lives and described themselves as unable to keep up with and control the demands placed on them. Without the central support person they had no one with whom to share the daily household tasks and child care. In addition, the husbands of these women typically discouraged their wives' professional involvements. In general, these husbands failed to appreciate the complexity of their wives' life-style.

One woman stated that a professional-wife-mother role was unworkable unless a woman's husband was supportive of it. She commented:

I never had any intentions of giving up my work, and my husband knew about that, and he approved it, too, because he knew that I have a commitment that I want to fulfill just for my own satisfaction, and this has been a difficult point, because he knows it and I know it. And he knows that I will just not be happy staying home, and we just haven't resolved that at all. It was a difficult thing to keep a house and go to graduate school. My husband isn't a very good housekeeper, and he really is one of those people who doesn't believe in woman's liberation at all. He just thinks that if women want to do more, it's their choice but they have to cope with everything in addition to what they want to do. So that has not helped at all. I just run around all the time and try to do my best. After the child came, the situation really got worse, and I just tried to throw everything in and say, "I give up."

Three women who were reluctant to describe their husbands' nonsupportive role did indicate that their husbands' lack of encouragement and participation in household and child care tasks was acutely distressing.

Some husbands evidenced both accepting and disapproving attitudes and behavior. One woman described her husband as accepting and understanding of her professional involvement but as still expecting her to fulfill the traditional wife-mother role. While appreciating his support of her career goals, she often found his expectations regarding their home life a source of frustration. She stated:

Sometimes he would help, sometimes not. He never liked it when I was working in the evening, if I ever had to be out at a meeting or anything. He never liked it, even when in medical school. When he was home, he wanted me to be home. If I was out pursuing my professional activity, which wasn't too often, he didn't like it. I felt the subtle pressure always to be home when he was there. I was free to do whatever I wanted as long as he was busy elsewhere. But when he was home, he wanted me to be at home too. I didn't like it, but I didn't fight it directly very much. I try to accommodate him and live with him. You know, I limit my professional activities as much as possible, both because I don't want to fight him and because I also don't like to work nights, and I don't like to be out odd hours. I probably would be a little more active professionally if my husband were willing to let me, if he were willing to step in without resenting it. Maybe I'd be a little more active, not a whole lot.

This woman compromised some of her career aspirations in order to fulfill her husband's expectations.

The six women who had no central support person were less able than the other women to tolerate the nonsupport, opposition, and criticism sometimes directed at them by peripheral persons. One woman complained:

You would think that people would be more liberal. Now, for example, when the people around here heard about my husband going to New York, they were up in arms. They said, "You're leaving and you didn't tell us." I said, "But I'm not leaving." The people around here sound like a bunch of male chauvinist pigs. They keep asking over and over again, "Why are you doing it?" In the first place, I don't think it's any of their business, and secondly, I'm just a little bit surprised by the women too and their attitudes.

These women were often angered by the negative attitudes of others and found it difficult to vent their anger comfortably. Although the negative attitudes of peripheral persons did not pose serious problems for women lacking a central support person, they did contribute to these women's overall feeling of frustration and defeat.

ROLE BALANCING STRATEGIES

Each woman reported that role balancing did not become an issue until her first child was born. With the addition of parenting responsibilities, the women's lives increased in complexity, and all the women had to alter both their routines and priorities in order to accommodate the constraints of their new situation.

Child care tasks quickly assumed priority over household tasks. The women all reported having to learn to live with more disorder than usual. It was simply impossible for them to accomplish all their household and parenting responsibilities simultaneously.

In addition to spending less time doing household tasks, the women attempted to accommodate their professional role to their parenting one. Prior to the birth of their first child, these women were professionally very active. Their work often included evening and weekend commitments, bringing work home, organizational activities, research, and publishing. After assuming the parenting role, the women had to abandon many of these "extra" activities in order to have sufficient time for child care. While some women decreased their professional activities in response to outside pressures, the majority did so in response to a desire to spend more time with their children. One woman described the controls she initially placed on herself in order to contend with the professional-maternal conflict. She commented:

As I told you, I had a great deal of anxiety during that first year that I worked, and I made rules that weren't necessary. I made a rule that I couldn't work, ever, overtime and that I'd always work just business hours; and I made a rule that I couldn't work on things at home while she was awake. I sort of really hemmed myself in, and I thought that this way I could meet the requirements of the child psychiatry textbooks and still work. Every day, after I went back to work, I would come home and look for signs of autism in the child [Laugh] and so on, and I was sure she was really going to be a mess. After about a year of this, I realized she was turning out all right and that this wasn't necessary, and I gradually began to do more work things.

Another woman referred to a shift in her priorities that had helped her resolve her sense of conflict. She stated:

I have different feelings about it now than I did then. Like my work is much less important to me now, although it's still important, you know, but not as important as it was. I guess it's really clear to me what's important in my life. You know, it's my husband and my child, and you know, if my patients are upset, or something, I feel bad about it, and I'm really sorry, but I don't go home and think about it like I might have before. I have too many other things to do.

Some women, although they considered the curtailment of their professional lives to be temporary, expressed frustration about the matter nonetheless. One woman said:

Well, as a professional, I'm frustrated because I had to move so many times and didn't finish my Ph.D. Therefore, there are limits on what I can do. Like, I'd very much like to be more involved in research, I think. I may yet finish that up. I don't get enough time to read, and I suppose that part of that is the family thing. People without a family can go home and read all evening. With me, forget it. I carry the bag home and put it in the corner and carry it back. There are real limitations professionally. But, I'm still very much into professional stuff, and it's very satisfying to me. I get a big charge out of it, and I wouldn't want to give up the professional thing because it gives so much to me.

Clearly, the curtailment of professional activities was one way these women dealt with the addition of mothering responsibilities.

281. Careers and Motherhood

Another way the women coped with the added role was to become better organized and more efficient. One woman described such a change in herself:

At the time, before my daughter was born, I was doing a lot of committee work for my profession, and I would use my evenings for that because my husband was often away. That changed after we had the baby because I felt that I wanted to devote time to her. We organized things a different way. For example, I got my work organized enough so that I could do my committee work there. And I made it a point to use my hours as effectively as I could and to not take any work home. I really made a point to do that. I found that the more organized I got, the more efficiently I did my work, anyway. I did all my administrative work, and I still made a point of talking to all my staff and students every day. Things really went like clockwork.

By becoming better organized, some women were able to assume a mothering role without compromising their professional role.

Child care arrangements can either facilitate or hinder a woman's ability to manage her various roles. Thus the women interviewed invested much time and energy in finding and maintaining suitable child care. Often they had to employ a series of baby-sitters before finding one that was both competent and reliable. One woman commented on the frustrating nature of this process:

I have had eight people in fourteen months. I have tried to get one by putting an ad in local papers, and I have had three or four people come, but none of them lasted. One was alcoholic; we didn't know when we hired her, obviously, but after she had come and I realized what was happening, I thought if we didn't have anything at home, she wouldn't have access to it. But she wouldn't stay, so we had to send her back. I had one girl that stayed for ten weeks, and then she wanted to leave, and I had one girl that came here, but she said that the only way she would stay would be that I find her a boyfriend. I don't have any resources for that; she wouldn't stay and she left.

Those women who were fortunate enough to find suitable child care rewarded their baby-sitters with praise, good pay, and loyalty. One woman credited her attitude toward her baby-sitter for the success of her child care arrangement. She explained:

I make a big point with my baby-sitter that I consider her as professional as me and that I think her work is as important as mine, because I do. Quite honestly, a major goal in my life is that my child should be raised successfully, and that I don't have to stay home to do it; so I make a point of telling her that I appreciate her and that I consider her every bit as professional as I, so we don't put baby-sitters down. I think that a lot of women tend to assume that if somebody baby-sits and they're working, the baby-sitter,

in some way or another, is ineffective, and that's why they're a baby-sitter.
And so, they don't pay much, and they don't show much regard, and
people come and go, and they're always changing. So I think it's important
how you approach baby-sitting.

Other women were able to arrange their working hours so that they could
be at home while their husbands worked and vice versa. The women whose
children were older and attended day care centers encountered fewer child
care problems because neighbors or older siblings filled in for sitters. Eventually, these children were encouraged to be responsible for themselves both
during and after school.

For the women interviewed, motherhood forced them to make an explicit
evaluation of their priorities. For many, this led to the subsequent rearrange-
ment of daily schedules, always in the direction of allowing more time for
child care. Typically, the women attempted to minimize the amount of
evening and weekend time devoted to work activities. On the other hand,
since career continuation was dependent on establishing satisfactory child
care arrangements, all the women in the study devoted substantial amounts of
time and energy to finding suitable day care facilities.

SELF-EVALUATION

Generally, the women had a sense of satisfaction with their various roles and
felt that they performed well. They expected much from themselves and
consequently had periods of self-doubt. They valued intellectual stimulation,
adult relationships, and personal feelings of self-worth. Although they also
generally valued the home and child aspects of their life, they found extended
periods spent in the home-maker role boring or unfulfilling. One woman's
comment is typical:

I enjoyed the creative aspect of it very much, and I still do. I cannot do it
full-time. I just get very neurotic. . . . I had trial periods of just attempting
to go to the park every day and go to the supermarket and have the house
clean, and I always had the feeling that I was waiting for something, and
I didn't know what. I was always waiting. The day, in itself, didn't mean
anything. I realized that I was waiting for T. to grow up, that I wanted
her to be more interesting because it was not stimulating enough to be
home all day. It was just like writing days off from the calendar. I didn't
want to write off those days. I love my life, and I love to live it as fully as
possible. I can play for half an hour or forty-five minutes, then I get bored.
So I had to accept that and feel that that's me, that there's no therapist
that's going to change that.

Another woman described a professional discontent that was representative
of the feelings expressed by sixteen of the women. She stated:

I like to study a lot. I don't have time for it though. I find that the personal demands on me are so great that I'm limited professionally. I am, have been, and will, for a number of years more. Energy that I have to devote to my work is quite heavily curtailed by my personal responsibilities. If I were free to work, I know I would study a lot, do a lot of reading, do something along these lines. I'm partly fulfilled professionally, not entirely. I'm more or less biding my time until my family responsibilities ease up. Then I don't know what I'll do. I don't even know if I can advance in it. I don't even know if I'll get tenure at the rate I'm going.

Most of the women planned to resume their former professional activity level once their children were grown.

   Their marital role was important to these women, and they enjoyed the comfort and stability that a marital relationship provides. But their degree of satisfaction with this role was not as high as that they experienced in the roles of mother and professional. They were disappointed that the time they spent with their husbands was limited. Most considered the strain caused by this lack of togetherness to be temporary, but four women had considered separation and divorce. Even those women who had supportive, cooperative, and satisfying marital relationships reported that their inability to spend more time with their husbands was a major problem. They recognized that their marital relationships sometimes got slighted in their attempts to maintain high-quality professional and parenting roles. For example, one woman stated:

I think we both regret, at this point, that there's not enough time to be lovers. There's always the feeling that the kids are listening. Can't have sex on Sunday morning because there are little feet on the stairs. So there isn't the kind of freedom you used to have. It's hard to keep a relationship going, being a parent, and being a professional. So, we keep on saying things like, "We have to keep it going well enough so that we won't feel terrible about each other when we're alone again." We have periods where we would go on with our routine without doing anything about it and then one of us will start and say, "What's been happening? We haven't been talking."

While distressed by the lack of time they spent with their husbands, most of the women regarded this disadvantage as unavoidable.

   All the women enjoyed the parental role very much. They believed that the time they spent with their children was satisfying and pleasant. For example, one woman said:

As a mother, the satisfactions are fantastic. I have four really great kids. They are no trouble beyond what kids normally are. They're healthy, both psychologically and physically. They're just beautiful. They're people; they're really people. I've never treated them as kids, you know. Kids are people, you know, and it shows. So I'm pleased with that.

The women who questioned their competence as mothers had concerns not unlike those of mothers who do not work outside the home. They worried: "Am I doing the right things for my children?" At times every woman doubted her decision to work and feared the impact her working had on the well-being of her children. The women devoted much thought to the conflict between the adage "a woman's place is in the home" and their chosen life-style. Over time they had reconciled this sense of conflict to some extent by noting the apparent health and well-being of their children. Some women found reassurance and support for their life-style in Women's Liberation literature and recent publications supporting maternal employment. One woman's comments demonstrated how important such outside support can be. This woman said:

I've found a little bit in the professional literature to make me feel better. In the last year, there was a series of two articles on working mothers in Pediatrics. Basically, the message is that the traditional teachings had to do with monkeys that were raised with stuffed stockings and babies that were raised in orphanages, and it's hardly a comparable situation when a child goes to a home where he's loved and cared for, and that people shouldn't necessarily believe the other teachings. When I saw those, I was very reassured, because independent as you may be, you always want to have some kind of evidence or writings or something to kind of support how you feel about things. That's good for me.

The women interviewed sought external affirmation that their professional commitments were not jeopardizing their children's welfare.

In general, these women were highly critical of themselves in all their roles. They wanted to do more in each role and often felt a need to apologize for or justify their various behaviors. In short, they expected themselves to be superwomen. It is therefore not surprising that they often neglected their own needs. Recognizing that they were not endowed with an endless supply of energy, they typically sacrificed some of their own needs in order to meet the needs of their families. One woman explained:

I like to mess around with different things, and I never have the time, and it's irritating when I can't. Anne Morrow Lindberg has used two similes about the need for having a retreat for yourself — that you can't let yourself be a sponge that's constantly being squeezed or a pitcher that you're always pouring out of. You have to reverse the procedure once in a while.

These women needed time for themselves but seldom found it.

In summary, the women found their lives full but cumbersome. They were confronted each day by people who expected certain behaviors from them and to whom they at times felt it necessary to justify their situations. Their full life-style imposed numerous constraints on them. Many felt professionally stalled at least temporarily, and had to contend with the attendant frustration. They were proud of their children and received much pleasure as they watched them grow and develop, but they suffered pangs of self-doubt about the long-term effect their choice of life-style might have on their children's well-being. The presence of a central support person was of paramount importance to these women as they struggled to meet the demands of their multiple roles. They derived satisfaction from their life-style to the extent that they could communicate with and depend on certain persons, particularly their husbands, to share or help blend these roles. In addition, husbands, family members, and friends were important sources of emotional support when they encouraged the women's professional endeavors and were sensitive to the problems involved in combining a career and motherhood. The women were appreciative of the practical and emotional support, both of which contributed to their satisfaction with the life-style they had chosen.

19. Becoming an Adult: From the Young Adult's Perspective. Susan H. Colgate

Previous chapters in this book have focused on the processes by which individuals establish, develop, and maintain particular roles *within* a family. This chapter focuses on the process by which young persons assume adult, independent roles *outside* their family of origin. In order to examine this process from the point of view of the young persons themselves, we interviewed twenty-two such persons, eight males and fourteen females, ranging in age from 19 to 25. These young men and women were divided into two groups: one group of fifteen had recently married, and a second group of seven, still single, had moved to new apartments or had taken jobs. Only one person — a young woman — was still living with her parents when interviewed, having postponed her plans to move out when her father died.

Two terms have commonly been used to describe the reorganization in family roles that takes place when adolescents move from childhood to adulthood. These terms are *emancipation* and *launching.* Emancipation is defined by Webster's dictionary as "the act or procedure of legally freeing from the paternal power . . . making the person released *sui juris."* To emancipate is defined as "to free from any controlling influence." Thus an adolescent moving from childhood to adulthood begins to be freed from both parental power and influence and to assume legal responsibility for self. The difficulty of achieving emancipation from parents in our culture is evidenced by the facts that (1) the new status is legally defined and codified; (2) it is an irreversible legal change; and (3) it automatically occurs when the child reaches a certain age if his actions have not already precipitated the change (the "emancipated minor"). Despite such legal codification in our society, confusion about the adolescent's status as emancipated is widespread because the age of emancipation varies from state to state, as does the age at which the adolescent may be allowed to

287

assume adult roles or adult privileges such as driving, marrying with and without parental consent, voting, or drinking. Some theorists have suggested that our society's confusion about the transition to adult status is a product of our highly specialized industrial technology, which requires that young people continue to be educated for several years after they reach physical and sexual maturity.

Webster's dictionary defines launching as "an act or instance of initiating" or "of public introduction: presentation." This meaning is perhaps derived from other definitions of launching: "the act or process of putting a boat in the water"; "a ceremony accompanying the launching of a ship"; and "the act or process of releasing a self-propelled device." These definitions imply a public act or ceremony of allowing an adolescent to commence an independent voyage during which he or she either sinks or swims.

The launching of a child into adulthood is not a single public event; young persons do not suddenly become self-propelled; nor do they remain that way. Nevertheless, despite our conviction, supported by our findings, that launching is a continuous process, we have chosen to use the term launching in this chapter because it symbolically represents the adolescent's severing of some of the ties that bind him or her to the family.

In childhood, our primary social responsibility is to the family. The family is entrusted with socialization of the child into society. In the family, we learn such things as language, acceptable social behavior, moral values, respect for property, and self-discipline. Society delegates these tasks to the family. But as children mature, they begin to acquire new social responsibilities outside the family. If they fulfill their responsibilities in a mature way, society begins to accord them adult privileges: they may choose to smoke, drink, drive, marry, hold property, and work. Most young people are ready to assume both new responsibilities and new privileges when society is willing to accord them. Their families, however, still unable to trust the young person's judgment, are often eager to assign more responsibilities while hesitating to allow adult privileges. The young persons, on the other hand, usually consider the responsibilities and privileges to go hand in hand and thus feel justified in demanding what they consider their rights.

In the process of assuming an adult role in society, the young person's self-image develops from that of a child to that of a mature adult. Usually the parents' image of the child also changes as they recognize that their child has become an adult. If this shift does not occur, it is difficult for the young person to behave like an adult while his or her family persists in treating him or her like a child. Parents and children alike may be fearful and reluctant to redefine long-established roles, but such redefinition is necessitated by the young person's inexorable maturation process. These necessary redefinitions of self and family roles cause a stressful and tumultuous period in family life. During this often-stormy period, both the young person and his family may lose sight of the fact that the process of advancing growth usually promises rich rewards for all members of the family.

FREEDOM FOR GROWTH: TERRITORIALITY

Typically it is the adolescent and not his or her parents who perceives the need for new roles as old ones become confining. The desire to leave the family in order to assume more adult social roles frequently arises from the adolescent's discontent with his or her family role. Adolescents may feel that family members still relate to them as the children they once were and that the family's protectiveness smothers their individual growth, their ability to assume adult responsibilities, and their freedom to enjoy adult pleasures. Freedom to grow sometimes seems impossible within the family context. Thus assuming an adult role frequently requires a physical move out of the nuclear household to establish a separate territory. Such a move can be accomplished by marriage, going away to school, or moving to an apartment. One young person cited this reason for moving away from home:

I wanted to have a place of my own, that I could call my own. I wanted to decorate it the way that I wanted. I wanted my own space kind of thing, you know. I wanted to have my own friends over. Just to be out . . . of the parental type of supervision, without having to check [with] them if everything was okay, if I could bring someone over.

The establishment of territory separate from the family home is one way of asserting independence.

Although in some cultures marriage does not commonly require that both partners physically move from their parents' homes, all the married persons interviewed set up married life in a home physically separate from the homes of both their parents (although the distances varied greatly). In our culture, establishing a separate territory is important in achieving recognition of new social roles as independent adults. One young woman referred to this need for establishing her own separate territory. She said:

His mother and me are so much alike that we just don't get along. . . .Some day, as soon as I get the rest of my china and crystal, I'll have both sets of parents over but then they will be in my territory.

Couples associate a place of their own with consolidating their couple identity vis-à-vis their parents.

SOCIAL LIFE: THE PRIVILEGE OF FREEDOM

Parental dominance is considered most intolerable when it infringes on social life. The individuals interviewed said such social infringement was the primary source of conflict between themselves and their parents. Although their responses varied, all the young persons seemed to feel that their parents were unwilling to let them pursue their social lives as they wished. When experimenting with and assuming adult social behavior patterns, the young persons came into conflict with their parents' expectations and attempts to discipline them. These parental attempts to control social behavior were one reason why the young persons moved out to live alone. The social behavior conflict concerned dating and family participation and responsibility. Some young persons spoke of actual arguments or discipline regarding dating behavior. One individual stated:

There was a lot of conflict about how late — I would come downtown a lot, and I wouldn't get home until late, and my parents had every right to worry, you know. I would be worried, too, but I just couldn't . . . take that any longer. I was just waiting to move out because it was just getting on my nerves. Every time I would come home, you know, let's say it would be at 3:30 [A.M.], it wasn't that I was, you know, trying to come home to prove, just to come home late or something. I just didn't realize the time when I was having a good time. And they would really, you know, if that happened an awful lot, they would get really upset. And I just couldn't handle that any more because I kept saying to myself, I'm going to be working, I'm going to be, you know, I'm out of school, although I'm still, you know, young and that, I just couldn't see always being, you know, yelled at and stuff like that.

By setting up an independent household, the young persons minimized parental control over their lives. Their moving out was frequently precipitated by a critical incident such as the one a young woman described in relating her sister's move from home. She said:

Int: Do you remember what the fight was about?

She: Yeah, about her staying out late one night. She came home like 4:00 [A.M.], I think. And she was what, 22. And he [her father] waited up for her to yell at her. So she told him off, and the next day she went out and got an apartment.

When adolescents think parental attempts at control are inappropriate, they often take dramatic steps to assert their independence.

Other respondents, although they had experienced no overt conflict with their parents about dating, had sensed an underlying tension and thus felt the necessity of moving out to avoid possible conflict concerning their social life. Such adolescents were reacting to their internalized version of parental expectations whereas the absence of actual conflict about their dating behavior may have indicated that their parents had changed their expectations to coincide with their perceptions of their children's maturity. Often adolescents do not perceive changes in their parents' expectations, and the frequency of family disputes about dating causes young persons in our culture to expect their parents to react negatively. Some of the young people interviewed said that moving out was a way to protect parents from the reality of social life, to avoid hurting or upsetting them, and to prevent conflict. One young woman stated:

290. The Child Rearing and Child Launching Family

*My older sister doesn't like the guy I go out with at all, and there's a lot of
things my parents don't know about him that she knows, and I felt that at
any time she was going to bring this back to them.*

Another person said:

*I think it's sort of better, you know, for both of us because my mother doesn't
know exactly what I'm doing — not that I do anything wrong. Her mind
is a little more at ease. I just like not having to worry about if I have to
make up a story when I get home or something.*

Since conflict about social life frequently precipitated the young persons'
move from home, it is not surprising that many of the individuals interviewed
reported a change in their social life after they had moved out. This
change usually meant an increase in the amount of time they spent with
their respective boyfriends or girlfriends or an increase in the number of
dates they had. A third kind of change in their social lives was related to
their new-found freedom from family responsibilities. One young woman
commented on this freedom:

*I don't really have anything to stay home for now. Before Mom would seem
kind of lonely, and I'd stay home with her, and here, you know, there's
nothing like that. If I want to go out, I just go out.*

The respondents viewed their responsibilities toward their parents as
diminished once they no longer lived at home. They regarded their moving
out both as a way of relieving their parents' concerns about them and their
own concerns about their parents.

The married respondents reported a conflict between their new roles and
their still-persisting family responsibilities, demands, or expectations.
One young man complained about his wife's telephoning her mother:

*He: Anytime she passes the telephone or thinks of something to say, she calls
her mother. I wouldn't mind if they sat on the phone for two hours and
talked, but they say hello, talk for ten minutes, [and say] yeah, you're
right, and goodbye.*

She: She calls at inopportune times.

*He: Twenty minutes later we will get a continuation of this conversation; so
instead of talking it out in a half hour, it's spread across ten visits during the
day.*

The conflict between new and old family responsibilities and commitments
also surfaced during holidays, when the parents demanded and expected
reunions with their married children, who in turn felt themselves caught in a
conflict between these demands and their own desire for privacy. Many of

the young persons said holidays were particularly difficult times. The parents thought holidays were appropriate times for family reunions, which foster temporary regression into former parent-child roles. Such regression may be comforting and satisfying and allow for positive redefinition of family roles and growth as parents recognize and accept their children's progressing maturity and independence. On the contrary, it may serve to reactivate smoldering conflicts.

MISSING THE FAMILY

Launching can cause internal conflict in most young people because the mere act of trying to do something new causes feelings of insecurity, inadequacy, fear of failure, and loneliness. These feelings combine to create a nostalgic yearning for the security of a known role in the family. The young persons interviewed felt an overwhelming desire to be "on their own," to be free of parental dominance, and to establish their own identities. They did not want to retreat to their families. Yet they were torn between the warm, secure support of their families and their desire for independence and freedom. They reported a sense of isolation and loneliness at being away from family, home, and friends. Two respondents remarked:

It was very rough going, I think. Not so much financially or anything but emotionally to adjust. You are alone, and you have to go out and make friends, you know, even though you don't know how long you're going to be there.

I missed the joking around and just having someone there at home; coming home to an empty apartment is not exactly fun.

The respondents clearly recognized both advantages and disadvantages of being launched from the family home.

Some young people indicated that this sense of loneliness and loss diminished over time. Their moves were almost like an acute grieving process. After they have been away from home for a while, they realize that they have not completely lost their families, and their grief subsides. One person stated:

My first night was the most traumatic; you know, I couldn't sleep. I never had been away from home, and I thought I'd never be home again. I was lonely. I missed my friends. I missed, you know, my family.

This sense of loneliness was not limited to single persons. The married persons also missed their families, particularly their parents. Two young men stated:

That's one of the roughest things, especially at first, is missing your parents. I found it really hard 'cause I wanted to talk to them and go over there, you know, they are my parents.

*They're my parents, and I love them. They mean as much to me as anyone
else — I mean more than anyone else. They're my family, and I'm sure
she [wife] feels the same about her parents.*

While the feeling of loss experienced by marrieds and singles was similar,
the issue of divided loyalties further complicated the separation process for
the married persons.

NEGOTIATING A NEW ROLE IN THE FAMILY

In the course of our interviews, it became clear that launching or emancipation is never complete. When identifying our sample, we tried to use various
specific indicators of establishing independence from the family, such as
finances, separate housing, or marriage. However, as the young people discussed their situations and their feelings about them, it became apparent that
moving away from home is a gradual process. No person interviewed ceased
to consider his or her family of origin a primary reference point. For better
or worse, the parents' home remained "home," even after a new home
was established. One young woman remarked:

*I'll tell you, in some ways I don't feel as though I've left home. Technically,
this is my legal address now. I live here, and I've lived here for about eighteen
months and, technically, this is my home, but you know, you still think
of that [parents' home] as being home.*

Persons derive security from and are somewhat dependent on their original
families throughout their lives even though at various stages they must
fight battles to force family members to recognize what social role is appropriate to them as a maturing member. This battle takes place even in
the absence of a parent or both parents. Children so internalize their parents'
conception of them as children that even in the absence of the parents or
after the death of the parent(s) the children behave in ways that they feel
might prove to the parent(s) that they are mature adults.

Our culture has no universal ritual or ceremonial event that clearly marks
the transition from childhood to adulthood. No sharp demarcation point
exists between these two stages of life. Instead, there is a prolonged and
gradual transition process by which many young people practice or ease
themselves into a particular independent act. In some instances, a young
person's launching may be so gradual that no launching event is identifiable.
Yet several events may be viewed as milestones in the transition. Once a
young person selects a particular event as a milestone in his or her launching
process, he or she may find that his or her parents refuse to accept that
definition of the event and refuse to participate in it. One young woman
described her father's reaction to her moving into her own apartment:

*He said, you know, I haven't said much about this, and you haven't asked me
for much advice, but I think you're doing the wrong thing moving out*

because you're going to fall apart or something like that. You're going to come running back home to us.

Another young woman described her parents' reaction to her new job and relocation:

My parents didn't believe I would do it. They just thought that's all talk; she won't get a job. I got the job down here, and I kept saying I'm going to move in the summer. And they kept saying no, you won't move, you won't move, you'll stay here. And then finally, I moved. They still kept saying, you won't find an apartment, you'll move back home.

Parents' refusal to acknowledge the significance of certain launching events can make the transition process more difficult.

Frequently, a family's initial denial or frank sabotage of a young person's launching efforts were followed by capitulation, cooperation, and help if the family realized the young person's resolve was unshakable. During the initial, often uncertain period of establishing an independent role, a young person may feel a strong need to avoid contact with the parents or to flaunt his or her new status. One recently married woman stated:

I think we'll get closer to them and we'll end up spending more time with them once we've got our own life set up and we feel secure in each other and have more time to be with them. I think it will develop gradually, and we'll end up seeing more of them eventually.

Even while actively asserting their independence, children anticipate wanting to reestablish closer relationships with their families.

INDEPENDENCE AND ADJUSTMENT

The young people interviewed described their launching as an ongoing process during which their degree of independence from the family and adjustment to mature roles fluctuated. They were never totally independent of or dependent on their families; at times they sought new adventures, and at other times they returned to their families to recharge their batteries, to get advice or material help, to rest, or to fulfill long-standing obligations. Their adjustment was equally inconsistent. At times they regarded adult roles or responsibilities as challenging, exciting, and gratifying; at other times they found them frightening, confusing, and frustrating.

The amount of contact the young persons maintained with their parents was one measure of their degree of independence and adjustment. Although the persons interviewed had a wide range of contact patterns, all maintained some contact with their parents, by means of visits and telephone calls. Such contacts were influenced somewhat by distance and even more by the financial resources of the young persons and their parents. Some families had regular contact schedules that included telephone calls three times a week, or once a week, or every two weeks. Nearby offspring often had regular visiting schedules that included Sunday dinners or Friday night bridge games. Nearly every person had contact with his or her parents on holidays, and every person had called on his or her family for help during crises. Such help was varied and included such matters as finances, moving to a new home, fixing a flat tire, caretaking during childbirth, or simply the provision of comfort, support, or advice.

The young persons sought and received such help from parents and siblings equally. In fact, once they had moved out of the home, the young persons developed new patterns of interaction with their siblings, especially when these siblings were older and had been launched previously. Such siblings were most often used as role models and sources of guidance. Siblings took an active role in helping launch each other. They offered mutual assistance in finding an apartment, checking security, moving possessions, alleviating financial need, and, last but not least, giving emotional support when there was a conflict with the parents. Often older siblings were frankly protective of adolescents trying to launch themselves. Younger siblings often supported a brother's or sister's launching attempt because they could either participate in it and thus advance their own launching (like the younger sister who came to spend one night a week at her sister's new apartment so she could go out without a curfew) or at least pave the way for their anticipated future launching. Many who had been living at home at the time of a sibling's launching felt that they had learned from the experience. On the other hand, one young woman felt that she had learned from her older sister's decision to remain at home. This young woman remarked:

I could see my sister — how dependent she is on my parents and the family, and I think that's another reason I moved, because I didn't want to get like that. I didn't want to be that dependent. I just, I think that really scared me, to be like that when I'm her age.

Thus the respondents viewed their siblings as both positive and negative role models.

Many of the young persons moved out of the family home gradually. One young woman described her step-by-step movement thus:

I was planning to move out last May, but I couldn't find a place. So they [her parents] were exposed to that idea for about the third time in May. I had mentioned it before and just not found a place or put it off because of school. In September, I said, well, I'm going to go out and look for an apartment. They didn't say anything, but they knew it was coming all along. I kind of left little hints here and there. I went out to buy dishes, you know, and I'd show them little things I bought, and they knew what it was for; so it wasn't a big shocking thing. I thought I would expose them, you know, little at a time so they'd get used to the idea. And they did; they got pretty used to it.

Another way the young persons gradually moved out of the parents' home was to move to the home of a sibling or other relative. Such a move was viewed as a transitional step between living in the bosom of the family and being fully on one's own. This step-by-step progression in independence was reflected in the actual physical distance the young persons moved away from their parents' home. Some first moved into another apartment in the same building or into a nearby building owned by the parents or other relatives. They then moved at a later date to a more distant location as marriage or the advancement of their careers demanded and as proximity to family receded in importance.

THE REWARDS OF GROWTH

Because the transition from childhood to adulthood is an inexorable process precipitated by an adolescent's physical maturation, young persons may feel themselves being thrust into adult roles while they are still hesitant to leave childhood behind. On the basis of advancing years and physical maturation, society assigns young persons new tasks for which they may feel unready. They may feel that their families are pushing them to do things that they doubt that they can achieve. For example, one young woman remarked:

When the girls left home, my sister and I, there was none of this, you know, running away from home to escape home life at all. It was with the blessing of our parents. It was actually in some ways with the urging of our parents. Not because they wanted to get rid of us but because they wanted to see us develop more as individuals and wanted to see us reach a certain plateau of happiness on our own without being affected by them and without living under their particular judgment. You know, they wanted us to get out on our own and be able to manage our lives carefully without a lot of parental pressure.

Like other young persons interviewed, this woman was hesitant to leave the security of home.

Yet young persons are more likely to be eager to try out adult roles and experiences. As childhood roles become confining, adult privileges and responsibilities become very compellingly attractive. For the young persons interviewed, the advancement into adulthood was considered to be challenging, exciting, and very satisfying. Doing something independently for the first time brought the young persons great satisfaction and pleasure, and this sense of personal accomplishment was the great reward for and stimulus to continue their growth. When asked what she liked most about living away from home, one young woman replied:

Just being on my own. It's really hard to explain. It's just a heavy sense of being able to do it. I think that's the biggest thing.

This sense of accomplishment was enhanced when the young persons measured themselves against the standards of their peers and felt that society recognized and approved their transition to the new role. They regarded their move to a new, more adult stage as a superior achievement, and therefore felt very proud.

The young persons' parents were also rewarded as the young persons grew in their new roles. When lines of communication were intact, the young persons were happy and proud to share their accomplishments with their parents. Parental recognition and sharing of achievements enhanced the young persons' sense of satisfaction. For example, one young woman stated:

My Dad sees it as you'll always have work because they need nurses everywhere. And he's right. I'm really pleased, and they're proud of my finishing school. They're happy about it. So I think I'm, you know, I'm not a disappointment to them.

Another young woman spoke similarly and expressed satisfaction that she compared well with her sibling. She commented:

They're really proud of me that I'm able to do this at my age. Because they look at my sister, and she could never do this.

On the other hand, when the launching produced such estrangement that the young persons and their parents no longer communicated, the rewards and satisfactions of achievement were diminished for both. The individuals whose values and life-style differed radically from those of their parents felt a sense of loss in that they could not share their life and satisfactions with their parents. For example, one young man said with regret:

I can't sit down with my mother and talk more than an hour because I may hit on something I don't want her to know, you know? A problem I've had or something. With my Dad I go a little bit further, because he's more — 'cause my mother's very religious. I'm a lot different from my mother now.

When parents did not feel pride in the young persons' accomplishments and share in the satisfactions of their growth, the young persons often felt guilty over having hurt their parents by leaving home. Adolescents need their parents to express pride and pleasure in their adult accomplishments. Parental recognition of adulthood is part of the goal of a young person's launching. Parental recognition helps young persons to feel secure in their new role and enables them to participate in family life in a comfortable way that is rewarding for all family members.

In conclusion, nurses who deal with young persons and their families should teach them to keep the launching process in proper perspective. Young adults may feel that a particular problem or conflict is going to last forever because neither they nor their parents will change or be able to compromise. Obviously, this need not be true. Parental recognition of a young person's maturity and achievements in one matter will change their perspectives on his or her behavior in other matters. Parental acceptance of a young person's need for independence will make him or her more able to fulfill parental expectations.

A young person's fluctuating level of independence and adjustment should be expected. An adolescent may amaze everyone with his or her sudden adult behavior at one moment, but such behavior may be followed soon after by utter childishness. Throughout life, we experience periods of dependency on the family. Such periods of dependency should never be considered unhealthy. Launching is a persistent issue throughout life because the child has internalized the parents' expectations.

Nurses should recognize that negotiation is an integral part of the launching process. Often family members can reconcile a conflict if they are willing to bargain for whatever is most important to them at a particular time. This bargaining should not be viewed judgmentally as manipulation; it is a necessary way of effecting change while keeping communication channels open.

When young persons leave home, they are often acutely and painfully lonely. They may even regret having left. This quite natural reaction subsides quickly. As young persons become established and secure in their adult roles, they will relate to their families in more satisfying ways.

At times both the young person and his or her family may wish that they had never given up the security of their former relationships. They may idealize the security, harmony, and comfort of those relationships. Such regret is natural because neither young persons nor their parents can foresee the satisfaction both will experience when the former successfully assume adult roles. As the young persons grow in self-confidence and pride in achievement, they and their parents should be urged to maintain contact and communication so that both can share in the rewards of continuing growth.

20. Becoming an Empty-Nest Parent.

Janice K. Janken and Kathleen Astin Knafl

This chapter focuses on parents who have completed their child
rearing tasks. We chose to examine such "empty-nest" parents whose children
were grown and no longer living at home for two reasons. First, we sought
to determine the accuracy of popular beliefs that the empty-nest state is a
difficult period in the lives of parents, a period that requires major adjustments in order to make life meaningful and productive. Recent articles have
claimed to address the needs of purposeless parents whose children no
longer require the majority of their attention. We thus chose parents for
whom rearing a family had been a positive experience and whose children
were for the most part economically independent. Our goal was to understand how these parents perceived and managed this period of their lives.
Second, we sought to determine how such parents carried out the parenting
role after their children had achieved independence. In contrast to the
wealth of information written about parenting of children through their
adolescent years, relatively little has been written about parenting after
children have been launched. Yet mothers and fathers do not cease being
parents simply because their children have left home.

Data were collected from 22 parents, ten married couples and two additional women, one who was divorced and one whose husband refused
to be interviewed. All parents were interviewed once, and the couples were
interviewed together. Demographic information about the sample is summarized in Table 2.

This chapter explores several dimensions of the empty-nest state. It
first examines the process by which parents launch their children. It then
examines the adjustments parents must make and the satisfactions they
experience after all their children have been launched. Finally, it explores
the way in which parents carry out the parenting role after their children
have achieved relative independence. In general, the chapter traces the

Table 2. Demographic Characteristics of Respondents

Number	Age*	Education	Occupation	Number of Children	Religion	Economic Level
1	F 58	Vocational training	Secretary	4	Protestant	Comfortable
	M 58	Some college	Stock broker		Protestant	Comfortable
2	F 59	High school	Service worker (housewife)	2	Roman Catholic	Adequate
	M 60	High school	Service worker		Roman Catholic	Adequate
3	F 61	High school	Housewife	1	Protestant	Comfortable
	M 61	Graduate school	Professional		Protestant	Comfortable
4	F 57	Graduate school	Professional	3	Protestant	Comfortable
	M 58	Graduate school	Professional		Protestant	Comfortable
5	F 73	Graduate school	Housewife	3	Protestant	Comfortable
	M 77	Graduate school	Retired controller		Protestant	Comfortable
6	F 43	College degree	Professional	2	Protestant	Comfortable
	M 46	Graduate school	Professional		Protestant	Comfortable
7	F 45	High school graduate	Clerical worker	2	Greek Orthodox	Adequate
8	F 61	Some college	Housewife	3	Protestant	Adequate
	M 62	Some college	Manager-proprietor		Protestant	Adequate
9	F 69	Some college	Housewife	2	Protestant	Comfortable
	M 70	Graduate school	Professional		Protestant	Comfortable
10	F 55	High school graduate	Manager	2	Roman Catholic	Comfortable
	M 58	Vocational training	Craftsman-foreman		Protestant	Moderately wealthy
11	F 51	Graduate school	Professional	3	Latter-Day Saints	Comfortable (divorced)
12	F 48	College degree	Professional	3	Protestant	Comfortable
	M 47	College degree	Professional		Protestant	Comfortable

*F = Female, M = Male.

transition parents experience as they assume and then adjust to their new empty-nest role.

THE LAUNCHING PROCESS

Launching is a term used to denote the point at which parents release their children from the family to lead relatively independent lives. Going away to college or getting married are common launching events. Although launching is often defined as the point at which children first leave the home, the parents interviewed perceived launching as a gradual process and not as a single event. The following quotes illustrate this point of view:

He: He kind of gradually left home. He went to three years of medical school and four years of college in Illinois. He was here, he stayed down there and came home for about a week or ten days, two weeks. Then, when he got out of there, he residenced in town, and he lived here and spent a year at the hospital. Then he went to another hospital and stayed there for a time, and then he got married. He was off and on during that thirteen years studying medicine, stayed off and on here, and then, when he got through, he went in the Army.

He: [Talking about a daughter who went to nursing school] The last year they could live out of the hospital; so she came home for that year.

She: And then she went back to school until she graduated, and then she came home until she was married. And then she left home.

He: It was so gradual. He went four years to regular college, and then he came home, and he worked summers, and he went to Wisconsin for business college to get his master's up there. And then he came home again, and he was working, and he was engaged. And so these things sort of occurred in little bits and pieces to the extent that when he was married, which was almost two years after his graduation from his first four years of college, it was prepared for. The stage was set, and so okay, he leaves the house, and he moves to a neighboring community, and it's not very far away. It was just really a bunch of general little knocks.

Each of these parents had experienced a time when their children left home to live independently, but in each case the parents tended to view their children as not completely launched and their home as the children's base. The parents only gradually became aware that their children had been launched. One instance of a child's leaving home did not precipitate immediate acceptance of the fact that that child was gone.

Yet the parents interviewed were able to identify one event during which they felt acutely aware that their children were leaving home. The following quotes refer to the point at which parental awareness of a child's leaving home was most acute:

She: She went away to school, and the bottom fell out of my world. The first

301. *Becoming an Empty-Nest Parent*

six months she was gone, I just didn't think I was going to get used to having her gone. She was a pal, a companion, and a great help to me. But she did go; she had to go.

She: Very difficult.

He: For her to leave home and go to college was difficult for us. Extremely difficult.

He: Well, I left that morning and went to work, and when he got ready to go, he just took his little bag and went down the alley to get on the train.

She: Yes, all I can remember is seeing him go down the alley with his little bag, which of course tore our hearts out, but there he went to serve his country in the war.

He: I guess we both went the first time he went to school. It was temporarily a very traumatic experience, a few lumps, a few tears shed.

She: I just couldn't talk. As soon as I turned away I started to cry. And all the way home, driving all the way home, I just felt so bad. I felt like just think what it must really be like when they go in the service. I mean this is a joyous thing for them [going to college]. So it really did break me up.

The experience of being aware of a child's leaving home was difficult and painful for the parents. They often used the word "traumatic" to describe how they felt about this event.

In general, the parents thought that a child's first departure was more difficult than those that followed. Because the majority of parents had sent their children away to college immediately after high school, they identified the first trip to school as the most traumatic event. However, whether the parents launched their children to college, marriage, an apartment, or the armed services, the majority indicated that a child's first departure was the most painful.

In contrast, two couples who sent their daughters away to college did not experience the acute and painful awareness of launching until a later time. These parents felt the pain of departure when their daughters married. One woman stated:

When your child gets married, you suddenly, well, while they are dating, you can still make comments, you can still say, "I don't think this is right" or "I don't think you should stay out late" or something on that order. But once they are married, it's wise to keep your thoughts to yourself. As a mother you feel free to express yourself, but once your child is married, if you're wise, you keep your thoughts to yourself because that's the way of acknowledging your daughter and her husband as a couple. . . . My youngest daughter [away at college] is still a part of our little group and until she gets married, I'm more or less hanging on.

Both couples' reactions to sending their daughters to college were insignificant when compared to the traumatic feelings they experienced when their daughters married.

In general, the parents reacted to the launching of children as a necessary but difficult and sad process. However, two couples reported that they were eager to launch one of their children and in fact had encouraged the child to leave home. In both cases, the parents thought the child's value system conflicted with their own. One couple stated:

He: By that time she was working and so independent that things were beginning to get a little difficult. She had her own friends, who were constantly here, for one thing, one fellow in particular. I don't remember specific disagreements with her.

She: She had time after graduating from high school to kind of look around and still have some kind of structure at home without having a tremendous amount of responsibility thrust on her right away. Then getting a job, then beginning to want to be more independent, pursue her own way of doing things. She became interested in nutrition. That was not necessarily a clash, although it was a different life-style because she was interested in organic foods and wanted to cook her own meals. At that point, the next step in her being independent was to manage her own finances, her own resources. So I think we encouraged the move.

The other couple said:

She: She was just plain rebellious.

He: Rebellious and resentful in her senior year in high school, and it's a good thing because by fall, when it was time for her to go to college, we were perfectly delighted to take her off to college and get rid of her. I think it's a perfectly natural and wonderful thing that the rebellion occurs at this point so that both parents and youngsters are glad to have a separation, and the separation comes very easily that way.

When these parents thought their children were pursuing a life-style different from their own, they were relieved to see them launched and did not experience the painful and traumatic departure event. However, both couples did experience the more common trauma when launching their other two children.

In spite of their marked response to each child's departure, the parents noted very little change in their family routine if younger children remained at home. The following comments are illustrative:

He: There was no difference as each child left for the first time. When K. left, R. and P. didn't act any differently than they did before. When R. left, P. didn't act any differently.

303. Becoming an Empty-Nest Parent

He: I think the kids each had their own circle of friends. They weren't chums or buddies with each other. They each had their own friends; so it didn't change the home life a great deal.

She: There was no difference in family living after our older one left.

In fact, the parents reported little change in their lives until their last child was launched. At this point, they were faced with having to restructure their family routine. They indicated that although it was difficult to see any child leave home, the real adjustment occurred after the last child was launched and they were left alone.

ADJUSTMENTS AND SATISFACTIONS

Launching a child engendered feelings of both anticipation and sadness in the parents. With the departure of each child, the accustomed activity and excitement of their family life diminished. As their responsibilities lessened, the parents gradually acknowledged and learned to enjoy the sense of freedom that accompanied their new situation. When discussing their lives since the departure of their children, the parents identified three broad areas of change. These changes related to routine daily activities, feelings of responsibility and personal freedom, and their marital relationship.

Patterns of Activity

Men and women reacted differently to certain aspects of the empty-nest state. The women reported experiencing the more dramatic change in their routine daily activities. Some described becoming an empty-nest parent as a gradual transition while others viewed it as an abrupt and wrenching break with a role and a way of life they had known and enjoyed. The men, on the other hand, reported only minimal change in this aspect of their lives. While some said they now had more time to pursue hobbies and various pleasurable activities, all said that the general pattern of their days had remained the same. When questioned about changes in his life since the departure of his children, one man replied:

Actually, it's pretty much the same. I have the same responsibilities and the same job pressures. I don't even have more free time. It's just that I have more flexibility in how I'm going to spend it.

The women thought that many activity changes were imposed upon them as a result of the departure of the last child from the home. One woman said:

You're so used to doing things when you have children at home that it was the biggest shock to me trying to decide what I wanted to do.

While the men perceived their lives as unchanged, the women felt a need to change the way they spent their days.

304. The Child Rearing and Child Launching Family

The women reacted to and managed these changes differently. Some enjoyed their additional free time and devoted more time to activities in which they were already involved. Those women who had previously worked or had established activities outside the home viewed the empty-nest state as a natural, essentially problem-free transition. For example, one woman commented:

Well, we were lonely when the children were gone; but we're both very active and have always been involved in many different activities. When they had left, I was doing substitute teaching and writing. I was looking forward to having more time to spend writing. My life was just too filled with activities to sit around and cry about their being gone.

Women who were genuinely looking forward to expanding their involvement in already established activities had little difficulty adjusting to the empty-nest situation.

Other women were distressed by the initial emptiness of their lives after their children left home. Because they did not have enough to do to fill their days, they experienced a longer, more painful adjustment period than the women who had outside interests. One woman described her reaction:

You have to analyze yourself. I was quite miserable for awhile. I didn't know quite what was the matter with me. Then I found some volunteer occupations that I could fill my day with. Since I've done that, my world is much better.

Four of the five women who had difficulty adjusting their daily routines to their new situation eventually resolved the problem to their own satisfaction. Three became involved in new activities, and the other woman gradually learned to spread her usual activities over a longer span of time. The woman whose adjustment problems remained unresolved had been an empty-nest parent for only a short time.

Activity changes were an important variable in the amount of adjustment the parents had to make. The men made relatively few adjustments since their daily work routine remained the same. Similarly, women whose daily routines included activities outside the home experienced few adjustment problems. Only those women whose activities focused exclusively on their families encountered problems. Rather than looking forward to devoting additional time to already established activities, they felt that circumstances over which they had no control had forced them to change their daily routine. Consequently, they regarded empty-nest parenthood as both more difficult and less desirable than the other parents regarded it.

Freedom and Responsibility

More subjective changes had to do with the nature and quality of the individuals' lives as empty-nest parents. Both the men and the women felt a lightened sense of responsibility and an increased sense of freedom. Only one woman viewed these feelings negatively.

305. Becoming an Empty-Nest Parent

The parents identified two broad types of responsibility inherent in child rearing. They differentiated physical tasks and emotional ones. The impact of no longer having to perform the various physical tasks of parenthood is apparent in the following comments:

She: I guess I just don't have the responsibility; so I don't have to do a lot of things. Like I don't have to get home to cook a meal or pick them up from something or drop them off.

He: With kids, you are always doing — fixing bikes, doing this, taking them here and there. It took a big part of my life. I could never go right home from work. I'd go right from work and pick up seven kids and drop them off here and there. I had a regular route that I dropped off kids. No one ever asked me. Mine would just say, "Dad will take you home."

The parents viewed life without children at home as simpler, with less time devoted to the obligations of parenthood.

The parents also reported a decreased sense of emotional responsibility for their children. Although they all cared deeply for their children, they no longer experienced the constant worries associated with children living at home. One man said:

There is no longer that worry of where are they every minute. When they're [living] with you, there is always that concern in the back of your mind. Where's B.? Where's J.? When will they be home? Who are they with? What are they doing? When they're gone, you can drop that. It's gone. It's no longer something you have to be concerned with.

Parents invariably identified adolescence, the years immediately preceding launching, as particularly worrisome. In comparison, they viewed their present emotional investment in their children as less intense and more fulfilling. The parents continued to worry about only those children who were not financially and domestically established.

The parents felt an increased sense of personal freedom as their family responsibilities lightened. Their newly acquired freedom allowed them greater latitude in how they managed their lives. For example, one parent said:

We're freer now to go out to a restaurant. Like maybe after church instead of going home we might go out to a pancake house. You're freer in your activities because you don't have the responsibility of having somebody at home. It's more relaxing. It's easier on both of us.

Although some of the women had initial difficulty adjusting to this diminution of responsibility with its resultant increase in freedom, they learned to appreciate this aspect of being an empty-nest parent.

The men and women linked their general satisfaction with being empty-

306. The Child Rearing and Child Launching Family

nest parents to their more focused satisfaction with the lives their children were leading. In short, they believed they had earned their more relaxed, freer existence because they had successfully fulfilled their responsibilities to their children. One woman remarked:

It just seems we have lots of time to do the things we like and want to do without worrying about responsibilities. We're satisfied with how the children have turned out, happy with the way things are.

Even though the parents had very little control over the diminished responsibility brought about by their children's departure, they still viewed their new-found freedom as well-deserved and therefore something to be savored.

Moreover, the parents saw themselves as having accomplished an important adult developmental task. In spite of the occasional adjustment problems they had experienced, the men and women described launching children into independent lives as a normal, healthy process. One man emphasized the normality of the process, saying:

There are major issues here. The umbilical cord should be cut and has been cut. Things are as they should be. They have their independence and there is nothing to dislike about the situation.

Even those women who had initial difficulty coping with being empty-nest parents stated that in their unhappiest hours they knew their children's launchings were essentially healthy occurrences.

The Marital Relationship
The marital bond of all but one couple was strengthened after their last child was launched. This strengthening was a function of having more time to spend together and fewer constraints on how that time could be spent. The couples communicated more with each other and, in general, felt closer to one another. The following quotes (the first by a woman, the second by a man) illustrate this shift in the quality of the marital relationship:

We are much, much closer. Like he would never go shopping with me and now he does. It's really different. We'll sit and talk with no interruptions. Before if you wanted to say something, maybe it was just something you didn't say in front of the children. Now we can just sit and talk for an hour.

I think we're a little closer as a couple. We don't have to devote all our attention to the kids. I think we have a little more concern for each other. I think we tend to do more things together than we did when the kids were at home.

These couples indicated that while their relationship had always been good, it was now much stronger and closer. They were communicating more often and in a more positive way. Problem-oriented discussions centered on the children gradually gave way to more relaxed exchanges. In short, these empty-nest parents had less complicated lives that allowed for more time to enjoy each other. Several couples compared this time of their lives with the period when they were young married couples without children.

PARENTING THE INDEPENDENT CHILD

Once the children were launched from the home, new patterns of contact and interaction emerged between them and their parents. These patterns reflected both a quantitative and a qualitative change in the parent-child relationship.

Patterns of Communication and Contact

The parents and their children maintained both direct and indirect contacts with each other. In addition to actually seeing each other, they stayed in contact through telephone conversations and correspondence. Interestingly, the parents reported less variation in the amount of indirect contact than in the amount of direct contact.

Regardless of the distance separating them, the parents and their children had frequent telephone contacts. Weekly telephone conversations were the norm for those parents whose children lived in the vicinity. Three women had daughters who contacted them daily. One woman noted:

Our oldest daughter calls me every day as soon as the kids are off to school. It's nice; there's always something to talk about.

Both the parents and the children initiated telephone contacts. The parents said that children who lived in the vicinity called them frequently and without hesitation. Yet they expressed some concern that their own calls might be regarded as an intrusion or interruption. One woman stated:

I don't often call the girls because I feel it's better for them to call me. My mother and I had a very close relationship. She always felt she would be interrupting my life with the children or something, so [she] seldom called. But I called her every morning. So the girls continue the practice and call me every morning.

Despite the parents' occasional fears that their own calls might be an intrusion, they offered no evidence that their offspring had ever responded to their calls in a negative way.

Telephone contact with children living some distance from their parents was slightly less frequent. These contacts were usually on a monthly basis, although they ranged in frequency from several times a week to several times a year. Often parents joked good-naturedly about astronomical phone bills. Usually, the parents and their children had informally agreed to alternate initiating long-distance calls. Long-distance calling was not limited to emergencies or special occasions. Quite simply, parents and children called each other as a substitute for visiting each other. One woman remarked:

*Very often I'll just get a call from her. In fact, just yesterday I got a call, and
she said, "What are you doing Mom? I was just thinking about you, wanting
to talk to you." Actually, I'm just so thrilled we have the telephone. I
don't know what I'd do without it.*

Clearly, the telephone was a crucial and regularly used means for maintaining
close contacts among family members.

The parents viewed writing as a less satisfying form of communication.
Except for one woman who made a point of writing to each of her three
children every week, letter writing was not the preferred mode of communication. More typically, the parents described both themselves and their
children as "not the greatest letter writers." The convenience and immediacy
of the telephone clearly made it the parents' favorite means of communication.

The responsibility for maintaining parent-child contacts was almost always
delegated to the woman family member. Mothers and daughters were in
especially frequent contact. Accordingly, all reported instances of daily
contacts were between mothers and daughters while the least frequent
contacts were between parents and their sons. The sons called their parents
less frequently than the daughters. Moreover, married sons delegated the
task of correspondence to their wives; any letters were written by mothers
and daughters-in-law. Only one father regularly initiated contact with his
children. Communication usually took place through the women to the
men in the family. One man described this phenomenon thus:

*The kids will be over, and I'll be out puttering around in the yard. They'll
be in talking to their mother, but they're there, and I know they're there,
and they know where I am. It's like when we're talking on the telephone,
my wife does 98 percent of the talking, but I'm listening. As long as there's
the communication, that counts for me too.*

Other men said that their wives would report on the content of telephone
conversations, selecting the most important information. All the men thought
they sustained close contacts with their children although they recognized
that this contact was frequently channeled through their wives.

Nine of the ten couples reported that the amount of contact was greater
between female than male family members. When describing their contacts
with their children, the parents would often initially say, "We're constantly
on the phone." When questioned further, however, they revealed that the
men would talk briefly with children and the women would talk in detail and
at great length, especially with their daughters. For example, one man noted
with pride that his daughter felt free to talk to her mother about anything.
He believed these talks were indicative of an open, close relationship between
this child and both himself and his wife. In other words, the women established the tone or quality of the relationship, which the men then generalized
to themselves. The women also talked to their sons on the telephone more

often and at greater length than their husbands did. However, the women reported less frequent telephone contacts with sons than with daughters.

The amount of direct contact the parents had with their children varied much more. Like telephone contact, direct contact was not primarily determined by distance. Parents and children who lived close to each other visited as frequently as several times a week to as infrequently as once a month. For example, one daughter who was busy with her job during the week and with her social life on the weekend had few opportunities to visit her parents. Nonetheless, she maintained close contact by calling them four or five times a week. Regular, frequent visits were the rule only if the parents and the child lived in the same immediate area.

Parents and children who were separated by great distances had only limited opportunities to see each other. One man commented:

It can be very difficult. You've got one in Pennsylvania, one in West Virginia, and one in Colorado, and getting together becomes difficult. Like this last Christmas, we took our one daughter out to Colorado with us to be with our son. Normally on Thanksgiving, she has driven here to be with us even though it's a 1,600-mile round trip. This past Christmas was the first time we haven't all been together. The one just couldn't make it.

In spite of the limitations imposed by distance, parents and children in this situation usually saw each other at least once a year. They regarded vacations and family holidays as welcome opportunities to be together.

Family members who want to maintain contact in a society as mobile as ours must supplement their direct contacts with other means of interaction. The parents interviewed all stressed the importance of the telephone in maintaining close family ties. These parents felt very much in touch with their children in spite of the great distances that separated them. Visits to children who lived out of town were major and very special events. Although they delighted in these visits, the parents recognized that such infrequent contacts were inadequate for maintaining close family ties. The parents thus developed a new view of their role as parents. They saw themselves as interested, caring persons very much on call to meet the needs of their children.

New Perspectives on a Role

When questioned about the role of the empty-nest parent, the men and women spoke in comparative terms, contrasting their present relationship with their children to their parenting role when the children still lived at home. Their discussions typically included both a general, reflective evaluation of their past parenting role and a description of their efforts to explicitly alter that role once their children were fully launched.

Evaluations of past performance were indirect. The parents never specifically evaluated what they had done; instead, they evaluated their children's activities and used them as measures of their parenting. They evaluated their children along two major dimensions: (1) their progress toward achieving financial independence, and (2) their progress toward establishing happy, stable home lives. The parents expected their children to accomplish these tasks and did not view them as fully launched until they had done so. The parents displayed different attitudes toward fully launched and partially launched children. For example, one parent said:

Now our oldest, I think we prepared him for manhood, and he's doing very well. He's very independent and has a good career. He's married with a wife and baby, and we have just taken a hands-off attitude. Now with the other two, well, they're not married yet; so that's a different story.

The parents fully expected that their children would accomplish the usual adult developmental tasks. All either defined their children as fully launched or well on their way to being so. Once the parents perceived their offspring as truly independent, the quality and quantity of their parental involvement changed.

These parents saw themselves as taking on a comparatively less directive and more supportive parenting role once their children were leading independent lives. They reported that they consciously shifted the orientation of their parenting once their children were fully launched. Supportive endeavors that had always been an element of the parenting role now became its prime focus. One man described this change in orientation thus:

As far as our relationship as parents, I would say that we are attempting to fulfill our conscience and be of any help we possibly can without interfering.

One woman commented:

I think as a parent I still have responsibilities to continue the relationship, to communicate that I still care without being an overly protective mother.

All the parents admitted that their parenting role should become and did become less directive once their children left home. The actual level of directiveness gradually diminished as the children moved toward complete financial independence and established stable home lives of their own.

Yet at the same time the men and women acknowledged the need to become less directive in their parenting behavior, they noted that this goal was difficult to achieve. After years of taking a very active part in their children's lives, most parents often found it difficult not to exert influence. One man said:

We have very strong feelings, and it's very difficult not to say what we think they should do, but they're all adults now, and they've got to make their own decisions.

311. Becoming an Empty-Nest Parent

One woman pointed out that treating her children as independent adults was particularly difficult when they returned home for visits. She said:

The minute they come home for any reason that same feeling is back again. When they go out at night, you worry where they are, what are they doing. When they aren't under your roof, you don't have to worry about them. But when they are back, you want to treat them just the same.

The parents' resolve not to cling to their children was apparent throughout the interviews. They viewed "letting go" as a very real responsibility of parenthood. Although most reported occasional difficulty in sustaining their resolve not to interfere, they overcame their tendency to be more directive. Possessiveness had never been an actual problem in their relationships with their children. Rather, it was a personal, internal matter that the parents themselves had to grapple with and overcome. For these men and women, empty-nest parenting was essentially parenting on call. These parents were available whenever their children needed them, but they maintained a comparatively low profile at other times. They were very interested in their children's lives and took great pride both in their children's successes and in the fact that they had maintained such close ties with them. They viewed their children's accomplishments as proof of their success as parents. They saw their present relationships with their children as essentially positive. No longer having to worry about the specific details of child rearing or its results, these parents at long last were able, quite simply, to enjoy their children.

This chapter has addressed two broad questions: first, is the popular image of the empty-nest state valid, and second, how do individuals parent an independent child? The popular image emphasizes the negative aspects of the empty-nest state. To a certain extent, this picture is misleading. The initial launching of children is painful, but after a relatively brief period, the parents interviewed not only adjusted to their new situation, but found it satisfying and enjoyable. One satisfied parent sensed the feeling of others:

You have learned nothing except that there must be many, many people who are completely satisfied as they get older. If you could interview most couples our age who have gone through our experience, you would find that they say, "It's good; we like it this way." It would be the very exceptional couple who didn't like it.

Clearly, many parents view the empty-nest state as a normal, healthy, essentially problem-free process. The parents interviewed maintained a high level of involvement in their children's lives, but the quality of this involvement changed as the children established their independence. Upon completing their child rearing tasks, the parents redefined their relationships with their children. Viewing their children as fully independent, they emphasize the supportive, nondirective aspects of the parenting role.

VI. The Family and the Nurse. When

planning the two chapters in this last part, we had two equally ambitious goals in mind. Chapter 21 places individual family roles in the context of a functioning unit that cuts across generations. As such, it presents a more integrated view of families than the other chapters in this book have presented. Chapter 22 discusses some of the pitfalls open to nurses who venture into research. Our own experiences provide the data used to consider the intervention versus observation dilemma of the nurse-researcher. While previous chapters have presented raw findings, the fruits of our various research endeavors, this final chapter looks at the subjective experience of doing research. It is therefore a highly personal chapter. In it, we evaluate certain aspects of our data and of our relationship to our research subjects. In it, we speculate about our findings and offer nurse-researchers valuable, practical insights into the substance and meaning of the research process for nurses.

21. The Family Across Generations.
Karen Skerrett

Earlier chapters have focused on various combinations of the
nuclear family, e.g., wife and husband, parent and child. This chapter focuses
on the larger family system. Obviously, families extend beyond the nuclear
unit. They include a grandparent generation and often an elaborate network
of kin. Indeed, family life begins at birth and ends at death. The nuclear
family is only one aspect of the family cycle. Each family member represents
a kinship link backward in time and a potential link forward into future
generations.

The term *generation* is complex and can be defined in two ways: generation
as cohort and generation as lineage. The two are separated only for ease of
analysis and do not exist apart in everyday life. Those who view generations
as cohorts define them as aggregates of individuals who have experienced together certain historical events, e.g., the generation of the Great Depression.
Those who view generations as lineage define generations as groups of individuals who are linked either socially or biologically in an explicit interpersonal relationship. The most obvious example of this linkage is the family.
In order to understand the dynamics of a given intergenerational relationship,
we must take four broad issues into account. First, each lineage member be-
longs to an age cohort whose value system is distinct. Second, any relationship exists in a particular sociocultural milieu. Third, each lineage member is
a developing individual whose set of concerns are unique to his or her own
personal developmental experiences. Finally, cultural and individual changes
occur within the life span of an intergenerational relationship that make it
a continuously evolving entity.

In order to fully understand the impact of one family member on another,
we must account for intergenerational relationships. Intergenerational interaction, the exchange of values, norms, and information, is a fascinating area for
investigation. However, very little work has been done to evaluate the quan-

315

tity and quality of the interactions between generations. Cross-generational interaction is a multidimensional process that raises a number of interesting questions. Are particular family members more influential within their own generation or with members of another generation? How does this influence come about? How is its impact felt? Does it really affect the way an individual behaves?

In order to best gain an understanding of intergenerational relationships, we put these questions to several families and asked them to answer in terms of their own extended family relationships. Specifically, we contacted families who had at least three generations of whom one of each was willing and able to be interviewed. Coincidentally, all the generational representatives were women, so this chapter evaluates intergenerational relations among women. One family constituted four generations; the grandmother had recently become a great-grandmother. In each family, we interviewed grandmother, mother, and daughter (so labeled throughout this chapter). Since we asked each generation essentially the same questions, we were able to identify common ways of perceiving the family. We sought to determine if extended families transact their business according to certain patterns and if these patterns can be identified by a member of each generation.

The ages of the family members interviewed were relatively similar; the grandmothers were in their sixties or seventies, the mothers in their mid-forties, and the daughters in their early twenties and beginning to establish their own families. Typically, the grandmothers were retired, and several had other grown children who lived out of state. The mothers were housewives either active in the community or doing part-time teaching. All the daughters were employed full-time. Although the families were few in number, they shared generously their thoughts and feelings, seemed to enjoy talking about their families, and gave the impression that the notion of intergenerational influence was a new idea and an interesting way for them to think about their family lives.

INTERGENERATIONAL CONTACTS

The frequency and nature of intergenerational contacts was the first pattern assessed. Each of the families was characterized by frequent contacts among the women. Shopping expeditions tended to be the most typical reason for contact. The generations always agreed in their descriptions of the frequency and nature of their contacts. The mothers either saw or talked on the telephone to their own mothers at least once a week; more telephone calls were made in the absence of a weekly visit. Mothers and daughters interacted frequently; one daughter whose mother lived close to her place of employment had the habit of visiting on her lunch hour to "watch the soap opera and eat with Mom." Contacts among all three generations were almost exclusively initiated by either mothers or daughters; grandmothers would occasionally call their daughters if they had not heard from them during the week.

The frequency of these contacts, in part a function of close proximity, seemed very important to both the grandmothers and the mothers and definitely related to whom each one felt closest to in the family. One grandmother, who described never having felt as close to a son as to a daughter, claimed she felt closest to the daughter interviewed because they saw so much of each other. She recognized the growing importance of such contacts since the rest of the family was "so splintered and out of touch." Her emotional distance from her son extended to his children as well. She remarked:

My other two grandchildren now . . . my two grandchildren on my son's side, I don't get to see — you wouldn't believe it. I haven't seen the oldest one in two years, and she doesn't even call me. That's where I'm trying to tell you the closeness comes in.

One mother, who cited another daughter as her favorite from birth, described how this favoritism shifted as her daughters matured. She was now much closer to the daughter interviewed, again because they visited so frequently, which the mother interpreted to mean that her daughter had grown more interested in her as a person.

It was difficult to discern to what degree these contacts were motivated by a sense of duty. This difficulty may be related to the unwillingness of family members to admit the obligatory element. When asked why she called her own mother, one mother replied:

I want to talk to her. It's a duty thing in a way . . . I mean I'm sure she'd be very upset if I didn't, but it's usually because there's something I want to get her opinion on or let her know something, because if I don't tell her what the children are doing, and she hears it later, she'd say, "Why didn't you tell me?"

One mother hinted that her frequent calls and visits to her mother contained a "shade of duty" but claimed that what may have begun as duty evolved into a "desire." Generally, because these families' contacts were motivated by a willingness and need to be close to each other, the pleasure afforded each was mutually reinforcing.

At the same time, each generation had a regard for the privacy of the other. Contacts were seldom spontaneous; if visits were made on the spur of the moment, they were always preceded by a telephone call. One set of grandparents who at one point began to drop in on their children unexpectedly got the message that such spontaneity was not appreciated, and these visits gradually ceased. Greater permissiveness was allowed between mothers and their daughters. Mothers were quite tolerant of daughters' occasional unannounced visits and made no effort to change this behavior.

As might be expected, aside from the shopping expeditions, the most frequent form of contact focused on family rituals and celebrations such as Christmas and birthdays. Each generation derived great pleasure from these activities, particularly as a result of the continuity and sense of stability they provided the participants. The women's descriptions of these occasions suggested a sense of awareness and appreciation of these festivities as symbols or statements of the uniqueness of their family lives.

The frequency and place of contact did shift noticeably over the life cycle of the families. Mothers reported seeing their parents more frequently when their children were small, particularly if the grandmother was providing child care during weekdays or baby-sitting in the evenings. These visits typically took place at the grandparents' home since it was "easier to bundle them up and take them there than have the gang here." As the children grew to puberty, family visiting took place at the homes of the mothers' generation. Daughters invited their parents to their homes infrequently and almost never invited their grandparents. No family member was able to remember why the change from grandparent to parent home had come about, but each generation was satisfied with the arrangement. Overall, these generations were content with their entire pattern of contact with each other. Only one grandmother verbalized a hope for change, wishing aloud that she could have such frequent contact with all her children.

PATTERNS OF INTERGENERATIONAL INFLUENCE

One of the most striking features of the process of intergenerational interviewing was the difficulty all family members had in talking about their influences on each other. They could respond to questions about the kind and frequency of their contacts, how they "got along" with each other, and, with a bit more difficulty, how they felt about each other, but the whole idea that they influenced each other was quite foreign. Frequently, the women would say that they gave or received "advice" or that they shared their "opinions," but they continually denied that they were either influential or being influenced. The women tended to attach negative connotations to the idea of influence; to them, the term suggested a conscious effort to manipulate others. They preferred to express opinions. They even made a distinction between solicited and unsolicited opinions, the former clearly being the more acceptable. In either case, the women did not equate expressing opinions with exerting influence. When asked to think of influence in broader terms, the women were better able to identify and discuss episodes that served as examples of influence being exerted among family members. They were also then able to differentiate between successful and unsuccessful attempts at influence.

No matter what term the women used to describe their relationships with others, the importance of kinship lines as the determinants of who could influence whom was clear. In each of the generations, in-laws appeared on the periphery of family influence in all quantitative and qualitative aspects of family relationships. Their behavior was either of less concern or was mediated through contacts with kin. Mothers, grandmothers, and daughters agreed that their spouses might be influenced by being present at family gatherings but that such influence was certainly indirect and of much less concern than their patterns of influence between each other. One mother described the single occasion when she tried talking directly to her son-in-law about a marital conflict. She stated:

I said that was "just between the two of us" though and she wouldn't know I'd talked to him and let it go at that. Well, of course, big-mouth son-in-law had to make a comment later; so I decided never to talk to him again in private if he was going to be that way.

This comment is a good example of the mutuality of the influence process. The mother's attempt to expand her kin boundaries to include advice to her son-in-law did not coincide with his definition of intergenerational relationships. His failure to keep the interaction private can be interpreted as an attempt to register his personal expectations to restore intergenerational family influence to exclusive kin boundaries.

The mother was clearly the most influential family member in terms of making an impact on others and receiving the influence of others. In each family, the mother emerged as a center of gravity or fulcrum that balanced the preceding and following generations. More connecting lines flowed from and toward her than connected any other dyads in the generational network. She was consulted concerning finances, home buying, furnishing, and decorating. She was the pacesetter in fashion and hairstyles. She was the interpreter of child care techniques and the guardian of health. One daughter who recognized her mother's role stated:

Well, my grandmother is a lot like my mother, not because my mother learned from her. My grandmother copies everything my mother does. My mother is in the middle. It never fails . . . my Mom will do something little . . . like if she had to make this centerpiece, the next time you go over there my grandmother has got the makings for it. Even stuff as small as that.

Although the mothers were most influential overall, the grandmothers clearly had the most lines of influence flowing downward from themselves to others. In other words, they attempted the most influence. Their opinions and advice, almost never solicited, focused on finances. This advice, usually connected to some action of other family members, such as buying a house or taking out more insurance, was occasionally precipitated by discussion of other issues. For example, one grandmother stated:

My daughter was here and said, "Oh, I'm so tired" and I said to her, "You're wearing yourself out running around too much. You should take it easy. You're always going out. Don't you think you should stay home and save money, too? All that winin' and dinin' adds up after awhile you know."

The financial issue for grandmothers always seemed to involve the mothers' and granddaughters' life-styles. Often grandmothers objected to money being spent on dining out or on entertainment when they thought the money should be saved. Grandmothers and grandfathers typically presented a united front on this issue although the grandmothers felt that because the children were "closer" to them, their opinions carried more weight than those of their husbands. As products of the Depression, the grandparents valued frugality as a necessary virtue and never seemed to genuinely trust their children's and grandchildren's belief that "things aren't that way any more."

Health was the only other issue about which the grandmothers consistently offered opinions. They advised their children and grandchildren to "take it easier, not work so hard, and be careful of their physical condition." Again, these patterns of influence reflected the grandmothers' stage of life. When the mothers were beginning their own families, they had solicited the grandmothers' advice about the care and rearing of the children. Similarly, the mothers whose daughters had just given birth spent a considerable amount of time in child-centered interaction. Sharing of motherhood roles was the one event that reunited the women in the family in a reciprocal bond of emotional reidentification, support, and help. Motherhood resulted in the greatest interdependence between second-generation mother and third-generation daughter. One grandmother explained these life cycle differences:

Well, years ago they relied on us more, you know. Because they were starting out. But now they're well established — like a business — they could do things on their own that they don't need our advice on. I don't think there's that much today they could turn to us for. Unless, you know, whatever the future brings we don't know.

At this point in their lives, the grandmothers were consulted for craft ideas or cake recipes but had little influence on matters of importance.

The mothers were most aware of how their own upbringing influenced their current values and determined the manner in which they reared their own families. Specifically, these women were dissatisfied with several traits of their mothers, such as their frugality and rigid discipline. They identified styles of "negative communication" between parents that they in turn were determined to change in their own marriages. They were less preoccupied with these issues than their mothers and reported a different quality of relationship with their husbands. Yet the comments of their own daughters attested to the difficulty the mothers had in trying to free themselves from established patterns. One daughter said:

Sometimes my Mom sounds just like Grandma. . . . She'll say, "You're not ready to buy a house yet" or "You spend too much money on clothes." Sometimes she even says "You go out too much," but they go out all the time.

In fact, the issues that were points of contention between the mothers and the grandmothers tended to be the same issues about which the mothers tried to be most influential with their daughters. The daughters were portrayed as "very open, free spirits" and "not hung up on much of anything." Thus it was difficult to assess the degree to which the mothers were attempting to balance or modify their daughters' differences from themselves. Although the mothers wanted to undo what they regarded as the mistakes of their own parents, they were still committed to their daughters' following life-styles and assuming values similar to their own. This kind of commitment, which also existed between the grandmothers and their daughters, further increased the distance between the grandmothers and granddaughters, who were not bound together in quite the same way as grandmother-mother and mother-daughter.

This difference in intergenerational ties may explain why grandmothers and granddaughters directed less advice toward each other and experienced lower tension levels than grandmothers and mothers or mothers and daughters. Typically, dissatisfaction with advice received was registered only between members of adjacent generations. The middle generation mother was obviously central. The mothers were the only generation with two generations dependent on them. One mother was even able to identify when the shift to having her mother dependent on her first occurred. She remarked:

I think after about 30, my mother more or less depended on me for advice. This happens, where she felt she wanted to know how I felt about certain things or how to do certain things. I think it just took a complete turn.

Mothers who disagreed with some of their own mothers' parenting had long since ceased discussing it directly. The only areas in which mothers attempted to exert an influence on their own mothers were finances and the use of leisure time. The messages were typically: "retire earlier," "take a vacation," "go out more," "don't worry so much," in other words, "be more like me." The acceptance of such advice indicated to the mothers that the grandmothers approved of the mothers' values and life-styles. The daughters seemed to follow their mothers' leads, although to a considerably lesser extent, in trying to get the grandmothers to take life easy. Similarly, the daughters' minimal attempts to influence their own mothers focused on the same themes: "take a cruise with Daddy" or "spend more money now."

Although the daughters extended little influence upward, the mothers definitely felt that they were more influenced by their daughters than by their own mothers. One mother summarized her attitude toward her mother's influence thus:

I think at this point in my life I pretty much know what I want to do. You know, I'll listen to her advice, but it seldom changes my way of thinking. I'll pretty much do it the way I want. Maybe when I was younger and didn't have much experience on my own, I might have taken more of her advice. But like with the children I feel I know them better than she does, and if I decided or my husband and I decided to let them do something, they'll do it.

On the other hand, the mothers listened to and occasionally sought out the opinions of their daughters. Several mothers felt their daughters were better home-makers and more up-to-date on current issues than themselves. The mothers were influenced by having their own attitudes and values reenacted and hence reinforced by their daughters. For example, one mother commented:

All of a sudden D. said to me, "Do you know how much I spend on groceries?"
or "Do you know how much my electric bill was?" I said I really enjoyed
hearing that because I never thought I'd hear it from her. I said, "Now do you
realize when I used to say this and that and you could care less?" I said you
realize now what I was trying to tell you — it made my heart feel good to
hear that out of her — she finally realized food costs so much or electricity is
so high or whatever.

"Reinforcing" and "broadens my perspective" were phrases frequently used
by the mothers to describe their relationships with their daughters. The grandmother-mother relationships were described as close but lacking in an enhancing, reciprocally supportive component.

   The daughters were unaware of the impact they had on their mothers. At
the same time, they thought their mothers greatly influenced their lives. Most
daughters claimed that their tastes in clothes, friends, home decorating, and
even general life-style directly mirrored those of their mothers. The daughters
had more difficulty pointing out patterns of influence or citing specific examples of such influence. Because the mothers and daughters were together
so much, a mother's influence on her daughter was perceived as having a kind
of pervasive or all-encompassing quality. These daughters tended to consult
their mothers before buying a new dress or piece of furniture. They usually
sought out their mother's advice before that of friends. The mutual admiration was striking. The mothers envied and took pride in their daughters and
the daughters emulated and boasted of their mothers. This mutual admiration
may reflect the general similarity between these two generations. The daughters adopted life-styles that were similar to those of their mothers, and they
expected to seek advice from their mothers when contemplating any radical
departures from the life-style they had been reared to embrace.

INTERGENERATIONAL STYLES OF INFLUENCE

One of the more fascinating patterns that these families exhibited concerned
the style of influence or how the different generations made their influence
felt. Different generations followed certain definite rules that dictated the
form in which influence could be acceptably exerted. The broad, overriding
rule followed by all three generations dictated against intentional influence.
Strong feelings about another's behavior were definitely subordinated to the
value placed on communicating to the others that they should be "living their
own lives." Family closeness and solidarity were important but not at the
expense of the freedom and individual privacy of family members.

   Each generation followed various other rules with varying levels of application within this general framework. Grandmothers, despite the fact that they
gave more opinions and advice, simultaneously seemed to qualify such advice
to the greatest extent. Typically, their method of offering opinions was the
least direct of all the generations. When asked how she went about giving
advice to her children or grandchildren, one grandmother replied:

*Well, to begin with, I think I find out first what kind of a mood they're in.
[Laugh] Then I, you know, talk to them real nice and I call them, "Now
honey, I want to tell you something. I don't want you to get mad, and if you
feel like I'm speaking out of turn I want you to tell me, and I don't want you
to feel like I'm trying to run your life or anything." And then I tell them what
I, you know, whatever it is I want to tell them.*

Grandmothers were the only generation who frequently inserted their
opinions while discussing unrelated topics or used closely allied situations
with friends as a platform for their own opinions. One grandmother told her
daughter:

*M.'s boy and his wife got into that high-rise, and the place folded. They lost
everything they had thinkin' it was such a good investment. I hope you and
J. never get into anything like that. You probably should save that extra he
got from his raise instead of taking that cruise.*

The mothers complained that the grandmothers' advice was often couched in
statements such as "your father didn't think you should have" or "your aunt
likes it when you drop her a thank you note." The mothers disliked this practice because they suspected their mothers were placing their own feelings in
the mouths of others.

The grandmothers tended to feel freer to exert influence in certain matters.
In matters of health, finances, home-making, and child care, the grandmothers
were more direct and seemingly more comfortable in sharing their ideas. For
example, the grandmothers volunteered: "I just come out and say, 'you
should quit smoking' or 'I tell her she lets her kids off too easy.' " But the
grandmothers regarded interpersonal relationships and particularly marital
and sexual compatibility as none of their business. In such matters, the grandmothers expressed the hope that their daughters had benefited from the home
life they had had and would know how to "please a man" and "keep him
content." They thought that the home life they provided was sufficient influence in these matters. However, they adamantly stated that if they should be
asked for help or told about a problem in the "family affairs" of their children, they would be more than willing to speak their minds.

The grandmothers evaluated the age and particular experiences of their
daughters and granddaughters when judging the appropriateness of influence.
Some of their advice was stimulated by a family member's recent experience;
other advice was deemed to be "just no longer needed." Almost echoing the
preferences of their daughters as their grandchildren grew older, the grandmothers shared fewer of their opinions about child care as they sensed that
what they said was ignored. "They're just a different generation, and they
don't know how the young kids think any more," mothers often said of the
grandmothers.

The mothers and daughters were less hesitant to offer each other advice than the grandmothers were to offer it to either of them. The openness that characterized relationships between these two generations extended into almost any matter. The mothers frequently commented that while sex had always been a taboo topic when they were growing up, they prided themselves on the fact that their daughters confided in them about sexual problems. Most mothers, however, said that this topic was discussed only if their daughters initiated the conversation. Similarly, any discussion pertaining to a daughter's marital relationship had to be brought up by the daughter. These cues came in a variety of forms, the mothers frequently relying on their intuitive sense to interpret their daughters' nonverbal communication. One mother said:

Sometimes, you know, I can just tell. She drags in here, and she has that look on her face, and I just know her. I have the feeling that maybe she and B. have had a little squabble. So I ask her, "What is it?"

The "permission" to act on such cues, particularly in intimate matters, did not apply to the daughters. They were in agreement that they did not try to influence their mothers and certainly not their grandmothers in any matters related to the marital relationship. One daughter said she might try, apparently by using the same intuitive sense, to get her feelings across indirectly, through humor. She commented:

Like if she mentions that she and Daddy had another fight, I'll say, "This is getting to be like divorce court" or something.

Mothers and daughters alike were direct and straightforward in offering and soliciting opinions about child care, household maintenance, health, and personal grooming. These messages were generally uncamouflaged: "Why don't you get a new, shorter hair style, Ma" or "That halter top shows everything you own." Finances were touchier and usually entailed a more delicate approach. Often a family council would convene that included the daughter and son-in-law and both parents. Opinions were broached more globally and tentatively if unsolicited. Although the mothers could clearly identify instances when their children chose not to take the advice given, they said that such rejection did not deter them from offering the advice. The daughters seemed to rely on a more casual, humorous approach or encouraged their mother's spending habits by being particularly supportive of a new dress purchase or parents' plans to travel.

The mothers offered advice most readily if the matter in question was within their own realm of expertise, such as home-making skills. The daughters sought out the mothers for advice about these same matters. This reciprocity seemed to afford each generation considerable pleasure. The time the three generations spent together, because it was so typically consumed in shopping, offered countless opportunities for spontaneous sharing of tastes that could be applied to the wide range of life-style behaviors.

The reciprocity and degree of intergenerational agreement was remarkable in light of the covert operation of such influence; at no time did the generations verbally and directly discuss how influence was received and used. Indeed, all three generations seemed "to just know." In the end, the social-shopping excursions accomplished more family business than the participants realized. For example, one daughter stated:

We just walk around, and without either of them saying anything, I'd look at something and say that's something Mom would like or that looks just like Grandma. And I think how they'd react to something I did or said a lot at other times, too, even when I'm alone, or I find myself reacting in the ways they might.

This reaction must be family socialization at its highest level — when one party no longer experiences a demand or influence as external to her own needs but as synonymous with them, as if they were inherent in the person. Despite the potential for errors in communication, such indirect styles of influence were the rule for these families. These patterns provided for the transmission of family priorities and contributed fundamentally to the maintenance of intergenerational solidarity.

Obviously, the family members interviewed were close, quite involved with and influential in each other's lives. Not all family members will be so. However, what these women shared about their lives and the patterns of influence between generations has several implications for nurses working with any family group.

First and foremost, our findings demonstrate that our definition of a family should be broad enough to encompass more than just the generation at hand. Whether we are confronted with an elderly man, a young adult, or a child, each of those individuals brings to the nurse a myriad of past and current relationships with other family members that continually exert an impact on his or her current behavior. The continuity that these women demonstrated from grandmother to mother to daughter helps us appreciate the pervasive influence of experiences in the family context on present behavior. Analysis of intergenerational family relationships highlights the complexity of individual change and the continuity of family behavior over time. Whether nurses are working with one family member or the entire family network, they must approach each individual from the perspective of his or her place within the larger system as it is operating at that time.

Perhaps this point has its greatest application in nursing assessment. In the initial data gathering, evaluation, and early problem solving phases of any family work, it is important to recognize that significant others, even when not physically present, can profoundly influence the individual in numerous subtle ways. Such recognition does not require that all family members be contacted or seen prior to any intervention, but it does mean that they must be highly visible in the mind's eye of the nurse so that they may be consulted at any time deemed appropriate or their potential influence on the individual's behavior borne in mind. The nurse who proceeds in this way is better equipped to identify influences on an individual's behavior that are embedded in past history and those that arise from his or her current family system, hence are perhaps less amenable to change. This practice results in greater awareness of the ramifications nurses' interventions always have. No matter what the setting, work with even one family member may have an untold impact on the lives of his or her kin.

Finally, although the notion of intergenerational influence was initially foreign to these family members, it definitely was a reality in each of their lives. However, the conditions under which influence was exerted remained more elusive. Since influence appeared to stem from trial-and-error learning that took into account not only the content of a statement but the manner in which it was presented, it is understandable that the phenomenon was implicit among family members. The challenge, then, is for the nurse to identify the conditions of family influence as they will affect nursing interventions and the family members themselves. Once family members become conscious of the various conditions under which they exert influence on others and can identify the methods they use to do so, will more effective intrafamily and intergenerational family relationships and more problem-free family living result? This question could serve as the basis of a research effort and an exciting exploratory process in which family members of all generations could become engaged.

22. Nurses and Research: Observation Versus Intervention.

Janice K. Janken and Katherine A. Cavallari

The research reported in this book was conducted by a group of nurses who met regularly to discuss the developing research project and to report advances in individual facets of the study. Although each group meeting began with a discussion of common research concerns such as reviewing interview guides and examining data, we group members inevitably began to discuss the problems that we, as nurses, were experiencing in our role as researchers. This chapter therefore examines the questions, problems, and issues that emerged as a result of our being nurse-researchers.

We found that our being nurses served as both an asset and a handicap to us in our role as researchers. We informed all our subjects that we were nurses at the time we arranged appointments for the interviews. Our subjects were often surprised to hear that nurses were engaged in any research, let alone research not based on an illness model. At the same time, they usually viewed nurses in a positive light and therefore were willing to participate in the project by being interviewed. In this instance, our being nurses was an asset to our research process. That is, our search for subjects was made easier because, in general, people viewed nurses as responsible, trustworthy persons with whom they were willing to share their points of view.

Our background in public health nursing also worked to our advantage. All of the research interviews were conducted in our respondents' homes. Thus we were working in our respondents' territory and had to adapt the mechanical aspects of the research to their surroundings. Although this point might seem trivial, at times it made a relatively simple procedure difficult. For example, we had to place the tape recorder in a location that would ensure pick-up of all voices and would allow the researcher to monitor the tape and change it when needed. In addition, during the interview, we had to contend with telephone calls, doorbells, pets, and children interrupting the proceedings. However, we chose to conduct the interviews in the homes of our respondents because this setting, as opposed to one of our offices, gave us a clearer picture of their life-styles and added to their comfort. More importantly, we felt that our public health nursing experiences, which had emphasized home visits, would contribute to our comfort in respondents' homes and improve our flexibility and adaptability in what might be considered trying conditions.

In spite of these advantages, we perceived our nursing background to be problematic in several respects, although, it is important to note, our respondents communicated no such problems. Throughout the project, we struggled to come to grips with the impact of our nursing background on the research process, or with the conflict we felt between our roles as nurses and researchers.

OUR CONFLICTING ROLES: NURSE AND RESEARCHER

Our primary problem was the conflict we felt between our nursing role — intervention — and our research role — observation. This conflict stemmed from the similarities between the research technique of intensive interviewing and the nursing technique of interviewing to assess patient situations. The goal of the research interview is to obtain information that reflects the respondent's own view of his or her situation. The goal of the therapeutic interview is not only to obtain such information but to begin to formulate plans and interventions to assist the respondent in his or her situation. Yet, although the goals are different, the techniques used to elicit information are similar. Consequently, on occasion we had difficulty keeping clear in our minds the boundary between the two types of interviewing. This difficulty in defining the boundary and our resulting conflict between observation and intervention will become clearer as we discuss the variety of questions that arose from this issue.

Although we had informed our subjects that we were nurses, we wanted to assume only the role of researcher while interviewing them. But what are the distinguishing characteristics of the nurse and the researcher? Our research was based on the assumption that we did not know the relevant variables and key issues in family development. In other words, as researchers, we were not claiming to be experts in the content to be discussed with the respondents. Yet nurses are expected to possess a certain expertise. Indeed, much of the content discussed during the research interviews concerned matters about which we, as nurses, had functioned as experts. As we proceeded with our research, we became more and more cognizant of the conflicting characteristics of the nurse role and the research role.

This book examines developmental stages that nurses identify as potential maturational crisis periods. Previously, when working with persons like our respondents, we were accustomed to being alert for crisis situations, giving anticipatory guidance, and if necessary, engaging in crisis intervention. However, as researchers, we sought not to impose the preexisting theoretical framework of crisis intervention on our subjects. Therefore, when our respondents communicated data that reminded us of crisis theory and triggered in us an obligation to intervene, we were ambivalent, torn between the need to suppress our theoretical knowledge and the urge to offer our customary interventions.

For example, all of us at some point in our nursing careers had been involved in counseling pregnant women about the adjustments that might be necessary as they developed in the mothering role. However, when we interviewed prospective mothers who made statements that reminded us of potential crisis situations about which we usually offered counsel, our only obligation in the role of researcher was to listen and elicit further data; our task did not include making a nursing judgment that these persons were experiencing difficulties common to pregnant women or providing customary support by acknowledging that the feelings they were relating were common or usual among expectant mothers. In fact, we were doing research to discover if indeed these were common and usual feelings. Thus we experienced conflict when our subjects shared information with us that reminded us of patient responses to which a nurse would offer support as appropriate intervention.

The conflict we felt between observation and intervention became even more acute when we perceived our respondents to be directly asking for support. Sometimes after respondents had related information, they asked: "Do other people feel this way?" or "You are a nurse. Have you heard things like this before?" Respondents who participated in more than one interview, particularly, questioned us about their health. That is, in subsequent interviews, the respondents seemed to feel freer about bringing up questions that tapped our nursing expertise. Whether research subjects direct such questions to all researchers or only to those with backgrounds like our own remains to be determined. The point is that we tended to interpret these questions as requests for supportive intervention. Consequently, we had difficulty responding to these questions and were aware of how hard it was for us to relinquish our nursing role of intervention.

We also suffered from our belief, characteristic of nurses, that we were not doing a competent job unless we found and solved a problem. We all remembered our student days when we were informed that all patients have psychosocial problems and that a nursing care plan is incomplete without at least one. Thus, as nurses, we were especially accustomed to examining behavioral and verbal interactions with a critical eye. But in order to remain consistent with our theoretical framework, as researchers we could not employ preconceived theoretical formulations in a critical examination of respondents' behavior or interactions. Usually, we were able to accomplish this research goal. However, on occasion, our respondents shared information or demonstrated behavior that if viewed from a disease orientation was indicative of problems that might be relieved by therapeutic intervention.

For example, six respondents admitted that they were drinking heavily and feared they were becoming alcoholics. Another respondent admitted that she was severely depressed. When our subjects shared such information or demonstrated behavior that would be problematic if viewed from a disease orientation, we again found ourselves wondering how to respond. We were caught between our research role of adhering to impartial observation and our nursing role of acknowledging that the person was experiencing pain and assisting him or her in seeking competent help.

THE EFFECT OF OUR ROLE CONFLICT ON OUR RESEARCH

The majority of interviews were without such role conflict. Nonetheless, we experienced role conflict frequently enough to become concerned about the effect it might be having on our research and on our respondents. In an attempt to begin clarifying differences between the research role and the nursing role and to formulate possible ways in which we might more comfortably handle these conflict situations, we addressed several other questions and issues.

Responses Elicited by Nurse-Researchers

First, we attempted to determine the degree to which our own behavior during the interviews might be causing such conflict situations to occur. Our concern was that our own role confusion had caused us to conduct the interviews in such a way that our respondents could not help but place us in a therapeutic role. In other words, we wondered if we might be collecting data by using interview techniques that were more appropriate for a therapist than a researcher. If this was the case, these techniques might unintentionally be indicating to our respondents that we were persons who were able and willing to provide interventions. In order to explore this possibility more fully, we reviewed the interview transcripts, closely scrutinizing the interviewers' statements and questions. This review revealed several instances in which our own behavior might have indicated that we were nurses first and researchers second.

Perhaps the most difficult instances for us to consider were those in which we had inadvertently slipped into the nurse role without being aware of having done so. When we began interviewing, we intended to assume only the role of researcher, and we made a concerted effort to maintain this stance. However, upon reviewing the interview transcripts we unexpectedly discovered that on occasion we had automatically assumed the nurse role. For example, in the following dialogue the respondent was misinformed about a birth control method. The interviewer automatically assumed the nurse role and not only corrected the misinformation but began to teach the respondent about alternative contraceptive methods:

She: [Talking about the intrauterine device (IUD) that she had considered using as a contraceptive] Especially something that's not supposed to be there, you know. It's considered a foreign body by your own uterus or your own body. So, I don't know about that. Then I've heard about some kind of an instrument that they inject into the uterus that secretes a hormone that makes the uterus think it's pregnant all the time.

Int: It's a type of IUD.

She: Is it a type of IUD?

Int: Umhum.

She: I thought, well, that is new.

Int: That's really new. That was just patented.

She: Yeah, I thought, well, forget it. So I think I will just stick with the gel.
I guess what it amounts to is that we're not — it's not that we don't want to
have children — I mean if it happens, okay, but if it doesn't, that's all
right too. I guess if I really wanted to be certain, we would use probably an
intrauterine device of some sort. But not the kind you could . . .

Int: Have you considered a diaphragm?

She: No. They're not safe 'cause they do have a tendency to slip.

Int: Usually, though, they combine them with a gel, which makes it safer.

She: Oh, really?

In this instance, the interviewer had clearly departed from the researcher
role and entered the nurse role. The questions of validity and reliability
raised by role departures such as these are discussed later. The question
raised here is: when we slipped into the nurse role and presented ourselves
as experts, were we implying to our respondents that we were willing to
provide intervention for a variety of problems? In turn, were we promoting
respondents' viewing us as nurses rather than as researchers? Unfortunately,
these questions cannot be completely answered. The actual impact of the
interviewers on our respondents requires further investigation. However, this
examination of our own behavior served to increase our awareness of the
difficulties we had in adhering to the research role. Consequently, we became
more cognizant of our own behavior during interviews and began to more
carefully monitor our responses. Our primary task was research, and we did
not want to impose nursing interventions on respondents as a result of our
own role confusion. We did not wish to inadvertently encourage our respondents to view us as nurses.

Interview Techniques of Nurses and Researchers

Second, we considered the implications of using selected interview techniques. To date, no real distinction has been made between interview
techniques that are appropriate to therapeutic situations, those that are appropriate to research situations, and those that can be employed in both settings.
Thus we wondered if certain techniques that we had used in therapeutic
settings and had transferred to the research setting might be partially responsible for implying that we might be able to help our respondents and
therefore for encouraging them to share their health concerns with us.

The interview techniques that we questioned most were those that required empathetic responses from the researcher. In doing so, we probably were reacting to the notion that empathy, a subjective experience, is at odds with research, which strives for objectivity. However, we eventually decided that empathy and research were not necessarily in opposition.

One such technique that we questioned was the use of subjects' nonverbal communication as a tool to elicit further data. As respondents spoke, we not only listened to what they said but also observed their speech, affect, and body language. Then, on occasion, we commented on the observed nonverbal behavior and asked the respondent to clarify its meaning. For example, if a subject looked tearful as he or she related certain information, the interviewer might say, "You look upset as you say that. How do you feel?" This technique required that the interviewer have an empathetic understanding of human behavior. The interviewer had to be able to piece together the verbal and the nonverbal behavior to obtain the personal meaning of what the respondent was relating.

A second such technique that we questioned was verbalization of the subjects' implied thoughts and feelings. The following dialogue, in which the subject discusses the events that led up to her divorce, illustrates the use of this technique by the researcher:

Int: *Another question I was concerned about is, you know, in your unhappiness for so many years, in fact, it sounded like the love for your children was very one-sided, that it came from you. You know, it sounds like your husband didn't . . . .*

She: *Right.*

Int: *He didn't show them affection. It was just from you, and you were very unhappy. How did that affect your ability to love them or to give love to them?*

She: *Oh, I gave them love. I gave them, you know, tons and tons of love. That was what I loved.*

Int: *Sometimes when people are very unhappy, it's kind of hard to give to somebody else when you're hurting so much yourself.*

In this instance, the researcher empathized by verbalizing the respondent's implied feelings of unhappiness, pain, and difficulty in giving love.

These techniques, which required that the interviewer have an empathetic understanding of the respondent, usually proved successful in evoking an elaboration of the respondent's feelings and points of view. However, in many psychotherapies these techniques are used not only to elicit information but to increase the client's self-awareness. Thus we wondered if these techniques might be more appropriate for therapeutic situations. However, we decided that a therapeutic interview and a research interview based on symbolic interactionism both try to achieve an understanding of the meaning of what people say. Thus we decided that empathy was not necessarily at odds with research and that we could legitimately use these techniques to elicit further data in the research setting. This decision is another example of the continual struggle we experienced in our attempt to differentiate our research role from our nursing role and to clarify in our own minds the boundary between the two.

Questions That May Raise Difficulty for the Nurse-Researcher

As a result of our concern that perhaps we were inviting respondents to place us in a therapeutic position, we noted that with certain respondents we felt apprehensive about asking certain routine questions. Prior to our asking these questions, the respondent had implied that the subject matter chosen might be painful or difficult to discuss. Thus we feared that by asking a routine question we might be encouraging the respondent to focus on his or her problems. Although, on the one hand, we recognized that all persons have problems and that it is human to feel and express emotions, on the other hand, we feared the consequences of opening a Pandora's box. When respondents shared their problems, we found adhering to the research role especially difficult. Thus we were apprehensive about asking certain questions for fear they might place us in the tenuous position of feeling compelled to intervene. At the same time, we realized that the question might not be as emotionally charged as we anticipated and that by avoiding it we would be losing valuable data.

For example, one subject alluded several times in the interview to the fact that she had been engaged to be married until recently. One of the final questions suggested on the interview guide was to ask if the respondent was dating anyone. Realistically or not, the researcher feared that asking this question might result in a tearful account of the events surrounding the broken engagement. Although the interviewer realized that there was nothing unusual about feeling distressed over a broken engagement, she also recognized that she might very well feel the urge to offer customary nursing intervention. Thus she felt ambivalent about asking the question. In this instance, the interviewer proceeded to ask the question, and the respondent, as anticipated, answered it by relating the details of the broken engagement. However, the subject's reaction to the question was not as severe as the researcher had imagined, and much data would have been lost if the researcher had succumbed to her initial fear of asking the question.

Ethical Considerations: Obligations to Respondents

Finally, we examined the ethical aspects of our professional obligation to respondents. We were aware of our professional responsibility as stipulated in the Nurse Practice Act. At the same time, we were aware of the legal factors affecting our research. Yet, when we felt a conflict between our nursing role and our researcher role, ethical considerations only increased our confusion by providing opposing guidelines.

On the one hand, the law describes a "breach of contract," which refers to violating the obligations to which persons have agreed either explicitly or implicitly. Our subjects signed consent forms agreeing to participate in the project and thus our contract was explicit. As researchers, we were obligated to elicit data as stipulated in the contract. On the other hand, the law describes "negligence," which refers to those situations in which the nurse does not have the duty to intervene but has the duty to act responsibly. As nurses, we were not obligated to intervene, but if our respondents could definitely benefit from intervention, we were obliged to act responsibly. We believed "to act responsibly" meant referring the person to an appropriate resource. Unfortunately, we often had difficulty determining if the respondent needed referral. In general, the legal guidelines delineating our professional obligations seemed ambiguous and were of minimal help in reducing our role confusion.

CLARIFYING OUR RESEARCH ROLE

It is probably apparent that we raised more questions than we could answer. Undoubtedly, we will continue reflecting on these issues as long as we continue to do research. However, during our discussions we did formulate several concrete ways that we as individuals could clarify our research role and more comfortably handle situations in which we felt our researcher role and nurse role were in conflict.

Before the first interview, our subjects were usually unclear not only about what questions to expect but also about what behavior to expect from us. To prepare them for the interview, we therefore found it helpful to explain what the project entailed and to clarify what our role as researchers would be. We did this to reduce the possibility of our respondents' later viewing us as nurses. We identified two actions that advanced our role as researchers. First, instead of merely handing the consent form to the respondents and asking them to read and sign it, we went over the salient points with them. Thus the respondents not only read but also heard that they were participating in a research study. Second, we informed the subjects that we were interested in learning about the ideas and feelings pertinent to their present family circumstances and that we did not presume to know what these important issues were. Thus we attempted to reinforce the notion that we were researchers and to deny expertise in the matter under investigation. In short, prior to the interview, we attempted to establish our role as researcher.

Although we attempted to de-emphasize our nursing background and instead stress our researcher role, respondents nevertheless asked us questions relating to health issues. At these times we tended to feel role conflict. In reaction to this particular conflict, we employed several additional measures to assist us in further defining our research role for our subjects and to help us more comfortably handle these situations.

The first method of responding to our subjects' health-related concerns or requests for nursing intervention was to deal directly with the issue as we, the researchers, perceived it. That is, the interviewer told the respondents that she was in a bind because, on the one hand, she would like to assist with the problem but, on the other hand, nursing intervention was not part of her job as a researcher. In this way, the interviewer again clarified her role as a researcher and avoided engaging in nursing intervention. Not all interviewers, however, felt comfortable employing this method and either refrained from using it or used it in combination with other measures. In some instances, we felt that we had a professional obligation to assist our respondents. Thus this technique, although most effective in advancing the research role, was not applicable to situations in which the interviewer felt it was appropriate to intervene. In addition, some members of the research group thought that this measure was too abrupt and might impede subjects' willingness to share their viewpoints. They therefore did not use this method.

A second method of responding to health-related concerns required the interviewer to inform the respondent that the issue could be discussed after the interview was completed. For example, during one interview, the husband and wife respondents were discussing the prenatal classes they were attending. During their discussion, they stated that they did not fully understand the purpose of the exercises and asked the researcher to explain their benefit. The interviewer responded by telling them that she would be willing to discuss the exercises more fully after the interview. In this way, she pointed out that teaching was not part of her research role — that is, if the interviewer agreed to intervene, she first established the fact that in so doing she was departing from the research role and entering the nursing role. This method was probably the one most frequently used to respond to subjects' health concerns.

The method of offering to discuss respondents' health concerns after the interview, thereby clearly separating the nursing role of intervention from the research role of observation, was a fairly comfortable method for the majority of us interviewers to employ. At the same time, we recognized that our use of this measure, as well as others that will be discussed, raises questions about the reliability and validity of our data. We had to ask ourselves what effect the nursing intervention had on the adjustment subjects were making to their various family roles. For example, did the nurse's intervention (e.g., explanation of the purpose of exercises) alleviate a concern that many prospective parents have and thus alter the couple's development in the parenting role? We also questioned whether the interviewer's consent to intervene in any way changed the quality or content of the data that was reported subsequently. To draw upon the same example, did the interviewer's willingness to teach the purpose of the exercises result in the respondents' offering more health-related data than they would report to other researchers and perhaps even cause health concerns to preempt discussion of other role development issues during the interview? These questions concerning reliability and validity we had to consider whenever we made a decision whether to intervene. If the decision was to intervene, we had to analyze the data in light of the possible effects the intervention might have had on respondents' behavior. Thus, although the method of discussing health concerns after the interview alleviated role conflict in the nurse, the same measure contaminated the research to a degree.

In instances like the one in which the subjects asked about exercises, it was relatively simple to first recognize that the respondents were requesting intervention and then to separate the nursing role from the research role. However, in other instances, the respondents' actual desire for assistance was less clear. For example, a respondent who admitted that she was severely depressed did not explicitly say to the interviewer that she expected or desired help with her problems. Yet the interviewer perceived that the respondent was asking for assistance and at the same time thought that perhaps psychotherapy would be beneficial. In instances in which it was unclear if the respondent was asking for intervention, we first asked the respondent if we were correct in thinking that he or she was asking for assistance. If the answer was in the affirmative, then we referred the respondent to an appropriate source. For example, the depressed woman was referred to a psychotherapist. Given the large number of interviews that the group of researchers as a whole conducted, relatively few cases of referral occurred.

In instances in which respondents became emotionally upset as they replied to certain questions, we did not continue to pursue the topic. Instead, we acknowledged that the topic was a difficult one for the respondent to consider at this time and that it could be explored at a later point after the problem was somewhat resolved. For example, in the majority of interviews, we asked respondents to talk about their parents. One subject tearfully stated that her mother had died the preceding week. Consequently, the interviewer did not pursue the topics of parents and family background. To have pressed for such data would have served only to promote a situation in which the interviewer would feel obligated to assume the nursing role and offer supportive intervention. Instead, the researcher acknowledged the subject's pain and said that this topic could be pursued during a future interview.

Another respondent related information about his children from a previous marriage. The respondent became tearful as he talked about the ambivalence he felt about not living with those children. The interviewer recognized that to pursue this topic would most likely result in her intervening and attempting to assist him in identifying alternative ways in which he might handle this situation. Therefore, she acknowledged his dilemma and then proceeded to a different question. During a subsequent interview, she asked how he had resolved his problem.

These, then, are the concerns we identified as we struggled with the conflict between our nursing role of intervention and our research role of observation. Although we strived to adhere to the research task of observation, at times we had difficulty doing so and felt obliged to assume the nursing role and intervene. The decision whether to intervene was a difficult one to make. We recognized the need to consider the potential effects that the intervention might have on both our respondents and our research. In the majority of instances in which we perceived our nursing role and research role to be in conflict, we opted to remain in the role of researcher. However, in those selected instances in which we chose to intervene, we tried to explain to our respondents that such intervention was not a part of the research process. In addition, we recognized that our occasional departure from our researcher role cast doubt on the reliability and validity of our study; consequently, we examined the data in light of these considerations.

THE EFFECTS OF OPPOSING VALUES AND SOCIALIZING ON RESEARCH

In examining the possible impact of our nursing background on the research process, we identified two other problems in addition to the conflict between our role as researcher and our role as nurse. The first problem was the effect on the collection and interpretation of data when the researchers and the respondents had opposing values. The second problem was the possible influence on the data of researchers socializing with the respondents. Both of these problems were addressed by the research group in the context of their effect on the validity and reliability of the study.

In regard to the problem of opposing values, we were particularly concerned about the effect of the feminist point of view shared by the researchers. That is, we were all women, and we were all very involved in our careers. In contrast, our sample included men and women, many of whom tended to view their roles from what is often considered a traditional point of view. Frequently, the woman's first priority was to tend to her home and family while the man's first priority was his career. Thus, the researchers and many of the respondents held opposing viewpoints about acceptable male and female roles.

Although we were most willing to accept our respondents' points of view on appropriate male and female roles, we could not help but question whether our own values influenced the data we received and the way we interpreted them. For example, did the fact that all the interviewers were female alter the data, or would the respondents have shared similar information with male interviewers? Also, would male researchers view the data in a different light and draw different conclusions? Of course, since no men were in our research group, these questions could not be answered. However, we had to evaluate this factor as a possible inherent bias in our research.

In addition, we questioned the possible effects of our careers on the data we collected. That is, it was apparent to respondents that we were committed to our careers by the fact that we were practicing nurses and that we were conducting research. Thus we wondered if the respondents recognized that our viewpoints on appropriate sex roles were opposite theirs or if they assumed that we shared similar viewpoints but were involved in careers by second choice. If they recognized that our viewpoints were different, they may have altered the content of what they said either by trying to align their statements with our opinions or by more vigorously trying to support their own positions. This question of the way respondents perceived us could not be completely answered. However, discussion of our own values as compared with those of our respondents increased our self-awareness of our biases. In turn, we tried to control our responses during interviews to lessen the chance that our respondents would realize that some of their values and ours were in opposition. Also, we attempted to take our biases into account as we examined the data. For example, if a working woman said that her husband rarely assisted with chores such as washing, cooking, and cleaning, we had to take care not to assume that she was complaining. We might believe that the husband could share such tasks, but we had to remind ourselves that the respondent's statement did not in fact indicate whether she considered his behavior acceptable or unacceptable. Thus we continually examined our values and evaluated the effects they might have on our data and the way we interpreted them.

We then considered the possible influence on the data when researchers socialized with respondents. After completing the interview, most of the respondents invited the researchers to stay for coffee. During the coffee period, two interesting phenomena occurred rather consistently. First, the respondents asked the interviewers questions pertaining to their personal lives. Second, the respondents offered information in addition to that discussed during the interview. The research group examined several issues in connection with these phenomena.

When the respondents asked us to stay for coffee and then asked us questions about ourselves, we usually felt somewhat ambivalent. On the one hand, we recognized that the respondents had revealed many personal experiences to us; thus we felt obliged to stay and share a few facts about ourselves. On the other hand, the notion of socializing seemed at odds with the usual conception of research as a formal, impersonal process. However, in considering this issue more fully, we came to the conclusion that we facilitated subjects' willingness to share their viewpoints with us by disclosing selected facts about ourselves. That is, if we refused to disclose information about ourselves, we could not expect respondents to be open about themselves with us. The questions that the respondents asked us usually pertained to our marital status, whether we had children, where we lived, and our career goals. It is interesting to note that these questions were abbreviated forms of those that we asked our subjects to explore in depth during the interview. We felt that our subjects were justified in asking us these questions, but we tried to answer them in as brief a manner as possible.

Although we felt it was necessary to answer the respondents' questions about ourselves, we had some indication that this personal information affected the data subjects related to us. For example, respondents added to their statements comments such as: "You are married; so you know what I mean" or "You have children; so you will understand this." Fortunately, not all of the interviewers were married or had children; so this bias was not constant in the research. Nevertheless, we had to be careful not to assume that we did indeed understand just because we were married, had children, or, in general, had shared an experience seemingly similar to that of the respondents. In other words, thinking that we had experienced similar situations did not mean that we shared similar views of the event.

When the respondents provided additional information pertaining to their family roles, we were not sure if they felt less inhibited when the tape-recorder was off, if they felt more willing to talk after we had shared information about ourselves, or if they suddenly recalled information that they had not thought of during the interview. Most likely, all of these factors contributed to the phenomenon. Regardless of the reasons it occurred, the phenomenon caused us to consider two questions about data validity.

First, we asked generally how much relevant data might have failed to surface during the interview. Although this question was impossible to answer, we attempted to allay our concern by asking the respondents at the beginning of subsequent interviews if they had had any additional thoughts on what had been discussed the last time. In this way, we provided them with the opportunity to relate additional data that they thought might be relevant. However, in those cases in which we conducted only one interview with a subject, we had to take into consideration the possibility that we had not obtained all relevant data.

Second, we questioned our accuracy in recording the additional data that were sometimes offered during the coffee period. That is, since the tape-recorder was no longer running, we were placed in the role of participant observers, where we had to try to remember the exact words of the respondents. In the usual participant observation situation, the observer, after many hours of practice, has developed the ability to recall almost totally long segments of conversations and relevant scenes he or she has observed. In contrast, we had not been trained to remember long segments of conversation and were frequently caught off guard when the respondents related this additional information. Obviously, our inability to recall the subject's actual words, coupled with our interpretation of what the respondent had said, introduced a source of error into this data. However, when the respondents offered additional information during the socializing period, the interviewers tried to record the data immediately after leaving the respondent's home in order to reduce the chance of forgetting and/or misinterpreting it after a period of time.

Another phenomenon, closely related to the issue of socializing with respondents, concerned the development of friendships between the researchers and the respondents. In most cases these relationships developed insidiously, emerging as a direct result of the numerous contacts between the interviewer and the respondents during the course of a long series of interviews. In the process of establishing an open and trusting relationship with the respondents, the researchers occasionally found that a friendship relationship had also developed. None of these relationships was allowed to develop such that the researchers and respondents socialized outside of the interview situation, but strong bonds of concern and mutual interest did develop between them.

In some cases these relationships developed without the researcher's awareness. In one instance, for example, only the illness of the interviewer brought the situation to light. The researcher had completed three interviews with one couple and then became seriously ill and was unable to complete the remaining two. A replacement interviewer was sent to complete the series. The researcher was quite surprised when she received a get-well card and a telephone call from the couple expressing their concern about her illness and regret that she could not complete the remaining interviews with them.

The development of friendship relationships with the respondents had some very positive results. The respondents began to look forward to the interviews and made a point of remembering details that they thought would be relevant. As a result, the quality and volume of data elicited in these interviews increased significantly. In addition, the respondents were more willing to put themselves out for the interviewer. For example, in one case an interviewer was quite far along in her pregnancy and was unable to travel to the respondents' home for the interview. Aware of the interviewer's condition, the respondents agreed to come to her home for the interview.

Admittedly, these friendships also had a potentially negative effect. By becoming friends with the respondents, the researchers were risking the loss of a certain degree of objectivity in the interview situation. Assuming the role of friend could alter their role as researchers and place them in situations in which they might make certain assumptions about the respondents and not properly explore certain relevant areas with them. The researchers attempted to avoid this potential hazard in two ways. First, they never carried the relationships beyond the interview situation. In addition, they attempted to become aware of situations in which friendships were developing or had been established. Thus aware of the situation and the limitations on the amount of information known about the subjects, they could avoid making unwarranted assumptions about the respondents and maintain the validity of the interviews. We also feared that friendships would create biases in the data analysis stage of the research. The interviewer was frequently involved in the analysis of the data she had collected. This problem never materialized, however, since the interviewer was never the sole person involved in the data analysis. At least two, and frequently three, people were involved in the coding, analysis, and interpretation of the data; so this bias was kept to a minimum.

These, then, are the questions, problems, and issues that emerged during the course of our involvement in the research project. Although some of these questions, problems, and issues reflect concerns shared by all researchers, others reflect our unique position as nurse-researchers. This uniqueness was apparent particularly in situations in which we had to decide whether to adhere to our researcher task of observation or to engage in our nursing task of intervention. However, even though our nursing background introduced several problems into the research process, we did not find these problems insurmountable. In fact, we viewed the contemplation of these issues as an important component of the research process. Therefore, we undoubtedly will continue to reflect upon similar concerns for the duration of our participation in both nursing and research.

Appendix: Interview Guides

Chapter 5: Joint Interviews

1. History of the Relationship

   a. Describe how you met, how you came to live together.

      Probe:
      How did you meet, and how did your relationship develop over time?
      How did you decide to live together?
      How long had you been dating before you moved into joint residence?
      Where had you been living at the time you decided to move?
      How long have you been living together?

   b. How have others reacted to your living together (parents, friends, work colleagues, others)?

   c. How about your friends? Are they living together, married, or single?

2. Description of the Relationship

   a. How would you describe your relationship?

      Probe:
      What are the advantages and disadvantages of living together (vs. marriage, vs. dating)?
      What are your thoughts about marriage for yourself? Have they changed with living together?
      What are the strengths and weaknesses of your partnership?
      How do you describe your relationship to others?
      What do you call each other when talking to others?
      How do you decide who is going to do what around the house (cooking, cleaning, other chores, etc.)?
      How do you handle finances?

   b. How does your relationship affect your relationship with others?
      Other men?
      Other women?
      Friends?
      Relatives?
      Work colleagues?

   c. Are your relationships with others the same as or different from before living together? How? Describe, giving examples.

   d. Has your relationship with each other changed with living together? How?

3. Views on Marriage as an Institution

   a. How do you feel about marriage as an institution?

   b. As compared to living together, what do you see as the advantages of marriage? The disadvantages?

c. How do you feel about your parents' marriages? Other relatives? Friends? (More in depth in second interviews.) Do you see any role models for relationships?

4. Future of the Relationship

    a. What do you see as the future of your relationship?

        Probe:
        Do you foresee marriage together? With someone else?
        Do you **see** children?
        Do you see any changes occurring in your life-style in the future? Explain.
        If you were to separate, would you seek to live together again with someone else? alone? legally marry? Why?
        Have you discussed as a twosome how long you plan to stay together? Have you discussed what issues might cause you to part?
        If one of you were to get a job promotion or transfer or wish to move, would you both go?
        Do you plan to have children? If so, could you discuss your plans?
        What would you do if an unplanned pregnancy occurred?

    b. Is there anything we have not covered that you wish to talk about?

Chapter 6: Joint Interviews During Engagement

1. How long have you known each other?

2. How long have you been dating?

3. How did you first meet?

4. What were your first impressions of each other?

5. Were you initially attracted to one another? Why or why not?

6. Describe your first date. Where did you go? What did you do? Were you alone or with other couples?

7. What do you remember talking about on this first date?

8. What impressed you most about him/her on this first date?

9. Was there anything you didn't like or that irritated you about him/her on this first date?

10. After the first date, what thoughts or feelings do you remember having about wanting to continue dating him/her?

11. Describe how your relationship developed after your first date.

Probe:
Did you continue to date regularly?
When did you begin dating each other steadily?
When did you begin to feel you were in love?
When did you begin thinking seriously of him/her as a permanent
    partner?
How did the decision to marry come about?
How was this set date decided?
How long were you engaged?
Describe taking him/her home to meet your family for the first time.
Have you had any disagreements since you started dating? Describe
    these. How resolved?
What kinds of plans have you been making for your wedding?
Who is doing most of the planning? Making most of the decisions?

12. What kinds of plans have you been making for after you're married?
    Honeymoon? Living arrangements?

13. How did your sexual relationship develop?

14. What place and meaning does sex have in your relationship?

15. If you could give one word to describe your relationship, what would
    it be?

Individual Interviews During Engagement

1. Background Information to Discern Role Development Within the Family

   a. Describe your mother to me. What are your most vivid memories?

   b. What do you like about your mother the most?

   c. What sorts of things about her irritate you the most?

   d. Describe your father to me. What are your most vivid memories of
       him?

   e. What do you like about your father the most?

   f. What sorts of things about your father irritate you the most?

   g. How would you describe the relationship between your father and your
       mother? How did they handle affection, disagreements?

   h. How do you see your mother's role in the family? What types of
       things did she manage?

   i. How do you see your father's role in the family? What types of things
       did he manage?

   j. Are there any ways in which you would want your marriage relation-
       ship to be like your parents? To be unlike your parents?

k. What sorts of things did your mother expect of you around the house?

l. Can you briefly describe the roles of your brothers and sisters as well as how you picture your role within your family?

m. What types of expectations did your parents hold for you? What did your mother and father picture you as becoming? What types of roles did they envision for you in adult life?

n. How do you see yourself fulfilling your parents' aspirations for you?

2. Development of the Concept of Family

a. Describe to me your ideas of what an ideal marriage would be like.

b. Describe to me your ideas of what an ideal family would be like.

c. How do you picture your fiancé(e) and yourself fitting into these roles?

d. Do you anticipate any problems in your marriage? In fulfilling the role of husband/wife?

Chapters 8 & 9: Joint Interview Six Months After the Wedding

1. Tell me something about your wedding, your reception.

   Probe:
   The meaning of these events for the respondents.
   The high and low points of these events for respondents.
   Whether or not these events were consistent with the respondents' expectations.

2. If the respondents went on a honeymoon, ask them to tell you about this.

   Probe:
   The meaning of the honeymoon to the respondents.
   The high and low point of the honeymoon for the respondents.
   Whether or not the honeymoon was consistent with the respondents' expectations.

3. What is a typical day like for each of you? A typical evening? Weekend?

   Probe:
   What they do for fun and relaxation.
   Shared interests and activities.
   Individual interests and activities.

4. How are you handling the housework, e.g., grocery shopping, laundry, shopping, cleaning, taking care of the car, etc.?

Probe:
How and when the division of labor was decided.
Each respondent's satisfaction with the division of labor.
Whether or not they see the present arrangement as permanent.

5. How are you handling the money?

   Probe:
   How decisions are made in this area.
   Whether they have joint or separate checking accounts.

6. How does being married fit in with work and/or school obligations and responsibilities?

7. Has marriage changed your friendships or your social life in any way?

   Probe:
   Patterns of socializing as a couple.
   Patterns of socializing as individuals.
   Any new friendships since being married.

8. What kinds of ties are you maintaining with your families?

   Probe:
   What do you call each other's parents?
   How often do you visit your parents? Is there a routine, or do you visit only on special occasions?
   Relative influence of each family on the couple's lives and life together.
   Any changes in the respondents' relationships with parents or in-laws since marriage.

9. What part does sex play in your marriage?

   Probe:
   Any changes in this aspect of the relationship since becoming married.
   The importance of this to the relationship in general.
   Sources of information and guidance, if any.

10. Do you have any thoughts or plans about having children?

    Probe (if appropriate):
    When? How many?
    Anticipated impact of children on their relationship.

11. What part does religion play in your lives, both individually and as a couple?

12. Have you learned anything new about yourself or about your mate since getting married?

    Probe:
    How this came about.
    Kinds of things they talk about with each other.

13. How do you handle disagreements?

Probe:
Specific examples.
Areas of agreement and disagreement in relationship.

14. Has anything unexpected or unplanned happened since the last interview that you consider important (e.g., births, deaths, moves, job changes)?

Probe:
Meaning of these things to the respondents.

15. What would you tell someone about marriage?

Probe:
Is it what they had anticipated? Why or why not?
Things (or persons) they found a help or a hindrance in preparing for married life.

16. Which of the following subjects did you and your partner talk about before your marriage?

a. Number of children to have.

b. How money would be spent.

c. Division of housework.

d. Child rearing responsibilities.

e. Religious observance.

f. Which partner(s) would work.

g. Political views.

h. Sex.

i. Feelings about each other's family.

j. Feelings about each other's friends.

Individual Interview After Marriage

1. How has marriage changed your life? How would you compare your life now with your life before you were married?

2. Now that it is behind you, how do you feel about your wedding and the events surrounding it? How would you describe that time of your life?

3. Have your friends or colleagues at work taken into account the fact that you are married? Do they ever make mention of this? Have your friendships or social networks changed since your marriage?

4. Assuming that your tastes and general life-styles were not identical before you married, how have you and your spouse gone about re-solving or coordinating differences in these areas?

   Probe:
   In areas of furnishings, food preference, daily routine entertainment, and free time.

5. How do you feel about the titles of husband and wife? How do you feel about being referred to by these terms? When do you use these terms in referring to your spouse or yourself?

6. Was the issue of whether or not the woman would change her last name ever discussed between you? Was this something you thought about or considered?

7. Are there any things that you used to do for yourself that your spouse now does for you? Are there things that you do for your spouse that he/she used to do for him/herself (e.g., buying clothes, servicing the car)?

8. Are there belongings that you think of as specifically belonging to either yourself or your spouse? Are there things that you regard as "ours"?

9. What kinds of decisions do you usually make on your own? What kinds of decisions do you usually leave up to your mate? What things do you usually decide together?

10. In the past we have asked about how you see yourself and your spouse as an individual. We would also like to know how you see yourselves as a couple. What kinds of things do you think make you a couple?

    Probe:
    For both intangible, feeling kinds of things as well as tangibles like opening a joint checking account.

11. Are there ever times that you feel like you don't really know or understand your spouse?

12. Are there ever times that you feel uncomfortable, embarrassed, ill at ease, or awkward around your spouse?

13. How about the sexual aspect of your relationship? How has that been going? Are there any problems along those lines? How do you feel about your spouse as a sex partner? Do you, personally, have any ideas or feelings about extramarital sex?

14. What do you think your life will be like when you're 30? 40? What kinds of goals do you have for your marriage? What kinds of things would you like to accomplish in the next few years?

15. How do your goals or hopes for your marriage fit in with other, more personal goals you might have?

16. What do you think are the most important things that have happened to you as an individual since you got married?

17. How would you compare your marriage with that of other couples you know? How would you compare your relationship to that of your parents?

18. Are there ways in which you influence your spouse? Do you ever give your spouse advice?

19. How do you feel about your spouse's appearance? Have your feelings in this area changed since you first met? How do you communicate likes and dislikes in this area? Do you think you influence your spouse's appearance?

20. Do you ever advise or try to influence your spouse regarding his/her work (school)? Does your spouse ever try to influence you on issues concerning your work (school)?

21. Does your work ever influence your personal life? Does your personal life ever influence your work?

22. How important is your work to you? Do you anticipate staying in the same occupation/profession?

23. How satisfied are you with your marriage in general? Are there any things you would like to change in the relationship?

24. How likely do you think it is that you'll still be married in 5 years? 10 years? 20 years? Why?

25. How do you feel about participating in this study? What kind of an experience has it been for you? What do you think about the kinds of questions that were asked? Do you and your spouse ever talk about either the joint or individual interviews after they are over? Do you think that being in this study has in any way influenced your relationship with each other? Do you feel more comfortable talking and giving your viewpoints in the individual interviews than in the joint?

Joint Interview One Year After the Wedding

1. Tell me about what's been happening to you both since we last talked. How have things been going? Has anything happened in the past months that has been especially important or meaningful to either or both of you?

2. Has the division of labor you set up for housework and finances changed since you were last interviewed?

3. Compare your relationship when you were married only one month

and now. What changes have taken place? Is there anything you'd like to change in your relationship?

4. Describe your present relationship to members of your own family.

   Probe:
   For specific relationship with parents and siblings.

5. How would you describe your relationship with your spouse's family?

   Probe:
   For specific relationship with spouse's parents, siblings.

6. Do your parents ever give you any financial help, gifts, etc.?

7. How would you describe your and your spouse's political views? Do you ever discuss political issues, how you are going to vote, etc.?

8. Have either of you ever had to miss work because of illness since getting married? How did your spouse react to your illness? Do you have a family doctor?

9. How would you evaluate your sex life? How satisfying is it physically, emotionally?

10. Are there ways other than sexual intercourse that you and your partner communicate your affection for each other?

    Probe:
    For touching; kissing "good morning," "goodbye"; public displays of affection.

11. Tell me about how you see others influencing yourself, your mate, and your relationship. Whose advice and opinions do you seek out? Who offers you advice?

12. What do you like most and least about being married?

13. Do you anticipate or plan for any changes in the near future?

14. The following questions relate to your feelings about participating in this study:

    a. Did the tape-recorder inhibit your answers at all?

    b. Were you more comfortable in later interviews than in earlier ones?

    c. Have you told others that you are in the study?

    d. Have you shown any of the articles to your friends? Did the articles ring true with you?

    e. Have you ever given misinformation or painted a rosier picture for us than was the case?

    f. Has being interviewed influenced your relationship at all?

Chapter 10

1. Historical Development of the Marital Relationship

   a. Tell me how you first met your husband.

   b. What were your first impressions of him?

   c. When you first went out together, what seemed to impress you the most about him?

   d. How do you think these impressions of him have changed over the years?

2. Background Information to Discern Role Development Within the Family

   a. Describe the way you saw your mother in the family.

   b. What type of things did she manage?

   c. How did your parents go about making decisions, such as when to buy something or where to live?

   d. How did they usually go about settling disagreements?

   e. Before you married your husband, what did you think your role should be in the family?

   f. Were there ways in which you wanted your marriage to be like your parents' marriage?

   g. Were there ways in which you wanted your marriage to be unlike your parents' marriage?

3. How the Black Woman Perceives Her Present Role in the Family

   a. What are some of the tasks you perform regularly for your family, let's say, each week (house, children, etc.)?

   b. How did you happen to take on these tasks?

   c. What do you feel should be the woman's responsibility in the family?

4. The Black Woman's Decision Making in the Family

   I would like to know how you and your husband go about making important family decisions.

   a. How was it decided that you should have children, or was this a decision?

   b. If you have decided to limit the number of children you will have, how was this decision reached?

   c. How is it decided when and how your child/children should be disciplined?

d. Can you tell me about some of the disagreements you and your husband have about the children?

e. How do you go about settling these disagreements?

f. Let's talk about your current residence.
How was it decided that you would move to this particular place?

g. How about major purchases?
How is it decided when new furniture, new clothing, cars, etc., are to be bought?

h. How do you feel about the way the decisions are made in your family?

5. Interpersonal Relations Between Black Men and Women

a. What kinds of things do you and your husband do together, say as far as going out together, entertaining friends, etc?

b. Why do you think you and your husband have been together for ___years?

c. How do you think your husband would answer this question?

6. What Are Some of the Factors That Determine the Relationship Between Black Couples

a. How do you think your children have influenced your marital relationship?

b. Do you believe that your economic condition has any influence on the way you and your husband get along? Can you explain this further?

c. How do you think religion has influenced the way you and your husband get along?

d. What are some of the other things that you feel have influenced the way you and your husband get along?

7. Black Woman's Perceptions of Male Acquaintances and Their Role in the Family

I read a report by Moynihan in which he implied that black men were irresponsible and incapable of assuming the role of providing for and protecting their families. How do you feel about black men as providers and protectors of their families?

a. Can you explain this further?

b. Among your married friends, would you describe the man as being weak or strong in comparison to the woman?

c. Can you explain this further?

d. What are some of the strengths that you see among these men?

e. What are some of the weaknesses that you see among these men?

8. The Black Woman's Perceptions of Status Among Married Acquaintances

a. Among your married friends, who would you say has the most authority as far as decision making is concerned, the man or the woman?

b. What are your feelings about this?

9. The Black Woman's Perceptions of Status in Relation to Black Men

a. In the family, do you think the black woman's position is superior, equal, or inferior to her husband's position?

b. Where do you think the authority or power should be in the family?

c. Can you explain why you feel this way?

10. How the Black Woman Socializes Her Children for Their Roles as Adults

a. What things do you think you do to prepare your son/daughter for marriage?

b. Do you see education as being important in a successful marriage today?

c. If you could only send one of your children beyond high school, which one would you send?

d. Can you tell me how you made this choice?

11. Do you have any other comments to make?

Chapter 11: Individual Interview

1. How long had you known your first spouse prior to marriage?

2. How old were you when you married for the first time?

3. Do you have any children from this marriage?

a. Age?

b. Sex?

c. Who has custody?

4. How old were you when you obtained your divorce?

5. Had you and your ex-spouse lived apart for any length of time before beginning the divorce procedure?

6. How would you describe yourself at the time of your first marriage?

7. What first attracted you to your ex-spouse?

   a. What characteristics were most attractive to you?

   b. What characteristics were least attractive to you?

      1. What did you try to do about these characteristics?

      2. What was the outcome?

8. As you look back on the relationship, how would you describe it?

   a. What areas of marriage were most enjoyable to you?

   b. What areas of marriage were most stressful to you?

      1. Did these areas come as a surprise to you?

      2. What did you do to try to reduce the stress?

      3. How did it turn out?

9. Would you term it a warm, intimate relationship at any time? Give an example.

10. What did you and your ex-spouse expect of each other?

    a. How did your ex-spouse think a husband should act?

    b. What things should a husband think about and do?

    c. How did you think a husband should act?

    d. What things should a husband think about and do?

    e. How did your ex-spouse think a wife should act?

    f. What things should a wife think about and do?

    g. How did you think a wife should act?

    h. What things should a wife think about and do?

    i. [If spouses' expectations agreed] Since the two of you agreed about how husbands and wives should act, how did you carry out this arrangement? How did the arrangement work? [If it didn't work] What did you do to try to change the situation?

    j. [If spouses' expectations disagreed] Since the two of you disagreed about how wives and husbands should act, what did the two of you do about the disagreement? Did you find this solution satisfactory? [If it wasn't satisfactory] What did you do to try to change the situation?

11. What interests did you and your ex-spouse share?

    a. What interests were not shared?

    b. Did you each pursue individual interests?

    c. What did you do together for recreation and entertainment?

    d. How was the decision arrived at?

    e. What happened when you each wanted to do something different?

12. How were the financial aspects of the marriage handled?

    a. Who paid the bills?

    b. Who made and kept the budget?

    c. Who decided on major expenditures?

    d. How did you arrive at this arrangement?

    e. How satisfactory did you think the arrangement was?

13. In your view, what was it that really made the marriage unworkable?

    a. What did you do to try to alter the situation?

    b. What was the outcome?

Chapter 12: Interview at First Trimester

1. Background of Respondent

    a. Tell me about yourself — the things you like to do, your personal interests.

    b. What has your married life been like?

    c. How close are you with your family (parents, siblings)?

    d. Tell me about your parents (ages, health, relationship with them).

    e. What things make you angry about your mother or father?

    f. What is your idea of what a good mother should be? Who comes closest to your ideal?

2. Current Situation of Being Pregnant

    a. How did you feel when you first suspected you were pregnant? when you were officially told by the doctor?

    b. In general, how are you feeling (appetite, cravings, altered affections or emotions, symptoms, sleeping, dreaming)?

    c. How do you feel about having a baby now?

d. How is your life different now that you are pregnant?

e. What sex child do you hope for (reasons; names yet?)?

f. What was your relatives' and friends' response to your pregnancy?

g. Any family difficulties going on now?

h. What was your husband's initial response to your pregnancy? his present feelings?

i. Were you planning to begin having a family at this time?

j. Is your married life any different now (relationship with husband, going out, entertaining, housekeeping, responsibilities, sex, plans for future)?

3. Opinions and Comments

a. Some people think women look their best when pregnant. What do you think?

b. Do you have any thoughts about breast feeding or natural child-birth at this time?

4. Are there any other issues or problems you would like to discuss?

Interview at Second Trimester

1. Tell me how you are feeling.

2. Describe what your life is like now. Working? Staying at home?

3. What things please you most now?

4. What situations most easily upset you?

5. How do you feel about the care you are getting?

6. What fears or concerns, if any, do you have now?

7. Whom do you speak to as a resource person for answers to questions/advice?

8. Recall all the thoughts and feelings you have had about "having or not having children," specifically in relation to pregnancy and being a mother: (a) when you were a little girl; (b) as you were growing up; (c) more recently.

9. What is your relationship like now with your parents? siblings? other relatives? friends?

10. Did your relationship with your parents affect your motivation to have a child?

11. Are there any family difficulties going on now?

12. What are your husband's feelings about the baby now?

13. What is your married life like now?

14. How do you feel about having a baby now?

15. How real is the baby to you now?

16. What meaning does your unborn child have for you as woman?

17. What effect do you anticipate or hope your child will have on your marriage?

Interview at Third Trimester

1. Tell me how you have been feeling since our last meeting.

2. Describe what your days are like now.

3. Do you dream much? If so, tell me about your dreams.

4. What things please or excite you most?

5. What situations upset or anger you?

6. What has your care been like lately?

7. Who do you speak to as a resource person for questions, advice, or support?

8. What is your relationship like now with your parents? siblings? relatives? friends?

9. Are there any family difficulties going on now?

10. What are your husband's feelings about the baby now?

11. What is your married life like now?

12. What kinds of changes do you think the baby will create in your household?

13. Have you noticed any differences in your behavior recently?

14. What are your thoughts about the baby now?

15. Recall all the thoughts and feelings you have had about labor and delivery: (a) when you were a little girl; (b) as you were growing up; (c) more recently.

16. What fears or concerns, if any, do you have now?

17. How do you feel about the way you look now (the weight you've gained, etc.)?

Interview After Delivery

1. How are you feeling now?

2. Tell me about your labor and delivery experience — thoughts related to security and trust; how labor began; stages of labor; immediate post-delivery period and hospitalization experience.

3. Describe what your early days of home-coming were like.

4. Tell me your thoughts and feelings about the baby now.

5. What kinds of changes have been created by the baby in your household?

6. Describe your family life now: (a) [First] between you, your husband, and baby; (b) [Then] relationships with immediate family (parents, siblings); (c) [Then] with extended family members (grandparents, aunts, uncles, cousins, etc.).

7. What are your thoughts about yourself in terms of being a woman and bearing your first child?

8. What kinds of expectations, if any, do you have of yourself now?

9. What are others' (husband, parents, in-laws, friends, neighbors, etc.) expectations of you now?

10. What fears or concerns, if any, do you have now?

Chapters 13 & 14: Joint Interview at Third Trimester

1. This Pregnancy

   a. How far along are you in this pregnancy? Due date?

   b. Are you hoping for a boy or a girl, or does it make any difference? Reasons? Names?

   c. How did you feel when you first suspected that you were pregnant? How did you feel when you were officially told by the doctor? When did your husband know? Did you tell him? How?

   d. In general, then, how has this pregnancy been progressing? How are you feeling? Changes in appetite, cravings, sleeping, dreaming, emotions? Any other symptoms?

   e. To husband:

   What have you been thinking about? Are there any physical changes or symptoms that you have experienced?

f. How has your life been different now that you are pregnant? Is it what you expected?

g. Is your relationship with your spouse any different? What about your social activities? Housekeeping?

h. Had you been using any form of contraception? What kind? Was it successful? What kind of place does sex have in your relationship? Has it been any different?

i. To husband:

   What has been your role throughout this pregnancy? Is it any different from what it is when your wife is not pregnant?

j. Some people think women look their best when they are pregnant. What do you think? How do you feel about your appearance?

k. Do you have any thoughts on natural childbirth? Breast feeding?

l. Since you have chosen to have a home delivery, can you tell me how you arrived at this decision?

   Probe:
   Previous hospital experience; influence of religion and friends.
   Once you made the decision, how did you proceed?
   What kinds of reactions have you received from your family and
      friends about this decision?

2. Parenting

   a. What factors influenced your decision to have a child? Timing?

   b. What is your ideal of what a good parent should be? Who comes closest to your ideal? Where do you think you got most of your ideas on how to be a parent?

   c. How do you think this baby will affect your household? Do you anticipate any problems?

   d. What kinds of preparations are you making for this child?

   e. Who do you speak to as a resource person for question-answering, advice, and support? What type of question-answering, advice, and support do you need either now or in the future?

3. Marriage and Family History

   a. Can you tell me about your family? What was it like?

      Probe:
      What mother and father were like.
      What their relationship was like.
      Respondent's role in the family.

Role of siblings.

b. How did you first meet? What were your first impressions of each other? Were you initially attracted to one another?

4. Is there anything you would like to add that we didn't talk about? Do you have any questions you would like to ask me?

Joint Interview Six Weeks After Delivery

1. Can you describe your delivery: the events leading up to and surrounding it?

   Probe:
   What it was like for each of them?
   Was it what they expected and, if not, how was it different?
   Would they do anything different?
   Significance of siblings' presence (if appropriate).

2. What has been the reaction of your family and friends?

   Probe:
   Influence.
   Incidence of unsolicited advice.

3. What kinds of changes have occurred in your typical day?

   Probe:
   Time element, having enough time to get everything you used to get done.
   Changes in division of labor.
   Changes in caring for other children.
   Changes in social life, feelings about leaving a child.

4. What things, if any, are different about your relationship as a couple?

   Probe:
   Sexual relationship.

5. To father and mother (if appropriate):

   How does having a child fit in with your work and/or school obligations?

   To mother:

   Do you have any plans to return to work? How do you feel about working when your child is young?

6. Has this new baby changed the way money is being handled or spent?

   Probe:
   Shifting priorities.
   Expectations about cost of child.

7. How has breast feeding fit in with your routine?

   Probe:
   Expectations.
   Physical problems.
   Anticipated length.

8. What has been the reaction of your other children to this new baby?

   Probe:
   Problems that have resulted, if any.
   Other children a help or a hindrance?
   Change in attention given to other children?

9. Do you feel like a mother/father?

   Probe:
   Comfortable holding and caring for child.
   Father's involvement in caring for child.

10. What responsibilities do you think you'll have as a parent in the first
    year? Later on? What attributes will help you meet these responsibilities?

11. Do you have any plans about having more children?

    Probe:
    When? How many?
    Would you have another delivery at home?

Individual Interview 8 to 12 Weeks After Birth

1. How has becoming a parent changed your life? How would you compare
   your life now with your life before you were pregnant?

2. Now that it is behind you, how do you feel about your pregnancy and
   the birth event? How would you describe that time of your life?

3. How do you feel about the titles of mother and father? How do you
   feel about being referred to by these terms? When do you use these
   terms when referring to your spouse or yourself?

4. Are there any things that you used to do for yourself that your spouse
   now does for you? Are there things that you do for your spouse that
   he/she used to do for him/herself (e.g., buying clothes, servicing the car)?

5. What kinds of decisions do you usually make on your own? What
   kinds of decisions do you usually leave up to your mate? What things
   do you usually decide together?

6. Are there ever times that you feel like you don't really know or
   understand your baby?

7. Are there ever times that you feel uncomfortable, embarrassed, ill at
   ease, or awkward around your baby?

8. How about the sexual aspect of your relationship? How has that been going? Are there any problems along those lines?

9. What do you think your life will be like when you're 30? 40? What kinds of goals do you have for your marriage? What kinds of things would you like to accomplish in the next few years?

10. What do you think are the most important things that have happened to you as an individual since you became a parent?

11. How would you compare your marriage and child rearing with that of other couples you know? How would you compare your relationship to that of your parents?

12. How would you compare yourselves with other couples who have just delivered a child in the hospital?

13. Do you anticipate any problems for the future (child rearing, returning to work, etc.)?

14. When you have questions, from what source or sources (relatives, books, etc.) do you find your answers?

15. How do you feel about participating in this study? What kind of an experience has it been for you? What do you think about the kinds of questions that were asked? Do you and your spouse ever talk about either the joint or individual interviews after they are over? Do you think that being in this study has in any way influenced your relationship?

Chapter 16: Joint Interview

1. Before your first child was conceived, what do you recall about how you felt about having children?

   Probe:
   What did you think would be the advantages?
   What did you think would be the disadvantages?
   Generally, how committed were you to having children?
   Did your friends have children? Did you see much of them?

2. What were the important goals or hopes that you held for your marriage at that point?

   Probe:
   What kind of spouse did you want to be?
   What kind of spouse did you want to have?
   How closely did you think you came to achieving these ideals?
   Have they altered since you have become parents?
   Before the child(ren) did you have ideas about what the ideal parent would be like? Have these ideas altered?

3. What did you think having children would be like?

4. How is it different?

5. What would you identify as being the important skills to be learned or tasks to be performed as parents?

   Probe:
   How did you learn the skills you needed to be a parent?
   Can you identify any people (or other sources of information) who served as models (negative or positive) for you as a parent?
   Have you seen parenting you didn't like?

6. How have you divided up the various tasks of being a parent?

   Probe:
   Are there set jobs for each?
   How did they come to be arranged this way?

7. As you think about how your relationship with each other has altered because of being parents, what would you identify as the major alterations? for the better? for the worse?

8. Have there been any alterations in your relationships with your relatives, friends?

9. What would you say your major areas of agreement or disagreement are about children or how to be a parent?

10. Based on your experiences, are there things you would do differently now if you could do them over again?

11. Is there any particular age at which a child is particularly easy to parent? difficult to parent?

12. How similar do you consider yourselves as parents to others in your neighborhood? others you know? your family of origin (own parents or siblings)?

13. How much of a role does religion play in your family?

14. If you had to say, who would you consider your important supports?

    Probe:
    Who would you go to for help?
    Who would you want to spend important holidays with?

15. Have there been any other influences on you as a parent that I haven't asked about that you consider important?

Chapter 18: Individual Interview

1. Prior to Marriage

a. Work (or schooling)
    Position
    Responsibilities
    Hours
    Feelings as a professional
    Career plans
    Colleagues' (or advisors') views
    Male vs. female-dominated profession — reactions
    Career plans

b. Nonwork aspects
    As identified by respondent (leisure activities, social, others)
    Responsibilities in living situation

c. How long working prior to marriage

2. Marriage

a. Date, age

b. Anticipated changes (as differentiated from actual changes)
    Work
        Hours
        Place
        Career plans
        Decision to continue/not continue
        Feelings about working
    Nonwork aspects
        Responsibilities as a wife
        Feelings about becoming a wife
        Leisure activities
        Relationships with friends, family

c. Actual changes
    Work
        Hours
        Place
        Career plans
        Feelings about working
    Nonwork aspects
        Responsibilities as a wife
        Feelings about being a wife
        Leisure activities
        Relationships with friends, family

d. Actions to contend with changes (solutions)
    Work
        Dealings with employer
        Rearranging schedule, career plans

Seeking emotional support from colleagues
Reactions of colleagues
Nonwork aspects
Scheduling of time — home, work, other
Delegations of home-making responsibilities
Seeking emotional support from husband, friends, family
Reactions of husband, friends, family

3. Parenthood

   a. Date, age

   b. Anticipated changes
      Work
         Hours
         Place
         Career plans
         Feelings about working
      Nonwork aspects
         Responsibilities as parent
         Feelings about being a parent
         Leisure activities
         Relationships with husband, friends, family
         Reactions of husband, friends, family

   c. Actual changes
      Work
         Hours
         Place
         Career plans
         Feelings about working
      Nonwork aspects
         Responsibilities as parent
         Feelings about being a parent
         Leisure activities
         Relationships with husband, family, friends
         Reactions of husband, family, friends

   d. Actions to contend with changes (solutions)
      Work
         Time off for delivery
         Other dealings with employer (e.g., conflict between child needs
         and work demands)
         Seeking emotional support from colleagues
         Reactions of colleagues
      Ranking of solutions in order of importance

4. The Present

    a. Typical daily schedule
       Schedule
       Leisure activities
       Time alone, with husband, with child/children
       Weekends

    b. Present delegation of home and child care responsibilities
       Housekeeping
       Child care
       Entertaining
       Financial matters

    c. Personal qualities
       As identified by respondent
       Commitment to career and/or family aspirations
       Drive, intellect
       Organizational abilities
       Energy level, sleep requirements

    d. Satisfactions and frustrations
       Professional, wife, parent
       Overlap and interference of one role to the other; examples

    e. Women's movement
       General reaction
       Effect on ability to combine roles
       Predicted effect on future women planning to combine roles

    f. Advice to others planning to combine roles

Chapter 19: Individual Interview

1. Family Background Information

    a. Describe your mother to me. What do you like most about her? least?

    b. Describe your father to me. What do you like most about him? least?

    c. How would you describe the relationship between your parents? How do they handle affection (disagreements)?

    d. What sorts of things were expected of you around the house? What sorts of things did your brothers and sisters do?

    e. Generally, how does your family get along?

    f. What types of expectations did your parents hold for you? How do you see yourself fulfilling your parents' aspirations?

g. What are your own personal goals and ambitions — what do you see yourself as becoming? How do you see yourself fulfilling those goals?

h. When you were living at home, how much time did you spend away from home? What did you do during that time?

i. Who was first to leave your family? Describe the situation.

2. Moving Away

   a. What were the events or reasons that led up to your leaving home?

   b. How did you make the arrangements? alone? with family? with friends?

   c. What were the feelings of your parents and brothers and sisters regarding your leaving home?

   d. What were the first few weeks away from home like? Was it what you expected?

   e. Describe a typical day. How is it different from being at home?

   f. How are you handling the housework?

   g. How are you handling the money and the bills?

   h. How often do you have contact with your parents?

      Probe:
      Frequency of contacts.
      Type and quality of contacts.
      Who initiates.
      Satisfaction.
      Relative amount of their influence.

3. Social Network

   a. Has moving away from home changed your friendships or your social life?

   b. Have you made any new friends? Are you dating anyone now?

   c. What do you like most about living away from home? least?

Chapter 20: Joint Interview

Most of what is written about parenting pertains, of course, to parenting children who are still living at home. One of the things we are interested in is being a parent after your children are no longer living at home. We'd like to talk with you about this time of your life.

1. Generally, describe your family life in the years before any of your children left home.

   Probe:
   Place or role of each child in family.
   Family division of labor.
   Discipline, limit setting.
   Handling of disagreements.

2. Describe the circumstances surrounding each of your children's leaving home.

   Probe:
   Had you thought about what it would be like before they left?
   What were the reasons for or events preceding the move?
   How were arrangements for the move made? child alone? with parents?
   How did you (your spouse) feel about this?
   How did other family members feel about this?

3. How often do you have contact with your children?

   Probe:
   Frequency of contacts.
   Type and quality of contacts.
   Who initiates.
   Satisfaction.
   How much do you see yourself influencing them?

4. Did you hold any general or specific expectations for your children? What did you see them as becoming?

   Probe:
   Fulfillment of expectations.
   Changing view of children since they have left home.

5. How would you describe being a parent now that your children are no longer at home?

6. Has your life changed since you no longer have children living at home?

   Probe:
   New or changed patterns of activities and relationships.
   Changed relationship with spouse.

7. Do you view yourself differently or see yourself as a different person since your children are no longer living at home?

   Probe:
   Sources of satisfaction.
   Problem issues or areas.
   Any changes in these areas.

8. What do you like most about no longer having your children at home with you? least?

Chapter 21: Individual Interview

We'd like to talk with you about intergenerational influence. We're interested in finding out about the kinds of contacts family members who are from different generations have with each other and the kinds of influences they have on each other. There are not right or wrong answers to any of the questions we'll be asking. We're interested in *your* opinions, ideas, and personal experiences.

1. Patterns of Contact

   a. How far do you live from your parent/grandparent/child/grandchild? How do you feel about this?

   b. What kinds of contacts are you maintaining with your parent/grandparent/child/grandchild?

      Probe:
      Type of contact — telephone, seeing.
      Frequency of contact.
      Quality of contact — formal, spontaneous.
      Respondent's feelings about these issues.

2. Nature of Interaction

   a. In general, what kinds of things do you do (talk about) when you get together with or talk to your parent/grandparent/child/grandchild?

      Probe:
      Respondent's satisfaction, reaction.
      Respondent's perception of relative's response and satisfaction.

   b. Does your parent/grandparent/child/grandchild ever give you advice? How do you feel about this?

      Probe:
      Area of advice giving: health, appearance, work, purchases, money, leisure, political-social, friends and social life, personal relationships.
      Specific examples — account of last time advice was received.
      Way in which advice is given — direct, indirect.
      Way in which advice is received.

   c. Do you ever give advice to your parent/grandparent/child/grandchild? How do you feel about this?

Probe:
Area of advice giving: health, appearance, work, purchases, money,
  leisure, political-social, friends and social life, personal relationships.
Specific examples — account of last time advice was given.
Way in which advice is given — direct, indirect.
Way in which advice is received.

d. Are there any other ways you feel your parent/grandparent/child/
  grandchild influences you? For example: Do you ever do something
  and think how they might react or feel that you are orienting your
  behavior toward this particular person?

  Probe:
  Area(s) of influence.
  Respondent's feelings about influence.

e. Do you feel you influence your parent/grandparent/child/grandchild
  in any way other than giving him/her advice?

  Probe:
  Area(s) of influence.

f. In general, how would you describe your relationship with your
  parent/grandparent/child/grandchild?

  Probe:
  Extent to which this person is seen as confidant or source of support,
    stress, joy, protection, etc.
  Extent to which respondent sees self as confidant or source of
    support, stress, joy, protection, etc., to this person.

3. Self-Concept

  a. Can you think of ways in which you are similar to your parent/
    grandparent/child/grandchild? How about ways in which you see
    yourself as very different?

  b. Are there any ways in which you would like to be similar to your
    parent/grandparent/child/grandchild? Are there ways in which you
    would like to be different?

Index

Adolescence
  family relationship, 288-291, 297
    298
  independence, 245, 255, 287-288
    legal, 287-288
    living quarters, 289-291
    social, 289-292
  peer influence, 242, 245
  problems for parents, 244-245,
    254-255, 268, 303, 306
  transition to adulthood, 29,
    287-288
  unwed mothers, 5
  value changes, 245
Adulthood. See also Middle adult-
    hood; Young adulthood
  definition, 287-288
  socialization, 15-20, 29

Baby. See Birth; Infancy
Birth, 177-178, 181-193. See also
    Pregnancy
  anxieties about, 173, 175-176
  cost, 187-188
  delivery. See below home delivery;
    hospitalization for
  as family affair, 3-4, 191
  father's role, 3, 259-263, 266.
    See also below home delivery
  home delivery, 181-194

    and child rearing, 195, 202, 211,
      221
    control and relaxation factors,
      165, 182, 189, 190, 193-194
    decision to use, 182-190, 203-
      204, 209
    doctor's role, 181, 187, 190,
      192-193
    families' attitude, 165, 189-190
    father's role, 3, 182, 183, 190-
      194, 210, 211-214
    positive reactions to, 182,
      191-193
    process, 190-193
  hospitalization for, 176, 184, 193,
    231-232
    delivery, 177-178
    fears for child, 178
    negative opinions, 165, 185-187,
      190
  interview questions, 359-360
  natural childbirth
    control factor, 182, 190, 193-
      194, 224
    description, 190-192
    doctors' viewpoints on, 260,
      262-263
    fears about, 175, 177
    and home delivery, 190, 225
    husband's participation, 177,
      182-183, 190-192, 259-263

and religion, 133
responsibility in, 106–109
role definitions in, 109, 120,
    128–130, 134, 249–252, 254
  by blacks, 139–144, 146–149
self-redefinition in, 20, 103, 105
sexual issues, 115–116, 130–131,
    132, 135, 284
social activities, 116–117, 134–135
social significance, 20, 58
success factors, 119–120
temperamental differences and,
    118–119, 120, 129–130,
    135–136
work and school careers, 134–135
Middle adulthood. See also Empty-
    nest parenthood
developmental tasks, 8–9
nursing guidelines, 4–5
Mother. See also Black wife; Mother-
    father interaction; Motherhood
-daughter relationship, 169–170,
    309–310, 316–317, 321–322,
    324
as generational influence, 319
as single parent, 5, 6
unwed, 5, 247
Mother-father interaction, 237–255.
    See also Father; Motherhood;
    Parenthood
on child rearing issues, 263–264,
    271–272
communication, 249, 253–254
conflicts over parenting, 252–253
on discipline, 244
household work division, 249,
    251–252, 253
  child's tasks, 244, 252
interview data, 238–242
interview questions, 363–364
role arrangements, 249–254
Motherhood. See also Father;
    Mother; Mother-father inter-
    action; Working mother
adjustments to, 217–218, 221
anxieties about
  during postpartum period,
      178–179
  during pregnancy, 168, 169,
      171, 173–174
breast feeding, 178, 182, 183,

204–206, 218–219, 220, 221,
    226
career secondary to, 165, 198–199,
    216
child, relationship with, 219–220
effects of, 216, 220–221
future, concerns for, 229
instinct for, 196, 216
as intergenerational bond, 320
preparation for, 216–217, 218
responsibilities, 217–218, 220–222,
    264, 270–271
social activities, 229
transition to, 216, 221

Natural childbirth. See Birth
Nurse-researchers, 327–340
ethical considerations, 333–334
interview guides, 343–371
interview techniques, 331–333
questioning difficulties, 333, 336
role clarification, 334–337
role conflicts, 328–331
socializing with respondents, effect
    of, 338–340
values, 337–338
Nursing. See also under specific
    family events and specific
    types of nursing
diagnosis and treatment, as
    function, 6
family-centered, 3–7, 12–13, 17,
    182
  economic conditions, as factor,
      255
individual approach (disease per-
    spective), 3, 5–6, 9, 10

Obstetrical nursing, 3–4
Occupational socialization, 17–20

Parent-child relationship. See Family,
    as concept; Family of origin;
    Parenthood; Young adulthood
Parenthood, 165–166, 195–286. See
    also Birth; Empty-nest parent;
    Father; Mother-father inter-
    action; Motherhood
and adolescence. See Adolescence
commitment and values, 195,
    198–199, 221–222, 246–255